MEDICAID POLITICS and POLICY

1965-2007

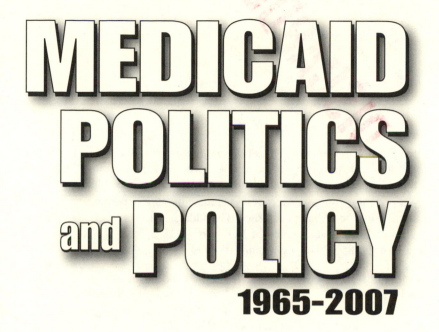

MEDICAID POLITICS and POLICY

1965-2007

David G. Smith
Judith D. Moore

Transaction Publishers
New Brunswick (U.S.A.) and London (U.K.)

Copyright © 2008 by Transaction Publishers, New Brunswick, New Jersey.

All rights reserved under International and Pan-American Copyright Conventions. No part of this book may be reproduced or transmitted in any form or by any means, electronic or mechanical, including photocopy, recording, or any information storage and retrieval system, without prior permission in writing from the publisher. All inquiries should be addressed to Transaction Publishers, Rutgers—The State University of New Jersey, 35 Berrue Circle, Piscataway, New Jersey 08854-8042. www.transactionpub.com

This book is printed on acid-free paper that meets the American National Standard for Permanence of Paper for Printed Library Materials.

Library of Congress Catalog Number: 2007033055
ISBN: 978-1-4128-0737-1
Printed in the United States of America

Library of Congress Cataloging-in-Publication Data

Smith, David G., 1926-
Medicaid politics and policy, 1965-2007 / David G. Smith and Judith D. Moore.
        p. cm.
  Includes bibliographical references and index.
  ISBN 978-1-4128-0737-1 (alk. paper)
    1. Medicaid.   I. Moore, Judith D. II. Title.
  [DNLM: 1. Medicaid. 2. Health Policy—United States. 3. Politics—United States. W 250 AA1 S645m 2007]

RA412.4.S55 2007
368.4'200973—dc22   2007033055

Contents

Preface   vii

Acknowledgments   xiii

1. Historical Background   1

2. Legislating Medicaid   21

3. Medicaid Implementation   59

4. Amending the Classical Model   95

5. Maturity and Trouble   145

6. A Critical Phase   227

7. Medicaid Under Siege   279

8. Devolution and Waivers   323

9. Past and Future   369

10. Postscript   405

Glossary   413

Bibliography   423

Index   433

Preface

One purpose of this book is to provide a connected narrative of the origins of the Medicaid program and its development over the last 40 years. There are some excellent books covering a specific period or aspect of Medicaid[1] but they do not provide an overall view that includes recent developments. We are frank to confess that we would not have undertaken this task if a number of individuals, better prepared than either of us, had chosen to do so. We have interviewed many of these people, and consulted on many occasions with some of them, so that the book has benefited from their recollections and insights.

Forty years after the enacting of Medicaid, witnesses to its origins and subsequent evolution are disappearing from the scene. Writing this book at this time was seen as an opportunity to preserve their memories of historic events and views of program changes as they developed.

History is important for understanding and evaluating the Medicaid program. One reason for thinking so—though not the only one—is the way in which the program was created and has grown over the years, by building on an established foundation, incrementally and by aggregation. Medicaid is not so much redesigned as added to or modified, so that understanding its working and its quirks requires knowing its past and, often, the successive historic changes in some part of the program.

The title includes "politics" and "policy," and there are reasons for stressing each and both. Medicaid as a program is especially subject to exogenous influences—the state of the economy, trends in federalism, developments in other programs such as Medicare and public welfare, along with the electoral cycle and shifts in the partisan balance nationally and in the state houses. A study of Medicaid politics helps understand how these influence Medicaid policy both in specific circumstances and over time. But politics and policy go together: a knowledge of policy helps to understand what is at stake; and a knowledge of politics what is possible. Together, they help to make this arcane program more accessible to the outsider and to those who know only one part of the program or one phase in its development. They are also helpful in deciding what to press for with respect to policy and how to go about it.

It is risky to say what the uses of a history as such might be. At a minimal level, though, getting acquainted with the layered complexity of the Medicaid program should help guard against easy optimism about how to "fix" the program or against despair that nothing can be done. Moreover, Americans often base arguments about policy upon origins and legitimacy of descent so that attention to history can help set the record straight and understand strengths and weaknesses of the program as well as some of the moral passion associated with both. As to where the program should go from here, we hope that this account will provide a modicum of guidance and add weight to some contemporary points of view.

The development of Medicaid, once enacted, can be roughly divided into three major periods or epochs. During the first , or "classical" period—which lasted from 1966 to 1981—the main effort was to get the Medicaid program firmly established and operating as conceived in the original statute: as essentially a categorically linked payer of claims (or reimbursable costs) for traditional fee-for-service providers and hospitals. The second period, which lasted from the beginning of the Reagan administration in 1981 until 1995 is one of growth and change in which categorical restrictions, payment mechanisms, and modes of service delivery became prominent topics for public debate and legislative action. It was also a period in which Medicaid "matured"—developed most of the programs and activities familiar today along with the controversies that surround them. The third period begins with the takeover of Congress by the Republican party in 1994 and is characterized as "critical" both because Medicaid is much criticized and because of the gravity of threats to the survival of the program.

A brief introduction to several major themes and underlying assumptions may be helpful in orienting the reader toward the following chapters, The most important unifying theme is that of Medicaid as a "weak entitlement"—both morally and institutionally. It is weak on moral grounds because of its association with public welfare. Also, unlike Social Security, Medicaid recipients have not paid into an account; and unlike the veterans are not owed because of war service or wounds. The entitlement is weak institutionally because, unlike Social Security or Medicare, the Medicaid statute does not use the language of entitlement and has neither a "trust fund," nor an administrative equivalent of the Social Security Administration with its large bureaucracy, corporate history, and political defenses.

This status as a weak entitlement, though not consciously intended, has been important because it allowed flexibility for the program to adapt and grow incrementally and, because it was an entitlement, to consolidate gains and keep them. Like the common law, Medicaid can grow in parts and without requiring comprehensive restructuring. But there is a downside: Medicaid grows unevenly and often uncontrollably over time, in different program areas or individual states, without direction or corrective action.

Because of its tendency to ratchet upward, the Medicaid program has grown fairly steadily in enrollment, benefits covered, total expenditures, and the share it consumes of state budgets. One result has been to sharpen differences between the federal government and the states, Democrats and Republicans, leadership states and the others, with Medicaid liberals promoting growth and laying on mandates, and conservatives and many states crying for an end to mandates, more "flexibility" or devolution, or even some form of block grant or disentitlement. In most of the years since 1994—more than a decade—the Medicaid program has been under siege, in large measure because of the lack of a workable resolution to this problem of unregulated growth.

Another important theme, running throughout the history of Medicaid, has been the unsettled status of national health insurance. For the most part, whenever national health insurance has seemed to be a robust prospect Medicaid has been neglected, largely because it was presumed that it would be reborn in splendor as part of the new scheme. For protracted periods, though, national health insurance would not be on the agenda and attention would shift to Medicare and Medicaid. That would still leave at issue the status of Medicaid and whether it should be aggressively expanded as part of a new march toward national health insurance or treated as a permanent fixture, likely to be around in some form or another.

Our view is that any version of national health insurance likely to pass in the next decade would be a limited and modest one, retaining Medicaid, though with significant reforms.[2] The main reason for thinking so is that the federal government, whatever political party is in power, will probably lack the unity and strength to take on any ambitious version. In an historic sense, it is "too late" for a comprehensive, unitary system of national health insurance: the forces supporting it have grown too weak and those opposing it too strong. Also, the task is complex and the country divided politically and much in debt. Of course, Medicaid could be displaced or radically transformed for other reasons. In the present context, we are only saying that we do not believe it will happen because of national health insurance and that the book is written from that perspective.

The preceding statement prompts the question of what role Medicaid should play in view of the dubious prospects for national health insurance. Medicaid may well be the closest the American poor will ever come to any kind of comprehensive health insurance. Some would see the role of Medicaid broadly expanded to include more of the uninsured and the working poor. We have reservations about this view, to be expressed later. But controversies about the role of Medicaid began early and have continued, over how expansive to be and what priorities to set in extending coverage—for instance, to the neediest, the uninsurable, the uninsured, and the working poor. This is a theme that runs throughout the book and has been central to recent disputes over waivers and demands for restructuring Medicaid.

Mention of the uninsurable and the uninsured opens up another central Medicaid issue, which is how to deal with the great divide between the frail elderly, the severely and chronically ill or handicapped and the rest of the population, which includes pregnant women and children, the working poor, and the curable. As a rough estimate, the first cohort, which amounts to only 30 or 35% of Medicaid enrollment, accounts for 70% of the total expenditures. The second group that is 65 or 70% of the Medicaid enrollment accounts for 30% of total expenditures. Many of this first group are, in fact, "uninsurable" because they are avoided by commercial insurers and health plans. Treatment for them is costly since it is long-term, often involves lengthy episodes of hospital or institutional care, expensive drugs, and customized services. They are often referred to as "vulnerable" because of frailty or inability to cope. Most of them cannot work and many do not vote. The other population, made up mostly of welfare or TANF recipients, the working poor and children are, on average, much less expensive to treat and are important investments in the future. Many are likely to vote.

This disparity was not so visible when Medicaid was first enacted, but it grew in size and importance during the 1970s, largely because of such factors as much larger numbers of the elderly, increasing coverage of persons with disabilities, and the costs of institutional care. Much of the Medicaid legislation during the 1980s arose from or was significantly shaped by this widening divide.

Medicaid policy from the 1980s to the present has been largely about two major issues. One is how to balance a commitment to the neediest and most vulnerable with a concern for the working poor and their children. The other has been about whether or how to sustain existing commitments despite rising costs, periods of recession, and fierce partisan differences. For a time, a Democratic Congress sought to advance both priorities with prescriptive legislation and mandates. States responded with demands for more flexibility and artful methods of increasing their Medicaid matching funds. Some governors even proposed ending the Medicaid entitlement and accepting less money in exchange for greater freedom to order their own priorities and methods of administration. A kind of resolution of this tension may or may not be possible, but understanding the fiscal and political dimensions of this division and the depth of the passions associated with it are important prerequisites for considering such a possibility.

Medicaid, along with other entitlements, has been under political attack for more than a decade, with various attempts to end its status as an entitlement or radically restructure the program. These efforts and how they played out is another unifying theme of this book. They are worth examining for what they reveal about Medicaid politics. One item they bring out, for instance, is that Medicaid, often regarded as politically weak, has hidden sources of strength and is politically tougher and more resilient than thought. Seeing why this is so is an important key to understanding Medicaid.

The book concludes with an effort to pull together some lessons or guiding principles that can be gotten from this history that might be applicable in thinking about Medicaid policy today and in the future. Though general and tentative in nature, they provide support for some "not to do's" and point toward some desirable policy directions. Our view, briefly, is to preserve and improve Medicaid, not end it. We believe that Medicaid has an essential role, probably even with the coming—if ever—of national health insurance; but that the direction of policy should be less toward expanding Medicaid and more toward improving quality and service delivery, equalizing coverage, strengthening the fiscal base, and seeking to reduce partisan and federal-state tensions.

Notes

1. Excellent books that deal with part of the history or particular topics are Robert
    Stevens and Rosemary Stevens, *Welfare Medicine in America*, New York: The
    Free Press, 1974.; Richard Sorian, *The Bitter Pill—Tough Choices in America's
    Health Policy*. New York: McGraw-Hill, 1988; Diane Rowland, Judith Feder,

Alina Salganicoff, eds. *Medicaid Financing Crisis: Balancing Responsibilities, Priorities, and Dollars.* Washington, D.C.: AAAS Press, 1993,; and Stephen M. Davidson and Stephen A. Somers. eds. *Remaking Medicaid: Managed Care for the Public Good,* San Francisco: Jossey-Bass Publs, 1998. Jonathan Engel. *Poor People's Medicine: Medicaid and American Charity Care since 1965.* Durham, NC: Duke University Press, 2006, covers the history since 1965 but does not go in depth into policy or politics.

2.   Cf. Richard P. Nathan, "Federalism and Health Policy," for an interesting argument that Medicaid might become an "appropriate and feasible" base or template upon which to build national health care coverage. *Health Affairs* Vol. 24(6) 2005, 1458-1466.

Acknowledgments

We can never repay our debts to the many individuals who helped make this book possible. Those who work in the field of Medicaid know how dependent they are upon others for knowledge and understanding of this astonishingly complex program and we, in attempting a history of the program from inception to the present, are deeply aware of our indebtedness to the many individuals who gave generously of their knowledge, insight, and wisdom. These acknowledgements can recognize their contributions. We hope that the book we have written may help to make them seem worthwhile.

We are grateful to the Robert Wood Johnson Foundation for its expeditious and generous financial support to meet travel and research expenses and to the National Health Policy Forum for use of facilities and released time for Judith Moore. We are also indebted to Nancy DeLew and to the CMS Oral History Project for their support. Although these organizations supported the research and writing, none of them sponsored these efforts or bear any responsibility for the content or conclusions of this book.

This book relies heavily upon interviews. Many of those we interviewed—especially those currently working as congressional staff, in CMS or other government agencies, advocacy and research groups—are not only busy and committed, but people who work in politically sensitive positions and have trusted us to represent their views fairly and with discretion. We have tried to honor that trust and hope that this book demonstrates that commitment.

Over 200 people were interviewed, many of them repeatedly, face-to-face and by telephone and e-mail. They are cited in the endnotes and index, though in a few instances no attribution is made at the request of the interviewee. Some individuals were especially generous and helpful: Gerald Adler, Robert Ball, Gordon Bonneyman, Charles Brodt, Sheila Burke, Howard Cohen, Jay Constantine, Stephen Davidson, Jack Ebeler, Christy Ferguson, Michael Fogarty, Peter Fox, Thomas Hamilton, John Holahan, Thomas Hoyer, Robert Hurley, Christopher Jennings,

Christine Koyanagi, Bruce Lesley, Cindy Mann, J. Patrick McCarthy, Karen Nelson, Lee Partridge, Sara Rosenbaum, Diane Rowland, Jennifer Ryan, Matthew Salo, Raymond Sheppach, Sarah Shuptrine, Wayne Smith, Rosemary Stevens, Sidney Trieger, Bruce Vladeck, Robert Wardwell, Henry Waxman, Alan Weil, and Marina Weiss.

We would like to acknowledge separately the contributions of three individuals for their continuing and exceptionally valuable contributions: Lynn Etheredge who helped launch this project, offered advice and help along the way, and read and commented on the entire manuscript; Andy Schneider for his truly extraordinary Medicaid expertise which he shared unstintingly on dozens of occasions; and Vernon Smith for unfailing wisdom and balanced judgment on many controversial topics.

With a subject as difficult and technical as Medicaid, we know that we will have committed errors of fact and judgment. We hope they are not too numerous; but we have no one to blame for them but each other.

1

Historical Background

Institutional Setting

Medicaid began as an add-on to public assistance, designed as much to help states pay for medical vouchers added to welfare categories as to provide medical assistance as such. It was essentially a program of "welfare medicine"[1] and in this respect inherited a long, if not rich, tradition of categorical welfare grants based upon local poor laws, charitable movements of the 19th century, and the "mothers' pensions" of the early 20th century. Much of the history of the Medicaid program could be described as rising above humble origins—but there is no denying such a heritage.

Medicaid was and has been a uniquely American system. More is meant than the fact that no other advanced country chooses to care for its medically needy in this fashion—although it is a fact worth pondering as to why Americans do so. Medicaid was, in its unique way, shaped by the weaknesses of American government and our cultural attitudes toward the poor, women, and racial minorities. It shared in the American "exceptionalism" described by Alexis de Tocqueville: a weakly institutionalized program created by a weakly institutionalized system of government.[2]

The American system of government was itself weakly institutionalized and intended to remain so—a historic legacy of continuing importance. The constitution contemplated was, according to James Madison, a "compound Republick,"[3] in which federalism and the separation of powers would operate together to check the accumulation of power, contain factionalism and sectionalism, and prevent political extremism.

This particular feature of the Constitution is important for Medicaid in several ways. It sets to work mutually reinforcing checks on government—typically replicated by state governments—that limit or fragment government and counter partisan politics. It also gives rise to a specialized "constitutional politics" of federalism that plays a large and constructive role in Medicaid policy and politics, both by setting the larger context for action and in specific policy outcomes. Most importantly, Medicaid is a state-based and administered program, so that federalism is itself one of the most important checks on power and of pressures for decentralization or devolution.

The characteristic of being weakly institutionalized is not peculiar to Medicaid. It is important, though, in accounting for programmatic and political adaptations that make Medicaid seem peculiarly American, especially in its incorporation of dominant social and political norms. A good example is the connection between public assistance and Medicaid. A combination of nastiness toward the poor relieved by selective generosity for other folk has characterized American social welfare. Much of this is because Medicaid was created, and has adapted and grown, by incorporating and building incrementally upon traditional categories of aid. Such an approach allies itself with the familiar and defensible, but like the common law, preserves much that is outdated, even retrograde, in custom and attitude.

Tocqueville noted, in accounting for American "exceptionalism," that these people were "born free, without having to become so."[4] They had no king or hereditary nobility and lacked the domestic or foreign policy that had in less fortunate countries strengthened the state, the army, and the bureaucracy. Instead, they had a love of the laws and a genius for local association, relied little on government, and were busy mostly with material pursuits and private activities.

Until the last decades of the 19th century, Tocqueville's appreciation would have fit the American democracy well. People lived apart, in small, individualistic "island communities,"[5] concerned mostly with local affairs. Neither the state nor the national governments dealt with domestic policy as we know it. Mostly, they collected taxes (or customs, excises), dispensed, licensed, and distributed patronage. They seldom legislated, except to codify the common law, modify the powers of an existing authority, or take action when a local government failed to perform. The Civil War and Reconstruction produced a temporary mobilization and expansion of governmental power, after which the "state of courts and parties" returned.[6]

Although formal government and public institutions remained relatively undeveloped, the private and voluntary sector did not. Tocqueville accused Americans of being absorbed in their own affairs with a kind of "virtuous materialism." That was true enough, as evidenced by the rapidity with which Americans occupied their vast domain and developed transportation, commerce, and local and national business enterprises. But Americans were also much influenced by religious movements, self-improvement activities, and benevolent appeals. And these collective impulses did get institutionalized—in charity associations, private hospitals and asylums, settlement houses, professional associations, universities and medical schools, libraries and museums. As contrasted with most other countries, the private sector—and especially the voluntary and charitable part—developed separately and more independently. It was often more responsive to need, better run, and more "enlightened," at least according to professional or otherwise informed opinion.

In the last two decades of the 19th century, Americans experienced a fundamental transformation of their society driven by concurrent revolutions in agriculture and industry, successive waves of foreign immigration, and rapid growth of urban populations. At the time, Americans boasted that they had achieved in twenty years what had taken Britain more than a century to accomplish. Whether true or not, this statement points to an important fact: that a vast amount of change was compressed into one short period of time. Moreover, these changes brought problems unfamiliar to a simpler, largely agrarian society—such as urban vice, crime and ethnic conflict; single working mothers and delinquent, vagrant or neglected children; industrial working conditions and child labor; cyclical employment and global markets.

Toward the end of *Democracy in America* Tocqueville prophesied that the American republic would survive the Civil War, which he believed would surely come, but was more pessimistic about the age of industrialism and the advent of mass society. No doubt, the republic survived, depending upon what one means by "survive" and "republic." In the present context, though, this crisis of transition probably reinforced some salient characteristics of both public and private benevolence: especially their separatism, categorical emphasis, and its multi-layered incrementalism.

One form of this separatism was a widening of the distance between private charity and philanthropy and public assistance, with the former tending to emphasize "scientific" charities, casework, and rescuing the poor from poverty and dependency and the latter taking primary responsibility for the traditional "poor law" welfare categories and some institutions, especially custodial care for the mentally ill, retarded, and elderly disabled.[7] One undesirable consequence was that public institutions, with the states' police and taxing powers and court jurisdiction were separated from some of the most active civic and professional leadership in the private sector. [8]

Another important legacy of the Progressive Era was to associate health and welfare policy with income security and labor legislation—a seemingly trivial matter, but important for the future. An example illustrates the importance of this association. In the first decade of the 20th century, there was talk of the German and British approaches to health insurance, but little prospect for anything of significance at the national level. One initiative from the American Association for Labor Legislation, though, was a model state law for employer-based sickness insurance.[9] Confined to industrial enterprises, the plan would insure only for lost wages, not for the costs of medical care. This initiative failed. At the same time, starting with the states and with industrial employment and income security (rather than health insurance) made sense as a way to avoid constitutional, political, and administrative difficulties that would attend a publicly sponsored proposal for health insurance.

A second example, more relevant to welfare policy and to Medicaid was that of "mothers' pensions." All during this era, there was concern about the plight of both women and children and how best to cope with working conditions, poverty, homelessness, neglect, vice, and delinquency. A category singled out for special attention was the single mother with children, who was often forced to work at night, neglect her children, let them wander in the streets, put them out to work, or give them up for foster care or adoption. One response to these problems was the mother's (or widow's) pension. Beginning around 1908 at the state level, these pensions provided for categorical payments to mothers for the benefit of minor, dependent children, not because these women were themselves poor or needy but to keep the family together and provide for the children. This kind of subsidy was justified not as "charity," but as support for a useful and needed activity that would help to hold families together and be cheaper than putting the children in an institution. As part of the scheme, it had to be established—often in orphans' court—that the mothers were truly needy and that they would maintain a proper home environment. Some states included only widows; others excluded divorced women or unmarried mothers, and married women usually had to be themselves "dependent," i.e., with husbands in prison, the insane asylum, deserting, or incapacitated for labor.[10]

Except for the war, there was little activity in health and welfare at the federal level. A lengthy campaign that publicized the high rate of infant mortality in the United States led to a White House conference on dependent children in 1909. That event helped to establish a Children's Bureau in 1912, located in the Department of Labor. Six years later, a Women's Bureau was created, also located in the Department of Labor. And in 1921, the Sheppard-Towner Act[11] passed. A substantial victory for the women's movement, this act provided federal grants-in-aid to the states to reduce infant mortality and protect the health of mothers and infants. It was upheld as constitutional by the Supreme Court,[12] but repealed under the Hoover administration.

These examples illustrate health and welfare policy made a century ago but in ways still relevant today, especially for Medicaid. Health and welfare were "local" issues both constitutionally and by settled tradition—matters for states and local government.[13] Government in general was not reliably competent or trustworthy, either in legislating or administering. There was also a strong presumption in favor of ordinary lawful business and the private ordering of affairs. The burden of going forward in law or administration was on the moving party. Under these circumstances, new public initiatives tended to depart cautiously from existing law or private arrangements, to build upon existing foundations, to proceed incrementally and categorically, and to percolate upward from locality to state and, occasionally, from the state to the federal government.

In a polity characterized by institutional weakness and corruption or incompetence, categorical incrementalism was a low risk and effective way of proceeding. It was a good way to focus energy and attention on a proposal, build support among advocates and clients, take advantage of some legislative niches, get some earmarked funds and monitor implementation. As a way of getting money, it was also highly adaptable and, because of latent support and roots in existing local institutions, likely to have considerable staying power.[14]

The "mothers' pension" example also illustrates negative aspects of categorical incrementalism, especially for welfare policy. Labels stigmatize people as, for example, "welfare" recipient or "delinquent" child. Establishing a category also tends to define the "problem"[15] and may determine the approach to solving it as, for example, picking the category of "dependent child" for mothers' aid or "industrial worker" for health insurance. The power to define is a strategic power of enormous consequence. Moreover, building upon past practices or categories of aid or service tends to ratify and even lock in outdated policies, practices, and ideology—for instance, the poor law categories and the kind of limited and tendentious philosophy that underlay the mothers' pension movement. It can also lead over time to a layered complexity in programs that makes major change a forbidding prospect, a feature that protects such programs but also inhibits reform.

The Social Security Act

The Social Security Act of 1935 was of historic significance for several reasons. It established the welfare state in America, by moving on from the alphabetic emergency agencies of the New Deal and giving to the successor agencies a firm institutional foundation on which future programs would build, such as disability insurance (1950), supplementary security income (1972) and Medicare and Medicaid (1965). Also of great and lasting importance are the many ways in which this heritage and the close association with social security has shaped the programs that were included as one or another of the titles of this omnibus legislation.

A curious fact is that the original title of this legislation, the "Economic Security Act," was changed, late in the process, by the Ways and Means Committee to the "Social Security Act."[16] The latter term was not in common use; but it was probably a better title, since it was less precise than "social insurance," (and more than social insurance was wanted) and not as categorically limited as "economic security" that had been the dominant theme. Also, "social security" was probably closer to what Roosevelt and much of the public had in mind[17] even though the provisions of Old Age Assistance and Aid to Dependent Children were pretty much straight welfare and those relating to public health and maternal and infant care had little to do with security except in the loosest sense. Some explanation is needed to account for these strange bedfellows.

In this instance, politics explains a lot. Today, most of the provisions of the Social Security Act seem, on their face, prosaic and uncontroversial. That was not true in 1934-35 when the New Deal leadership and Roosevelt's appointed Committee on Economic Security[18] were considering what should be included in the legislation. They were deeply concerned about whether they could do enough to mollify Harry Hopkins, their own Federal Emergency Relief Administrator, and to counter the appeal of populist "share the wealth" schemes such as the Townsend Plan, Huey Long's "Every Man a King," and the End Poverty in California

(EPIC) movement. On the political right, there were the South and the southern senators, the manufacturing and agricultural interests, and the American Medical Association. For the time, this act was a major achievement, which the work of the Committee helped make possible. But if it looked easy, it wasn't—the political and constitutional issues[19] were formidable and much of what was adopted or left out of the act can be largely explained by looking to these constraints. In a larger historical perspective, these titles help identify areas of institutional strength and weakness that have lasted.

The main titles of the original Social Security Act can be divided into three major parts: those that deal with social insurance proper (Old Age and Survivors Insurance and Unemployment Compensation—Titles II and III); those that provide matching funds to supplement state funding for the traditional "welfare" categories (the aged, dependent children, and the blind—Titles I, IV, and X); and two titles providing grants and matching funds for maternal and child services and for public health (Titles V and VI). Of particular interest are the differences in the ways these separate categories were treated.

A striking aspect of this legislation, especially in its development and statutory expression, was the emphasis given to the social insurance titles (II and III) in contrast to the titles dealing with health and welfare. That difference resulted in part from a primary concern of both Roosevelt and the Committee on Economic Security to get a system of social insurance in place that would assure income security for workers and retirees and give them a stake in this system.

A secondary objective was to reach toward a larger vision of "social security" by including some form of health insurance and long-term provision for the poor. No great surprise—the social insurance titles took precedence and place with minimalist provisions made for the health and welfare titles. Still, some details are useful to illustrate the effects of relative political weakness upon health and welfare policy.

One of the most important features of both unemployment insurance and old age and survivors insurance was that they were based on payroll taxes with both employer and employee sharing the burden. Both elements of this statement were of great future importance. Roosevelt was especially interested in the contributory aspect, emphasizing repeatedly that these benefits should not be a "dole," but something that the beneficiary had paid for and that "no damned politician" would be able to take away.[20] The payroll tax also offered other advantages, including political acceptability,[21] and ease of eligibility determination and collection. A second point is that the payroll tax tied these programs—as well as others that might be built upon them—to that fraction of industries included. Initially, the Committee had thought in terms of all industries employing four or more, which would have made these systems broadly inclusive. In the course of passage, though, the minimum was changed to eight. Furthermore, government employees, agricultural and domestic workers, and employees of charitable and educational institutions were excluded.[22] One reason cited was the difficulty of keeping records, a consideration that had merit. But another was the desire, especially in the South, for cheap agricultural and domestic labor. In this way, the Act itself tended to create a divide between an entitled working class that "deserved" its benefits and a large, indeterminate number of working poor without entitlement and the "undeserving' poor on welfare.

Some form of health insurance had been generally regarded by Roosevelt and the Committee as an important part of social security in the larger sense, though probably not as part of the initial legislation. The Committee deferred action but resolved to study the issue and included health insurance as one of the special topics for its staff. The Committee also appointed a Medical Advisory Committee—along with similar committees for nurses, hospitals, dentists, and public health. Initially, the medical community was divided on the health insurance issue, but the AMA—under the leadership of Dr. Morris Fishbein—managed to unite the physicians in opposition to the any such proposal. In achieving this unity, the AMA made some important concessions, agreeing to accept the child health provisions of the Act and endorsing schemes for voluntary health insurance. The strategy of the administration had always been to defer consideration of health insurance until passage of the less controversial titles seemed likely. With changed circumstances, Roosevelt chose a quick and largely assured victory over a lengthy and uncertain battle. Consideration of health insurance was postponed until after passage of the Act. Two months after passage, the Committee recommended to the newly constituted Social Security Board the establishment of a national health insurance plan based on shared responsibility of the federal and state governments. No action was ever taken on the proposal.

With national health insurance off the table, the Social Security Act dealt narrowly and obliquely with health care in Titles V and VI. Title V was a restoration, in weakened condition, of the Sheppard-Towner Act, providing a 50% dollar-for-dollar match for maternal and child health and child welfare block grants, but with less money and with a means test. Even this was strongly opposed by the AMA because it might impinge on (i.e., compete with) the private practice of medicine. The Association argued for an extension of public health as a preferred alternative and was partly mollified by an increased appropriation under Title VI for the Public Health Service, primarily intended for states in which public health had lagged, especially the South.

Not only did the Social Security Act make little provision for health care for the poor, it also mortgaged the future by explicitly and implicitly favoring "welfare" medicine as the option for them. Title V maternal health and child services were means tested; and public health services were mainly intended for rural areas. Otherwise, the Act offered matching funds for the traditional public assistance categories. In other words, welfare recipients could pay out of their own pockets. There was, of course, no bar against states augmenting the monthly cash assistance, but no separate provision for matching funds was made.[23]

Another omission, along with health insurance, was provision for long-term unemployment, whether occasioned by disability or because the private sector failed to generate enough jobs. The Committee was keenly aware of these issues and produced studies and recommendations on both—though nothing that became part of the legislation. Fifteen years later, in the 1950 Amendments, "permanent and total disability" was included. As for unemployment, the Social Security Act dealt only with unemployment insurance that provided income security for a few months and was designed to cope with occasional spells of intermittent unemployment. In separate actions, the Federal Emergency Relief Administration was terminated and public employment programs, such as the Works Progress Administration and the Public Works Administration established, representing a considered movement beyond emergency relief, but not a lasting solution.[24]

At an early stage, there was some hope within the Committee on Economic Security that the social security legislation could be a vehicle to deal with this issue of long-term unemployment, but a general opposition to the continuance of public relief and Roosevelt's commitment to contributory programs and dislike of a "dole" worked against that option. When the public works programs ended, their absence left a large gap between the federally sponsored programs for an upper stratum of workers with good and steady jobs and the marginal workers who, in hard times, had nothing but "welfare" for support. This "stratification"[25] not only left that lower level badly off, it created a large and historic divide in the development of future policy.

As a part of the wider concept of social security, both Roosevelt and the Committee intended to make some provision for the indigent elderly, not covered by OASI, and for needy women and children. Aid to the blind was not initially included in the Committee's report but was added in the course of legislation at the instance of the Senate Finance Committee.[26] Permanent federal aid for these programs was, in itself, an important step. Equally important was the way in which it was done—by the use of categorical grants-in-aid with matching funds, intended to support and enhance *existing* state welfare categories rather than to create new programs.

As initially recommended to the Congress, these programs included several features that were important precedents for the future. These additions were primarily directed at protecting the program from spoils and patronage, though with a sub-text of racial issues. One set of provisions mandated the designation of a single state agency and a state plan, federally approved, that would be in force statewide (in "all political subdivisions").[27] Another set required cash payments, confidentiality of records, and the right to a "fair hearing." These items may seem quaint and formalistic today, but they made good sense as attempts to assure program integrity in jurisdictions rife with spoils and racial discrimination.

These provisions were met with strong and nearly unanimous opposition from southern representatives. Most important was the state plan provision, which southern senators, led by Harry Byrd of Virginia, denounced as an interference with their handling of "the Negro question" and a federal effort to decide to whom pensions should be paid and how large they should be.[28] As a result of this controversy, the state plan provision was substantially weakened, leaving eligibility and benefit levels up to the states, so long as age, residence, and citizenship requirements were no more restrictive than those prescribed in the statute.[29] To this day, eligibility and benefits remain primarily matters for the states to determine, both for welfare programs and for Medicaid.

Authority over approval or withdrawal of state plans was sharply curtailed, largely over fear that the Social Security Act was aimed at forcing a civil service merit system upon southern states.[30] The operative language, provided by the Ways and Means Committee, authorized the Social Security Board to provide for such methods of administration as necessary for the efficient operation of the plan, "other than those relating to selection, tenure of office and compensation."[31]

Another major issue was the limits, if any, to be put upon payments to public assistance recipients. In this matter, the Committee on Economic Security tended to be generous and the Congress less so. Initially, the Committee considered not imposing any specific limit. Later, it proposed a formula used by New York and Massachusetts requiring a level of assistance that "when added to the income of an aged recipient [would provide] a reasonable subsistence compatible with decency and health." Southerners especially objected that this formula would authorize federal officials to write the terms of individual old age pensions. The Ways and Means Committee struck that provision and substituted for the aged and blind a specific sum ($30) as a limit on the amount the federal government would match.[32] For aid to dependent children, Congress adopted a federal limit of $6 for the first child and $4 for any additional ones, though later allowed higher numbers of $18 and $12. However, the match for ADC was set at 33 1/3% rather than the 50% that applied to the aged and blind.

Means testing and similar requirements such as providing a "suitable home" were not mentioned in the original legislation. The term "needy" was used in describing the intended recipients of public assistance, though not in the context of eligibility criteria. The reason for this omission, according to one observer,[33] was Sen. Byrd's successful campaign against a definition of, "need" in the Act. Also, both the Committee and Congress saw their role with respect of public assistance as rescuing state programs rather than revising them.

The issue of means testing as a federal requirement came up when some states sought to pay uniform monthly allotments to all over 65, as opposed to paying on the basis of need—which most states had been doing and continued to do. At the time, the General Counsel of the Social Security Board said that "it cannot be stated without question" that a state plan had to provide for a means test.[34]

But the Social Security Board believed that the Act intended this requirement, based upon the history of the legislation and the preamble to the public assistance titles.

Title IV, Aid to Dependent Children (ADC), which was seen initially as neither important nor contentious, became over time one of the most controversial and vexatious social programs in American history. Within the Committee on Economic Security and during the consideration of the

Social Security Act, the lead on children's issues was taken by the U.S. Children's Bureau and members of the child welfare reform movement. They backed primarily maternal and child health grants (a resurrected and enlarged Sheppard-Towner Act) and an array of federally supported child welfare services for the homeless, dependent, neglected, and potentially delinquent juveniles. Some categorical aid for crippled children was added, in part since it would have special appeal to Roosevelt, who had been a victim of polio or "infantile paralysis." Child advocates were enthusiastic about this program—so much so that they were willing to accept small initial authorizations. On the other hand, there was little interest in ADC, either in the child welfare movement, the Committee, or the Congress. Edwin Witte, the Committee's executive director, believes that nothing at all would have been done about ADC had it not been included in the Committee's report,[35] and thought that the smaller match of 33 1/3% reflected the "complete lack of interest' in the subject.[36]

With no significant debate, Congress endorsed the "mothers' pension" approach, leaving the details of implementation to the states. It would be hard to find a more fateful step taken with so little thought for future consequences. It was, in a small way, a step forward. The matching formula and payment rates, though stingy, were better than nothing. Congress also expanded the definition of "dependent child."[37] At the same time, the category of general assistance was not supported—a step that symbolically and practically omitted any kind of residual support for the working poor. Of course, much of the purpose of the Social Security Act was to get out of the business of "relief" or of public works. But this step left a gap in federal welfare policy between Title IV and Titles V and VI—between one measly program for needy dependent children and the maternal health and child services programs, which were largely data gathering and stimulative in nature.[38] This omission eventually put a substantial burden on a number of weak and unevenly developed state programs.[39]

In 1935, the year in which the Social Security Act was passed, 45 states had mothers' pensions legislation; but typically localities could choose whether to establish programs or not. In two of the 45 states (Arkansas and Mississippi) legislation existed but the programs were inoperative. In four others, programs functioned in 5% or less of the counties (Kentucky, Louisiana, Tennessee, and Texas). Local communities contributed 85% of the funds and administered the programs locally, sometimes through a county department of welfare but often through local orphans' courts or citizen volunteers, that provided their own interpretation of "fit mother" and "suitable home," applied their own means test and decided whether the applicant could or should work.[40]

The system suffered from the "double handicap of permissive legislation and local financing."[41] Counties were frugal, took care of "their own," and indulged local mores about whom should be supported. Some figures help convey the results. Less than 3% of families headed by single women received mothers' pensions. Most recipients of aid were white widows, with only 25% unmarried and 3% of African-American descent.[42] In 36 states deserted wives were eligible, but divorcees in only 22 states, and only 3 states explicitly included unmarried mothers.[43] Almost all states had provisions for means testing, and "fit mothers" or "suitable home" requirements. Both mothers *and children* were often required to work. Monthly grants ranged from a high of $69.31 in Massachusetts to a low of $4.33 in Arkansas. Under such conditions, mothers often had to give up their children for foster care or adoption—an outcome that would seem to defeat the purposes of such programs.

Some of these provisions had no direct relevance to the Medicaid program, established thirty years later—for instance, the fit mother and suitable home requirement—nor did welfare workers monitor homes of Medicaid recipients for signs of immorality, drunkenness, or a "man in the house." Yet Medicaid began as a program of categorical eligibility for the poor and indigent. It included means and assets test. And it inherited the stigma and indignity associated with "being on welfare". These features have persistently diminished Medicaid's acceptability among its recipients.

Later developments have tended to marginalize ADC (renamed AFDC in 1962)[44] even further and to confirm its identification as the American "welfare system" with the negative connotations that terminology has acquired. In 1950, a disability insurance program was added to OASI, the premier social security program—a step that began the elevation of "disability" as a category. When the Social Security Amendments of 1972 federalized the "adult" categories of aged, blind, and disabled, that left AFDC as a state responsibility and the one program especially associated with "welfare," deficient administration, and indignity.

The Social Security Amendments of 1950 authorized federal matching payments for vendor payments to providers of health care for welfare recipients. Vendor payments (in lieu of cash) had been used in the states because of a belief that welfare recipients might not know how to purchase services for themselves or would spend their cash assistance on whiskey or other non-essentials. So far, no specific federal provision for health care expenses had been made for the public welfare recipients as such, although state officials lobbied for some kind of aid. During 1950, health insurance was also on the agenda and these vendor payments were being pushed by the AMA as an alternative to national health insurance. Adopting them weakened the case for national health insurance, made possible direct payments to health care providers in the states, and—most important in the present context—directly linked federal support for health services to the public assistance categories and started the money flowing through these categorical conduits—a step taken with little attention to ultimate consequence.[45]

Another development of major and continuing importance for Medicaid was the growth of private and employer sponsored health insurance and pension plans. In the absence either of national health insurance or of a strong public health tradition, health insurance developed in the private sector, at first during the Great Depression, then more rapidly during and after World War II.[46] Eventually, over 70% of the working force was covered by employer sponsored insurance and over 50% had private pensions. This growth in the private sector had a number of consequences, several of them especially important for Medicaid.

The important and even dominant role of employer sponsored health insurance is one aspect of what Jacob Hacker has termed the "divided welfare state." Within it, most workers rely primarily on private and especially employer sponsored health insurance while publicly supported programs, such as Medicare and Medicaid or public health clinics, exist largely as alternatives or supplements to private insurance.

The practical consequence of this division for Medicaid is enormous, for it separates most of the working class with good jobs and health insurance—and especially organized employees in large corporations who can rely on their collective efforts and market position—from the poor who are relatively powerless and may lack both jobs and health insurance. This privileged status can work against publicly supported health insurance or health care. Organized labor has more than once helped to defeat national health insurance proposals on the ground that a particular proposal might be an improvement, but wouldn't make organized labor much better off than they were. In much the same way, labor leaders have seldom weighed in heavily in favor of Medicaid programs or other species of "welfare medicine" since they didn't see these as programs for them and their families.[47]

Another consequence of this strong, antecedent development of employer based insurance was to leave uncovered many who were poor risks, lacked access to insurance, or could not afford it. The retired elderly, for instance, found individual insurance difficult to purchase. Private insurance companies screened out pre-existing conditions and bad risks. Small businesses, agricultural and domestic workers, and the self-employed had little or no access to group health plans. And the unemployed or poor couldn't afford health insurance. Thus, one major role for Medicaid has been to insure the uninsurable—those that private insurers would not cover. Put another way, the good risks are taken by private insurers, most of the bad risks left to Medicaid.[48]

Employer supported health insurance implies employment in a particular firm or organization and therefore dependence upon the fortuitous circumstances of where one works and who or what gets included in the particular plan. For instance, are spouses and children covered? part-time employees or retirees? Are preventive care, rehabilitation, or long-term care included? The point is that employer sponsored insurance is variable and leaves gaps in eligibility and coverage that are especially hard on the marginal employee or the working poor. Typically, these problems are at their worst in marginal industries where employers are hard pressed and often unable to do more and employees have few resources or alternatives for employment or coverage. Their situation adds moral urgency to a Medicaid role of filling gaps where the private insurance system is deficient or unresponsive.

An employer based system of health insurance can also leave large numbers of unemployed workers without health insurance when they need it most, because of structural changes in the economy, global competition, or a lengthy cyclical downturn. As noted above (*supra*, 9), the Social Security Act did not address that situation, and no permanent provision has been made that does so. In default of a better solution, Medicaid has often become, especially in recent years, a form of health insurance for the unemployed so that employer sponsored insurance renders Medicaid highly sensitive to the state of the economy—a perversity in the sense that the capacity to help is likely to be weakest at the time the need is greatest.

Conclusion

A theme developed in this chapter is the importance of an "American exceptionalism" noted by Tocqueville and others as distinguishing this country from European ones: the absence of an aristocracy, an established church, or strong institutions of central government and yet the presence of a developed and dynamic civil society. To keep it that way, with power dispersed and decentralized, Americans devised a weakly institutionalized system of government with the dual protections of separation of powers and federalism that would guard against concentration of power or tendencies to an extreme.

A characteristic of American welfare (and health) policy has been the comparative weakness of public institutions and the relative strength of private ones, for instance, the role of private philanthropy or the organized political power of American medicine. The latter is, in itself, a major reason[49] that the United States, alone among advanced nations, still lacks national health insurance, and has Medicare and Medicaid instead. Moreover, we owe to politically organized medicine the fateful linking of health care for the poor to the categorical welfare system for the aged poor, the blind, and dependent children. This particular misalliance associated Medicaid with the tight-fisted stinginess and gratuitous meanness toward the poor that has characterized public welfare in the United States.

For much of its history, policy making for Medicaid followed a style characteristic of public welfare, especially for the aged, blind, and dependent children, which was to build incrementally upon a traditional, categorical base, linked to state welfare eligibility. Because of institutional weakness and lack of political clout both public assistance and Medicaid policy tended to be responsive rather than proactive and to percolate upward from locality to state and state to nation, with professional and advocacy groups pressing for changes that would be more generous or more remunerative, though typically along categorical lines.

Medicaid also remained tied to welfare eligibility, which excluded most of the poor and uninsured,[50] and associated Medicaid with the complexities and indignities of welfare eligibility determination and means testing. Though formally de-linked in 1996, this association with welfare and its stigmata continues—in the minds of both the public and Medicaid recipients—and is a significant barrier to enrollment even today.

Another part of the tale is what this incremental growth neglects or fails to achieve: the interstate variations that persist; the categories of poor or uninsured not covered; exemplary programs that are not replicated; and failures to assure access, increase equity, improve quality or maintain program integrity.

At the same time, the Social Security Act, by incorporating Old Age Assistance, Public Assistance, and Aid to the Blind among its titles and establishing them as entitlements with open-ended authorizations and generous federal matching, created the possibility of vigorous growth. Despite its mean heritage, the Medicaid program has developed from an add-on to some narrow and stingy welfare categories into the largest health insurance system in the United States—with SCHIP included, covering 60 million people.[51] In the course of this evolution it has taken on new roles of supporting preventive care for children and mothers, covering "uninsurable" categories and services, supporting the safety-net providers of last resort, and increasingly providing health insurance for the poor and uninsured.

Much of this success, we will argue, has been possible because of a creative use or adaptation of these inherited Medicaid traits of pluralism, categorical incrementalism, generous matching, and entitlement. But it was and is a partial success, marred by its welfare legacy, uneven development, institutional vulnerability, and lack of systematic reform.

Notes

1. As appropriately titled by Robert and Rosemary Stevens, *Welfare Medicine in America.*
2. A strongly institutionalized program, such as Old Age and Survivors' Insurance, within the Social Security Administration, would typically have a solid statutory base, adequate authorizations, good staffing with recruitment, training, and advancement policies, capacity to maintain program integrity, and ability to defend against private sector encroachments, mobilize support, and seek program modifications important for survival.
3. *Federalist No. 10.*
4. Alexis de Tocqueville, *Democracy in American* New York: Vintage Books, 1955, Vol. 2, 108.
5. Morton Keller, *Affairs of State—Public Life in Late Nineteenth Century America.* Cambridge, MA., Harvard University Press, 1977, 285
6. Stephen Skowronek, *Building a New American State—The Expansion of National Administrative Capacities,"* Cambridge, MA,: Harvard University Press, 1982, 39.
7. This separatism reflected a deep division of philosophy that remains with us to this day. However, for a sense of the times, compare some of these statements by some well-known personalities back then. George Washington Plunkett was a Tammany leader, who believed that the poor needed help *now* rather than long-term redemption:

   If a family is burnt out, I don't ask whether they are Republicans or Democrats, and I don't refer them to the charity organization society, which would investigate their case in a month or two and decide if they were worthy of help about the same time they are dead from starving. I just get quarters for them, buy clothes for them if their clothes are burned up, and fix them up till they get things running again. It's philanthropy, but its politics too—mighty good politics.... The poor are the most grateful people in the world." As quoted by Walter I. Trattner, *From Poor Law to Welfare State—A History of Social Welfare in America, 2d ed.* New York: Free Press, 1972, 84-85.

Contrast this statement with that of an advocate of "scientific" charity in a handbook entitled *How to Help the Poor*:

The old method of working for the poor always left him in the swamp but threw him biscuits to keep him from starving. The new method is to throw him a plank. He cannot eat the plank but he can scramble out upon it and have his share of the labors and reward which the experience of life brings to both high and low." As quoted by Robert H. Bremner, *American Philanthropy.* New York: Alfred A. Knopf, 1980, 205.

An early and perhaps the greatest advocate of the new philanthropy was Andrew Carnegie, who regarded wealth as a stewardship to be used efficiently and effectively for good. According to Carnegie, philanthropy must avoid giving that had "a degrading, pauperizing tendency upon … recipients." and choose instead projects that would "stimulate the best and the most aspiring of the poor of the country to further efforts for their own improvement." The philanthropist's responsibility extended only to the "industrious and ambitious," those "most anxious and able to help themselves." The "inert, lazy and hopelessly poor" was the province of the state. As quoted in Bremner, *ibid.,* 221-222.

8. One result was that public institutions for the care of the sick and poor fell behind those in Europe, a tendency noted shortly after the Civil War.
9. Robert J. Myers, *Medicare.* Homewood, Ill.: Richard D. Erwin, 1970, 4; Colin Gordon, *Dead on Arrival: The Politics of Health Care in Twentieth-Century America.* Princeton, NJ: Princeton University Press, 2003, 2.
10. Richard Ely, *The Labor Movement in America.* New York: Crowell, 1886, 254-55.
11. Infancy and Maternity Act, the first grants-in-aid program for health, though as a grants program preceded by education.
12. *Massachusetts v . Mellon,* 262 U.S. 447 (1923).
13. Public health was something of an exception, especially when interstate waters and seaports were involved.
14. Medicaid has, for example, been likened to crabgrass— it grows anywhere, especially in areas where other grass does not, it is hard to uproot or get rid of, but provides cover of a sort.
15. Describing a situation as a "problem" may suggest, sometimes intentionally, that the situation has a "solution,' while nothing better than an awkward compromise is possible. Cf. T. D. Weldon, V*ocabulary of Politics.* London: Penguin Books, 1953, esp. 76.
16. Edwin E. Witte, *The Development of the Social Security Act.* Madison, Wisc., University of Wisconsin Press, 1962, 97.
17. Arthur J. Altmeyer, *The Formative Years of Social Security.* Madison, Wisc.: University of Wisconsin Press, 1966, 3, 12.
18. Novel for its time, the Committee on Economic Security was created following hearings on an unemployment compensation proposal (the Wagner-Lewis bill, HR 7659, 73d Congress, 2d Session) and Roosevelt's decision that the issue of social insurance and its alternatives needed to be considered more broadly. The Committee was charged to do that, but also to come up with a proposal that the

president could take to Congress. They had six months—about half the time we would regard as minimal today. The Committee (five cabinet level appointees) was supported by an executive director and a staff that worked on special topics and produced technical papers. There was an advisory council that worked closely with the Committee, a technical board and a National Conference on Economic Security to broaden perspectives.

19. For a brief summary of the constitutional issues see Altschuler, *The Formative Years of Social Security,* 20 ff.

20. Altschuler, *The Formative Years,* 11; Witte, *The Development of the Social Security Act,* 119; and Colin Gordon, *Dead on Arrival: The Politics of Health Care in Twentieth Century America.* Princeton, N.J.: Princeton University Press, 2003, 92.

21. Especially as compared to a general tax; note also that the American Association of Labor Lawyers "model law" took this approach.

22. Witte, *The Development of the Social Security Act,* 53.

23. For further discussion, *infra* at   .

24. At the same time Roosevelt created the Committee on Economic Security he also established the National Resources Board, which was to work closely with the Committee in mobilizing resources to assure maximum employment. But little was done to create a long-term solution other than establishing the Works Progress Administration (WPA) and the Public Works Administration. Witte, *The Development of the Social Security Act,* 6, 11.

25. Cf., Linda Gordon, *Pitied But Not Entitled—Single Mothers and the History of Welfare.* New York: Free Press, 1994, 254.

26. Witte, *The Development of the Social Security Act,* 191.

27. Intended to ensure "equity" as between different areas of the state—a serious matter, considering both the temptations and possibilities for differential distribution of funds by county and locality along political and/or racial lines. Note also the importance of such provisions as cash payments and confidentiality in relation to patronage and how it works.

28. Witte, *The Development of the Social Security Act,* 143-4.

29. *Ibid,* 144.

30. *Ibid.,* 145.

31. This did not settle the matter. The struggle for a merit system and against "spoils" and patronage uses of old age assistance for electoral advantage continued for years and led to numerous administrative audits and, in Ohio, to a withdrawal of welfare payments and the electoral defeat of Gov. Davey. Arthur Altschuler, *The Formative Years of Social Security,* 75 ff.

32. An even lower limit of $15 had been suggested, although $30 was at the time being granted to widows under the Veterans' Pension Act. Witte, p. 163. Note that $30 added to a $30 match would be $60, not a princely sum, but more than $30.

33. Altschuler, *The Formative Years,* 61.

34. *Ibid,* 61.

35. Witte, *The Development of the Social Security Act, op. cit.,* 164.

36. *Ibid,* 164-165.

37. Congress raised the upper age limit on eligibility from 14 to 16, broadened the definition of absence or incapacity of a parent, and permitted the child to live with a wider range of relatives. Winifred Bell, *Aid to Dependent Children.* New York: Columbia University Press, 1965, p. 27.

38. Gordon, *Pitied But Not Entitled,* 24-25.

39. Winifred Bell comments: "Since many states either failed to provide residual programs to ensure minimum support to all needy children or made less generous

provision for families receiving general assistance, ADC has a vast potential for upsetting the traditional relationship between the legitimate and the illegitimate, the Negro and the white." Bell, *Aid to Dependent Children*, 28.

40. *Ibid.,* 10-11.
41. *Ibid,* 15.
42. In Michigan, in 1934, 1226 of the recipient ADC women on the rolls were widowed, 325 deserted, 175 divorced and 249 had imprisoned or incapacitated husbands. *Ibid.,* 200n12.
43. *Ibid.,* 8.
44. Aid to Families with Dependent Children.
45. Stevens and Stevens, *Welfare Medicine in America,* 23.
46. This development was enormously accelerated by wartime decisions. A 1943 ruling of the IRS held that group health insurance payments were not subject to the income tax. The War Labor Board also exempted fringe benefits (including health insurance) from wage and price controls. Jacob S. Hacker, *The Divided Welfare State—The Battle over Public and Private Social Benefits in the United States* (Cambridge Univ. Press, 2002), 121, 217-218.
47. See Gordon, *Dead on Arrival, ,* esp. Ch. 2
48. Blue Cross and a few other not-for-profit health insurance plans community rated for a time, but by 1950 most of these were experience rating, at least partially.
49. Although clearly not the only one—Cf. Gordon, *Dead on Arrival.*
50. Cf. Joe, Thomas C. W., Judith Meltzer, and Peter Yu, "Arbitrary Access to Care: The Case for Reforming Medicaid," *Health Affairs* 4 (1) 1985, 59-74.
51. In 2006, 55 million in Medicaid and another 4-6 million in SCHIP (4 million at a point in time; 6 million in SCHIP over the course of the year).

2

Legislating Medicaid

When passed, as part of the Social Security Amendments of 1965 (P.L. 89-97), the Medical Assistance program—more commonly known as Medicaid—was not high profile legislation. Unlike Medicare, there was no strong lobby pushing for its enactment.[1] Its inclusion as one slab of the "three-layer" cake was almost fortuitous. A legislative draftsman said that he doubted that more than a half day was devoted to consideration of its provisions. Nor did it occasion much discussion in committee or floor debate.

As legislation, Medicaid was often characterized as an "afterthought"—a casual and belated inclusion once the main business of Medicare was settled. Yet, within a few months after its initial implementation the program was being described as a "sleeping giant,"[2] because of its phenomenal capacity for growth. Although casual afterthoughts can often have big, unforeseen consequences, these two views of Medicaid seem in conflict. Yet each reflects a truth about the program. Though Medicaid came late in the legislative process, after other major structural decisions had been made, for Wilbur Mills—chairman of the House Ways and Means Committee and the most important legislative sponsor—the Medical Assistance Program was a significant benefit for the poor and structurally important as part of his overall design for health benefits in the Social Security Amendments of 1965.[3] Medicaid was considerably more than an "afterthought" for him. And for Wilbur Cohen—the most active and influential member of the administration—Medicaid was the culmination and ratification of a project begun almost twenty years earlier: to create a health benefit for the poor by incremental expansion, using the Social Security Act as a legislative vehicle.

Medicaid was more than an afterthought for some of the most knowledgeable and powerful legislative figures of that time.[4] Moreover, when regarded from a longer perspective, as a program intended to survive and grow, the Medicaid legislation had about it considerably more design than generally supposed. Much of this design developed over time and was crafted with external circumstance and political environment more in mind than program administration. It also shows that Medicaid was more "forethought" than afterthought and helps explain its staying power and robust capacity for growth.

When Medicare and Medicaid were enacted into law, in the spring and summer of 1965, the political environment was unusually favorable and—it is important to add—quite unlike the harsh conditions under which the Medicaid program has survived and grown. Following the election of November, 1964, the Democrats controlled both the House and Senate, with a super-majority in the House. Lyndon Johnson had won a landslide victory with a strong mandate to complete the unfinished work of the slain president, John Kennedy. For Democrats, this was the largest window of opportunity since the New Deal administration of 1932. In these circumstances, it was no great feat to include Medicaid as part of the "three-layer cake."[5] But that perspective loses sight of the extent to which Medicaid was already in being before it was enacted and specially adapted to survive in a hostile environment.

After the War

The years immediately before and after World War II were important for health policy then, and ultimately, for Medicare and Medicaid—not so much because of what was accomplished as for what was not. Coming out of the war, there was a deep and pervasive desire to return to "normalcy," to demobilize and cut back on wartime government and regulations, and to get on with careers and raising families. At the same time, the war had created an awareness of the need for improved health care,[6] of shortages in medical "manpower" and health care facilities,[7] and the future importance of modern biomedical science.[8] The war also brought an upward surge in national spirit, a confidence in what could be accomplished by collective effort, and a sense of obligation to those who had contributed to the war effort—and there was an strong desire to pick up on this agenda as well.

An administrative entity historically significant in linking the New Deal with post-war health and welfare policy was the Interdepartmental Committee to Coordinate Health and Welfare. This Committee was originally established in 1935, during the legislative consideration of the Social Security Act to do just what its title implied: coordinate activities.

In 1937, largely at the prompting of its chairman, Josephine Roche—who as assistant secretary of the treasury, had jurisdiction over the Public Health Service—and the support of Arthur J. Altmeyer, chairman of the Social Security Board,[9] the Coordinating Committee undertook a comprehensive survey of the health needs of the nation and developed a number of recommendations for action.[10] Historically, they were picking up where the Committee on Economic Security and the Social Security Act of 1935 had left off.

The Coordinating Committee's report was endorsed by a National Health Conference in July 1939 and sent on to President Roosevelt as an appropriate basis for a National Health Program. The recommendations were important enough for future developments to be noted individually:

1) Expand the Public Health and Maternal and Child Health titles of the Social Security Act.
2) Federal grants-in-aid to the states for hospital construction and initial operating costs.
3) Federal grants-in-aid for state programs to treat the medically needy.
4) Federal grants-in-aid to support programs for general medical care, including compulsory insurance programs.
5) Federal program to compensate for wage loss and temporary or permanent disability.[11]

There was a brief, euphoric period when the National Health Conference leaders believed that their program might pass,[12] but President Roosevelt sent the program on to Congress for "careful study" rather than action. Meanwhile, the American Medical Association voiced strong objections to the health insurance proposal and the midterm elections of 1938 indicated a weakening of political support for the administration so that, ultimately, the president endorsed only the provision for hospital construction.[13] Despite this discouraging response, Altmeyer persuaded Senator Robert Wagner (D., NY) to introduce a bill incorporating the Coordinating Committee's recommendations.[14] The bill failed to win much public backing and was not reported out of committee. Nevertheless, such efforts helped keep both national health insurance and a number of other specific social insurance proposals on the national agenda.

The vagueness of the terminology, "national health program," is worthy of note, since it left unspecified whether the health program would be primarily insurance or health: whether the primary thrust would be support for health care and facilities through federal grants-in-aid or an insurance plan, presumably national and compulsory. As for "compulsory insurance," Senator Wagner said that would be up to the states.[15] There were related questions of the extent to which a national health program should be about insurance alone or include health care, practical issues of whether health insurance should precede the building of capacity and quality or the other way around, and the administrative issue of which agency should bear primary responsibility.[16]

Unifying language such as "Interdepartmental Coordinating Committee" and "National Health Program" brought people together; but it also blurred or concealed important differences. Leading the vanguard of the National Health Conference were Arthur Altmeyer—chairman of the Social Security Board with a mission of expanding social security—and Thomas Parran—surgeon-general of the Public Health Service and the chief health officer of the United States—who was equally devoted to the improvement of health delivery capacity and quality. They marched together for a brief period, but increasingly, their paths diverged, with some unexpected consequences.

That national health insurance became associated primarily with social insurance rather than health care delivery may have made sense both programmatically and politically, but it did so largely because of circumstance rather than logic. In 1942, when the Roosevelt administration was beginning to think about postwar domestic policy, the idea of comprehensive social security got a big impetus from the Beveridge Plan in England.[17] The Social Security Board capitalized upon this opportunity by endorsing an earlier report similar to the Beveridge Plan and including in its *Annual Report* a comprehensive scheme for an extended and unified social insurance system.[18] Although neither of these initiatives received much attention at the time, later in the year, President Roosevelt associated the Social Security Act and the Four Freedoms of the Atlantic Charter. He urged that social security coverage be greatly extended and that it "provide protection against the serious economic hazard of ill health."[19] He never specifically endorsed national health insurance, but he did—with the encouragement of the Social Security Board—strongly associate health insurance with the expansionist thrust of social security.

When Roosevelt failed to actively support the Social Security Board's recommendations, a delegation from the Social Security Administration again waited upon Senator Wagner and asked him to introduce the bill they had prepared.[20] Some months later, he did introduce a modified version, the Wagner-Murray-Dingell bill, which in its various iterations was for many years the centerpiece (and lightning rod) of Democratic health policy and much of its social policy as well. The bill was, according to his biographer, the most ambitious of Senator Wagner's legislative proposals and the most comprehensive domestic proposal introduced by anyone during the war years.[21] It was compendious, running to over two hundred pages, and dealing with every part of the social security program. It was also sweeping and controversial: reaching into new territory such as compulsory national health insurance and short-term and long-term disability insurance. Moreover, it proposed to *nationalize* a number of programs that had previously been seen as largely giving encouragement to state efforts.[22] Senator Wagner had little expectation that his bill would succeed any time soon. President Roosevelt, who had a war to win and a conservative, isolationist Congress to contend with, wished the senator "good luck," but gave the bill no support.[23] Senator Wagner kept the issues alive through an "Informal Conference Committee" of labor and liberals that met in Washington to plan strategy for the postwar period.[24] The bill also quickly became and remained a rallying symbol and manifesto for health care activists and the liberal press.

As World War II drew to a close, the traditional restraints upon raising controversial domestic issues ceased to bind, and a number of major proposals for veterans' benefits, reconversion, and peacetime social and economic reforms began to sprout, among them old and new programs for social security expansion and national health insurance. After lying dormant for two years, the Wagner-Murray-Dingell bill was re-introduced in May 1945 as an amendment to the Hill-Burton hospital construction act.[25] In September of that year, Senators Wagner and Murray got President Truman's endorsement of the health provisions of their original compendious bill, which he recommended to Congress in November 1945 and to the American people in a nationwide radio address in January 1946.[26] This reincarnation of W-M-D was denounced in the *Journal of the American Medical Association* as "the attempt to enslave medicine as first among the professions, industries, and trades to be socialized."[27] Medical societies again levied special assessments upon their membership to fight the legislation. So fierce was the opposition that no hearings were ever held in the House and Senator Murray was unable to get his bill reported out of the liberal Education and Labor Committee, which he chaired. Nevertheless, in Harry Truman the cause of national health insurance had acquired a strongly committed and stubborn champion. He knew from early experience in small towns and rural Missouri the importance of health care for average American families and the poor and the difficulties local communities had in meeting their needs for facilities and practitioners.[28] He was appalled by the revelations of the Senate *Wartime and Education* hearings that fully one-third of potential draftees had been unfit for service because of physical or mental deficiencies.[29] Unlike the Roosevelt administration, that largely ignored health insurance after the passage of the Social Security Act, Truman became the first president to feature national health insurance in his domestic agenda and to campaign vigorously for it.[30]

Year after year W-M-D was introduced in Congress and routinely blocked in committee by conservative Republicans and southern Democrats. Only once, in 1949, after Truman's successful campaign against the "do nothing" 80th Congress[31] and Democratic victories in House and Senate, was there a credible hope for success. Again, the bill failed to be reported out of committee. Then, in 1950, Democrats lost heavily in the mid-term elections,[32] in part because of a lethally effective campaign orchestrated by a California public relations firm and funded by AMA special membership levies. Other factors were at work, such as the Cold War and reaction to the New Deal and wartime mobilization, but this history of failure with national health insurance strongly suggested that it might be time to try "Plan B."

Following the 1949 W-M-D debacle, the administrative leadership of the Federal Security Agency—Arthur Altmeyer, Robert Ball, Wilbur Cohen, and I.S. Falk—developed a proposal that became the basis of the later Medicare bill: limited hospital insurance for the beneficiaries of OASI. Their strategy was to strip down the health insurance proposal in a way that would maximize political support (health care for the deserving elderly) and minimize opposition (by restricting insurance to a limited hospital benefit).[33] This version came to be known as the Oscar Ewing bill—after the Federal Security Administrator who was charged with moving it forward.[34]

This proposal, and others like it, were described as "incremental," especially within the FSA, to distinguish them from comprehensive or universal health insurance schemes. In this respect, one point that should not escape notice is that the Ewing Plan covered only OASI *beneficiaries*, not eligibles or the elderly as such, whether poor, deserving, or neither. Nor did it include dependents, as W-M-D would have.[35] The strategy was to get a bill that might pass and then extend social security based coverage and add a plan for the poor.[36] For the time, though, federal support for health insurance was off the table. And with President Eisenhower's firm opposition to health insurance, that remained the situation for almost a decade.

Health insurance may have been off the table, but there were other postwar agendas, such as subsidizing health care delivery more directly. One example was the Social Security Act itself: with two of its titles dealing with social insurance and four of them with public assistance, maternal and child health, and public health services. The National Health Program of 1939 also had this same duality in approach, as did the first Wagner bill. Had this duality between insurance and service delivery ever been resolved we would, no doubt, have had a more integrated health care system. It is important that it was not.

The Public Health Service during the New Deal and World War II was, like the Social Security Administration, an elite service and ably led. It was also the sole agency that inclusively represented health affairs within the federal administration. In this position, it bore an important responsibility to think ahead and be proactive.

Almost as early as the Social Security Administration, Thomas Parran, the Surgeon-General, and the PHS leadership were planning and organizing for the postwar years. The PHS had been actively involved in the *Wartime Health and Education* hearings and in documenting the needs for health services and facilities. The war itself greatly accelerated the pace of medical discoveries, innovations in medical practice and health care delivery, and trends such as specialization and group practice. These developments had a momentum of their own that would require response and adaptation. They could also be important resources in taking the next great step in medicine itself—to move on from infectious diseases to the great killers and cripplers—heart, cancer, and stroke; and long-term diseases and disabilities. Parran and his associates foresaw a postwar era with far-reaching changes in the orientation of medicine and health care delivery and, accordingly, in the kinds of resources, training, and organization that would be needed.[37] Late in 1943, they began working on the various elements of a postwar plan.

The centerpiece was the Mountin-Parran "Integrated Hospital Plan." This plan was influenced to some extent by wartime experience with regionalization and integration of hospitals in Great Britain and by the American military. It also had roots in the Bingham Associates,[38] the

Committee on Costs of Medical Care, and organized delivery systems such as the Mayo Clinic.[39] Under this scheme, health care would be primarily organized around a central or base hospital, surrounded by affiliated community hospitals and local, government supported public health stations or clinics. Regionalism would be promoted by comprehensive surveys and construction grants. Care for the poor and chronically ill would be subsidized by an array of categorical grants-in-aid for such conditions as venereal disease, tuberculosis, mental illness, cancer, and heart disease.

A second major element was increased investment in scientific research and the training of health care professionals. In part, this was an effort to catch up for the wartime years. Even more, it was the animating element of the Integrated Hospital Plan—staffing the facilities, and equipping the next generation of health care professionals with the knowledge, skill, and motivation to take on the major killing and crippling diseases.

A final part of the strategy was to use the National Institutes of Health and its grants-making capabilities to enlist the scientific community, the medical schools, and leadership groups within medicine and elsewhere as allies in the conquest of dread diseases.[40] In a small way, the PHS had engaged in this kind of mobilization and constituency building for many years, especially since the establishment of the National Cancer Institute in 1937. Now, they proposed to give it a major role in their programmatic development. An important expression of this aim was the establishment—in the Public Health Service Act of 1944—of National Advisory Councils for the National Institutes of Health and the National Cancer Institute to advise on general policy and approve grants awarded by the NIH.[41] Another important provision of the Public Health Service Act was Sec. 405 of Title IV which, except for construction grants, authorized "all other necessary expenses in carrying out this title," in other words, an open-ended authorization for the Cancer Institute, relieving it of periodic authorizations and making the funding for this worthy; (and politically popular) enterprise much easier.

Like national health insurance, the postwar plan of the Public Health Service was one of those historic failures that shaped the future in both negative and positive ways. The Integrated Hospital Plan quickly lost its hierarchical, integrated aspect to become the relatively innocuous Hill-Burton Hospital Survey and Construction Act, with control decentralized to levels at which local and state leaders could dominate.[42] Proposals to subsidize medical education—in contrast to support for research—faced the adamant determination of the AMA to hold down the number of physicians being educated. Not until midway through the Eisenhower administration would the AMA even consider a subsidy to the medical schools, let alone direct support for training health professionals.

For the poor in need of health care the postwar plan contemplated a combination of public health "stations," an array of categorical and project grants, and an increased general health grant for the states.. This part of the plan seemed outdated and unimaginative, especially in relation to the historic challenge of conquering the killing and disabling diseases. Yet even this modest step failed repeatedly and dismally because it was seen as an encroachment on the private practice of medicine and contrary to traditional notions of federalism.[43] Even the most meager attempt to enlarge the public support of health care was seen as too radical.

One lesson to take away from this short history is which elements of the PHS postwar plan got political and financial support and which did not. Subsidies for construction and research got support. Public funding for professional training or provision of health services— especially any that threatened professional control—did not. As a way of extending health services to the poor, public health seemed even less promising than health insurance or public assistance.

One development that resulted in part from President Eisenhower's lack of interest in either health services or medical progress was a major breakthrough in the funding of biomedical science, engineered by an informal coalition of DHEW and NIH leaders, Mary Lasker and the Lasker Foundation, and a handful of appropriations sub-committee chairmen.[44] In essence, their aim was to subsidize and channel biomedical research, professional training, and service delivery along the lines of the "big categories" of the killing and crippling diseases. Their efforts helped create the premier biomedical research establishment in the world and rapidly accelerated biomedical research and its application to health care. At best, though, it was an expensive and indirect approach to meeting the needs of the poor and could easily divert attention from their needs to biomedical conquests.

The postwar years were a time in which private, especially employer sponsored, health insurance grew rapidly (*supra,* 15). This development also diverted attention from the plight of the poor and medically needy. Many of those with employer sponsored insurance saw little need to fight hard for national health insurance or make common cause with the uninsured poor since they and their families were adequately covered.

Moreover, the elderly—who were notoriously difficult to insure and also sympathetically perceived—had plenty of champions and no need to ally themselves with a stigmatized group that had little to contribute.

During this era, "welfare medicine"[45] was marginalized rather like a poor relation that is sometimes "taken in" but never fully included and has to survive on leftovers. Their cause had champions but they were not effectively heard in a political system that favored entrenched and well-organized interests.

Kerr-Mills

Medical Assistance for the Aging—more popularly known as Kerr-Mills—was enacted in 1960 as part of the Social Security Amendments of that year.[46] It is of historic importance because it provided the template for Medicaid in 1965. The developments that led to Kerr-Mills also provide an instructive example of incrementalism in health policy, revealing both the potential of categorical incrementalism as well as some of its noxious properties.

For health and social policy, incrementalism was much in fashion in the 1950s.[47] Efforts at comprehensive restructuring failed or were unpopular, in part, because of a return to "normalcy" after the New Deal and the war years. The Cold War and McCarthyism deepened the conservative mood and encroached upon the domestic agenda. It was also a time of divided government, a president with a minimalist domestic agenda, and of legislative committee "baronies" controlled by southern Democrats. Under the circumstances, incrementalism in domestic policy made sense. And creatively employed, it could be a powerful engine for change.

An important element in accounting for the latent power of incrementalism was the nature of the Social Security Act and its strategic position with respect to social legislation. In 1960, the act had eight substantive titles that covered most of federal health and welfare policy, except for the Public Health Service and the Food and Drug Administration.[48] Because it was largely an aggregate of different titles, it lent itself readily to tinkering with individual programs, adding a paragraph, a subtitle, or even a whole new title. Much of its purpose was to get timely payments to individual beneficiaries, so it had a periodicity and a "must pass" element that invited its use as a vehicle for related legislation.[49] The Social Security Act fell under the jurisdiction of the House Ways and Means Committee which virtually assured its passage.[50] Such a bill, when passed by Congress, was almost "veto proof," since no president wanted the onus of holding up twenty million Social Security checks.[51]

The election of 1948 was important background for the Social Security Amendments of 1950 that led, in turn, to Kerr-Mills. In 1948, Harry Truman was re-elected president and the Democratic Party regained control of the House. A dominant theme of the new administration was "unfinished business," referring both to the renewed mandate and to the urgency of completing New Deal commitments sidetracked by the war.[52] Leaders of the Social Security Agency strongly supported this agenda, and prepared draft legislation for health insurance, extension of Old Age and Survivors' Insurance (OASI) to include "permanent and total disability," and amendments to the child welfare title of the act.[53] A separate bill contained major amendments of the social security and public assistance programs.

The health legislation was another iteration of Wagner-Murray-Dingell, but this time health insurance was separated from the social security and public assistance legislation. Arthur Altmeyer, under whose direction the bills had been prepared, says that he recommended this approach to the president because of the "extremely contentious" nature of the bills, which might "delay, if not imperil … less controversial recommendations."[54] Another reason seems to have been that the health bill was almost certain to fail. According to Robert Ball, "No one expected it to pass, except for the AMA."[55] Edwin Witte, from the sidelines, said the bill had "no prospects of passing." He went on to observe that he thought the only health bill that had a significant chance was the Taft bill, which anticipated the later Medicaid legislation in essential aspects.[56]

The Public Welfare and Social Security Amendments of 1949, drafted separately from the health insurance bill, were more actionable and, for the Social Security Administration, more urgent in some respects. Social Security was stagnating, with no major amendments or expansions since 1939. At the time Arthur Altmeyer advised President Truman that the contributory system was seriously at risk and liable to be replaced by some kind of unsound or extravagant general pensions scheme, such as the Townsend Plan.[57] As fortune—aided by some advance scheming—would have it, Altmeyer and Cohen had a plan, already endorsed by the bipartisan Social Security Advisory Council.[58]

The proposal of the Social Security Administration would have picked up on the "unfinished business" of the New Deal and then some. The major provisions are worth listing in detail, since they illustrate the largeness of the vision of this leadership as well as some of the ways and means of realizing it.

1. Old Age and Survivors' Insurance
   a) Extend coverage to include agricultural and domestic workers; employees of not-for-profit institutions, and state and local governments; inclusion of Puerto Rico and the Virgin Islands.
   b) Inclusion of benefits for both temporary and permanent and total disability.
   c) Liberalization in definition of employees; of eligibility requirements; and of earnings limits.
   d) Increase the wage base for benefits and contributions from $3000 to $4810; raise level of benefits by 66 2/3%; increase monthly benefit by 1% for each year of coverage.

2. Public Assistance and Welfare

   a) Include public assistance for the permanently and totally disabled; include caretakers as part of Aid to Dependent Children; include Puerto Rico and the Virgin Islands.
   b) Authorization of matching for direct payments to public medical institutions and for medical care in addition to cash assistance.
   c) Extension of federal matching to include public assistance to all needy individuals regardless of category.
   d) Liberalization of all matching ratios and relating them to fiscal capacity of each state; 75% match for administrative costs associated with public assistance and welfare.

Perusing this list, it is not hard to see why the Social Security Act was termed a "legislative train" or an "incremental engine."

The newly constituted Ways and Means Committee held lengthy hearings and worked over the bill so thoroughly—starting in February—that it didn't reach the floor and pass the House until October, leaving no time for the Senate to consider it in that year. In the following year, the Senate considered the bill exhaustively and with roughly comparable number of days of hearings—rare for the Senate. The whole episode was also noteworthy because of the measure to which the Ways and Means Committee bought into this bill, developed confidence in their relationship with the Social Security Administration, and thereafter took possession of Social Security as one of its principal concerns.[59]

There were holes in the ultimate legislation.[60] Disability insurance failed to pass. Domestics were not included and only regularly employed agricultural workers were covered. With respect to Public Assistance, the major loss was the provision for federal matching for all needy persons, independent of categorical eligibility and relating this match to state fiscal capacity.[61] Another was a failure to eliminate residency and citizenship requirements for eligibility.

Despite these omissions, both President Truman and the Social Security leadership considered the 1950 legislation to be a significant triumph. It liberalized and enhanced OASI benefits and added 10 million eligible workers to the rolls. Major changes affecting the needy were the addition of a new category of the "permanently and totally disabled,"[62] and—vitally important for Kerr-Mills and Medicaid—authorizations of federal matching funds for direct payments made by the states for medical services for those categorically eligible for public assistance.

The Amendments of 1950 were important in a larger strategic sense of breaking a ten-year legislative deadlock and revealing some of the cumulative potential of incremental changes. Sometimes called "salami slicing" or "salami tactics" by its chief Social Security exponent and practitioner, Wilbur Cohen, an incremental strategy was combined with strong technical work and advice, close collaboration with advocacy groups and congressional committees, and skill in developing policy options with bipartisan appeal. Beginning with the 1950 Amendments, this combination helped the Social Security program to thrive for the next decade and to grow dramatically in both numbers and political popularity despite an era of divided government under the Eisenhower administration and a socially conservative Congress.[63]

Wilbur J. Cohen deserves special mention because both he and his brand of incrementalism were critical for the historical development of Medicaid. Beginning his career as a research assistant to the Committee on Economic Security, he became a "technical adviser" to Arthur Altmeyer and, in effect, his legislative adviser and liaison with Congress. Cohen was often the effective broker of deals, representing the SSA's views and negotiating with major interest groups and the congressional committee chairmen and members. Dedicated and tireless, his knowledge of legislation and of administrative detail was profound and his ability to come up with actionable proposals legendary.

Cohen's homely metaphor of "salami slicing" to build a sandwich was disarmingly simplistic. He had, in fact, an artfully pragmatic and theoretically sophisticated view of incrementalism.[64] He saw it as a good way to compartmentalize complex or intractable social problems, minimize partisan or ideological antagonisms, and make small, often strategically important, gains when an opportunity offered or could be created. Incrementalism helped, in his view, to understand the nature of the problem itself and correct for unintended consequences; and it was important to consolidate gains, encourage acceptance of change, and create receptiveness of additional steps forward [65]

Cohen's incremental strategy toward policy was neither unanimously nor enthusiastically shared by other administrative leaders of the Social Security program. All of them pretty much accepted gradualism as a prudent and politically acceptable way to proceed, especially given the American political system.[66] Still, they remained aware of their own unfinished agenda and of being part of an international movement toward comprehensive social insurance.[67] In Robert Ball's view, incrementalism was the policy only when or because they couldn't do any better; and, certainly, the SSA had shown itself ready and willing to act boldly when opportunity presented—for example, with the Wagner bill of 1943 or the Public Welfare and Social Security Amendments of 1949. Altmeyer accepted incrementalism, but did not celebrate it. Robert Myers, the actuary, regarded it as disreputable, since it tended to conceal ultimate goals and therefore to be manipulative and unfair.[68]

Wilbur Cohen is closely associated with Kerr-Mills and with the origins of Medicaid largely because both of these programs were incremental add-ons to the existing categorical Public Assistance programs; and they were that because incremental tinkering with the Social Security Act was the easiest and perhaps the only way to get such legislation passed. As legislative liaison, he saw the openings and made the most of them.

As matters stood, prior to 1950, the Social Security Act made no provision for medical care for Public Assistance recipients. States could include an allowance for medical care in the Public Assistance cash allotment, but limits on the federal match were low,[69] so that, in practice, such expenses would be subtracted from the recipient's budget, diverted from other funds (which were not matched), paid out of state or local general funds, or absorbed by the providers. In addition, assistance allotments had to be paid in cash—a strong and cherished principle intended to protect the dignity and independence of the recipient.[70] This arrangement may have sounded good, but in practice it meant that allowances were inadequate, that recipients found care where and if they could, and the costs of care often fell upon hospitals and physicians, public institutions, local welfare authorities, and so forth. The situation pleased almost no one except those who opposed any public assistance at all.

According to Wilbur Cohen, the push toward a program resembling Medicaid began in 1942, when Rhode Island sought to use some Public Assistance funds for direct payments to "vendors" of medical care. At the time, the Social Security Board ruled that such payments were not lawful under the Act.[71] But the need continued; and the Social Security staff studied vendor payments along with the more general issue of medical assistance. Their recommendations were forwarded to the bipartisan Social Security Advisory Council of 1947-48 and became part of the proposed Public Welfare and Social Security Amendments of 1949.

The public assistance part of these amendments—the Public Welfare Act of 1949 (HR 2892)—would have authorized federal matching for medical assistance and vendor payments for medical care, in addition to Public Assistance cash payments. All of this was part of an attempt to put public assistance on a larger footing and, if it had passed, would have established the essentials of a Medicaid program a decade before Kerr-Mills. It would also have abolished categorical eligibility, a reform not fully achieved to this day. [72]

The Public Welfare and Social Security Amendments were too ambitious, by some margin, for the Ways and Means Committee. Nevertheless, a reduced and more incremental version , the Social Security Amendments of 1950, did pass by large majorities in both houses on August 15, 1950. Though much reduced in scope, this legislation took several steps of vital importance in advancing both Social Security and medical assistance. For good or ill, it also linked medical assistance to public welfare and committed it to an incremental path.

The vendor payments of 1950 were a first legislative installment. In 1954, Cohen worked with Nelson Rockefeller—then undersecretary of the Department of Health, Education, and Welfare in the Eisenhower administration—to develop a Medicaid-type proposal for the needy.[73] In the Social Security Amendments of 1956, he was able to get a provision for a separate medical assistance match and an averaging formula helpful to state administrators.[74] Both in 1956 and 1958, the matching formula was liberalized. By 1960, four-fifths of the states had availed themselves of the medical vendor payment option and these payments had grown from an estimated $81 million[75] to $514 million.[76] This level of expenditure was far from meeting the need, but vendor payments for medical care nourished a growth industry within the states and created an appetite for more.

Wilbur Cohen was criticized for brokering an unholy alliance of welfare and medical care. Nevertheless, this exercise in incrementalism[77] could be described as both ingenious and beneficial. The support provided by the voucher payments was needed and was an important stimulus. Between 1945 and 1960, it was one of the few health care initiatives that succeeded.[78] It smoothed a transition from vendor payments to Kerr-Mills to Medicaid. Yet several baneful features should not be missed. Medical assistance came with the categorical limits of Public Assistance, the interstate variations and penurious standards, the indignities of eligibility determinations and means and asset testing. Another consequence was that medical assistance as a political cause, budget line, and administrative subdivision was subsumed under public welfare and separated both from the Social Security Administration and from the larger issues of medical care and health insurance for the population at large. Indeed, this separation—by supposedly providing for the indigent—may have substantially weakened support for national health insurance.[79]

Wilbur Cohen defended his approach, saying that it was the only kind of intervention that would have worked. He thought, rightly, that there would be enormous possibilities for building incrementally upon this foundation. He also said that he believed that both a Medicare and a Medicaid program were "necessary and desirable" and would not conflict with each other. [80]

With respect to domestic affairs, the fabulous fifties were a decade of prosperity and contentment for most people. This circumstance left Democrats searching for policy issues during the popular Eisenhower administration. Older Americans were one group, though, that did not share equally in these good times and for whom health problems, medical care costs, and lack of insurance were increasingly troubling. Accordingly, once disability insurance passed in 1956, a small group of health policy activists[81] prevailed upon Aime Forand (D., R.I.), a member of the Ways and Means Committee, to introduce a health insurance bill that was a revival of the scaled-down "Oscar Ewing" approach of hospital insurance for Social Security beneficiaries that had been developed after the defeat of Wagner-Murray-Dingell in 1949.

Except for the AMA—which mounted another campaign—Forand's bill received little attention.[82] But John Kennedy (D., Mass.) was planning a run for the presidency and looking for issues. Wilbur Cohen—who had considerable talent for picking winners and cultivating relationships with them—helped persuade Kennedy that health care for the elderly would be a good campaign issue.[83] Others also thought so. In 1959, the Senate established a Subcommittee on Problems of Aged and Aging[84] ostensibly to make a comprehensive study of these problems but, more pragmatically and politically, to raise national consciousness about problems of the aging and stimulate some action with respect to them. The highest ranking Democrat on the Committee was Sen. John

Kennedy. The chairman was Sen. Pat McNamara (D., Mich.) a close friend of Wilbur Cohen's.

The report of the Committee (SRpt 1121) of February 1960 was comprehensive and searching, dealing with issues of income, employment, discrimination against the aging, housing, nursing homes and social services, health status, and the financing of health care. The plight of the indigent elderly was discussed with insight and thoroughness, but with little said about how to meet their needs. With respect to the financing of health insurance, the report focused—as would be expected—on an extension of OASDI, with an additional payroll tax. As for health care for the indigent, the report lacked enthusiasm for either premium subsidies or regulating the insurance industry but mentioned as options expanding public health or incrementally increasing federal participation in public assistance.[85] As with the Social Security Act of 1935, the Report left open the choice between these options, though it flagged as an "issue for consideration" the extent to which it would be "necessary or desirable" to provide "medical care to aged people through public assistance."[86] That issue was largely determined by a complex interaction of the presidential campaign of 1960 and the personalities and political interests of Sen. Robert Kerr (D., Okla.) and Wilbur Mills.

In 1960, Sen. Kennedy and many of the Democratic leadership in Congress were pushing health insurance as an issue and struggling to get some legislation passed, which would almost certainly be vetoed by President Eisenhower, but would serve as good campaign material. In 1959, the Forand bill had failed to clear the Ways and Means Committee in large measure because of the opposition of Wilbur Mills. In 1960, his support was solicited, but he preferred to let others take the initiative.[87] When separate proposals supported by Kennedy and by Eisenhower had been defeated in Ways and Means and Finance, Mills was approached again, this time by a three-member delegation of Walter Reuther of the United Auto Workers, Speaker Sam Rayburn, and Senate Majority Leader, Lyndon Johnson, urging Mills to get a bill out of committee. He promised to do so but then—to their considerable surprise—reported out his own minimalist version, which was little more than an increased subsidy of voucher payments for the indigent elderly.[88]

In the Senate, Robert S. Kerr played a role roughly similar to that of Wilbur Mills in the House. Like Mills, Kerr was a small-town lawyer—from Ada, Oklahoma—but he had branched out into oil well drilling and production and owned a mid-sized (Kerr-McGee) oil company.

He served as governor of Oklahoma from 1943-47 and, in 1960, was in his third term as senator. There, he was chairman of the Public Works Committee, an important power base within the Senate, that enabled him to benefit his home state of Oklahoma and the southwest region. A determined man and a forceful debater, he was also effectively the leader of the Senate Finance Committee.[89]

In 1960, a presidential election year, health insurance was shaping up to be the leading domestic issue, with the Forand bill as the centerpiece. Senator Kerr did not like the Forand bill. Like Wilbur Mills, he was against financing health insurance by expanding Social Security,[90] and reportedly said he would "lose every doctor in the state" if he supported the Forand bill.[91] He saw no reason to help out Kennedy—who as a Roman Catholic would lose Oklahoma—as opposed to his good friend, Lyndon Johnson, who was also in the race for president.

Yet Kerr wanted to offer some kind of benefit for the voters of Oklahoma. So he consulted with his director of Public Welfare, Lloyd Rader, whom he relied upon in such matters. Upon his advice, Kerr hired Wilbur Cohen[92]—paying him out of his own pocket to work with Rader and others on a compromise bill that would also appeal to Oklahoma voters. That, Cohen proceeded to do, arguing with supporters of the Forand bill that Kerr-Mills should be supported either as a step toward Medicare, which might fail, or as an addition to Medicare, which made no provision for the indigent elderly.[93] Whether because of Cohen's arguments or because of poor alternative prospects, Kerr's Bill (HR 12580 as amended by Senate Finance) passed the Senate by a vote of 91-2.[94] The conference committee changed little, except to drop the Long Amendment, which would have made vendor payments for public mental and tuberculosis hospitals eligible for reimbursement.[95]

In retrospect, Wilbur Cohen was right in his prophecy that Medicare and Medicaid would ultimately be joined together, although that union took place five years later. At the time, no major group—other than the AMA--thought that Kerr-Mills was a positive achievement except as a placeholder and possible way station on the road to Medicare. Aime Forand said at the time that Kerr-Mills did no harm but that it did no good either. It was, he said, "a mirage that we are holding up to the old folks to look at and think that they are getting something."[96] Like most sweeping judgments of Medicaid or its antecedents, he overstated the case: Kerr-Mills did some good; and it did some harm.

Kerr-Mills most important innovation was to extend medical benefits to a new category generally known as the "medically indigent"—persons over 65, not receiving Old Age Assistance, but whose incomes would be "insufficient to meet the costs of necessary medical services...." Qualifying people not because of eligibility under a Public Assistance category but because they would be reduced to poverty by their medical expenditures was an idea pushed for years by Wilbur Cohen. Both House and Senate bills included this new option along with an authorization "for each fiscal year" of a "sum sufficient to carry out the purpose" of this new provision. Initially, the House version limited this sweeping authorization by the proviso that neither the benefits nor the matching ratios could be more liberal than those under the Old Age Assistance program, but the ultimate legislation deleted this requirement and provided for this new option a "Federal Matching Percentage" of 50% as a lower limit and 80% as an upper limit, which would vary within these limits inversely with the square of the per capita income within the individual state. Initially, this formula applied only to the new option, "Medical Assistance for the Aged," but eventually it became the basis for the Medicaid program.

These changes were important breakthroughs, in establishing a new concept of the "medically indigent," which loosened the categorical linkages with Public Assistance, and introducing a relatively simple, semi-automatic matching formula with no global cap that distributed payments in a politically acceptable way as between rich and poor states. Eventually, this new option, with its matching formula, would become a powerful means of expansion within the Medicaid program. More immediately, it was highly beneficial to the states of Oklahoma and Arkansas. By a rough calculation, Kerr-Mills would increase the number receiving medical assistance in Oklahoma by an additional 180,000 to 270,000, four times as many as were then receiving health care, an attractive feature to Senator Kerr in an election year.[97]

The most important negative was that Kerr-Mills integrated medical assistance for the poor even more firmly and pervasively with Public Assistance. With this step, medical assistance was burdened with the social stigma and political disadvantages associated with a "welfare" program. Some of the damage was more specific and insidious than that. As with Public Assistance generally, the determination of eligibility standards and benefit levels were left, with minimum restrictions, to the states. As with welfare, means and asset testing were administered by local welfare offices. Generally, the poorer the state the poorer the welfare program. For the neediest, a likely (and perhaps intended result) would be a program that continued to inflict indignities upon the poor while benefiting primarily the caretakers—physicians, hospitals, and local health facilities that could now be paid for what had been unpaid or charitable services.[98]

In the debates, Senator Kerr had spoken expansively of the ten million recipients potentially eligible to benefit from his proposal.[99] Yet by 1963—half-way through the program—only 28 states, three territories, and the District of Columbia had signed up.[100] At the end of the first year, 60% of the enrollees and almost 90% of the expenditures for the "medically indigent" were in three states: New York, Massachusetts, and California.[101] This distribution changed somewhat toward the end of the program, yet even in 1965, the same three—New York, California, and Massachusetts—accounted for 45% of the recipients and the top five states for 62% of the total.[102] In 1965, only 40 States had implemented Kerr-Mills, though three others had authorized it. Far from Senator Kerr's ten million or even the more realistic early estimate of two million, Kerr-Mills covered 264,687 in 1965—less than 2% of the elderly.[103]

Particularly striking about this pattern was the number of states for which participation was token or minimal. Generally, these were the relatively poorer states from the South and Southwest and rural or sparsely populated areas. Several of these states—such as Texas, Mississippi, and Arizona—did not participate at all; and for many more, the number of enrollees was one thousand or less compared, for instance, with New York or Massachusetts, each with more than 30,000 recipients. Equally as striking was the range in annual Medical Assistance payments per recipient—from a high of $430 (Illinois) to a low of $11 (Nevada). Against a national average of $190 per recipient, the stronger states paid out an average of $265 per recipient and the weaker—not counting non-participating States—an average of $123. One conclusion is that Kerr-Mills, despite its open-ended cost-sharing and income adjusted matching formula, did not succeed as a device for distributing money to the areas of greatest need.

As with the Public Assistance program, Kerr-Mills left coverage and eligibility almost entirely up to the states, except for specifying that there had to be some "reasonable standards, consistent with the objectives of this title." Given the shared interest in establishing a concept of "medically indigent" and the inclusive listing of services eligible for coverage, states might have been reasonably expected to move toward more generous requirements for eligibility and more expansive coverage of medical services for the elderly. Some did; but many did not. For instance, fourteen states established income levels for eligibility that were more restrictive and set lower dollar limits than for Old Age Assistance.[104] Only five states had "comprehensive services" as of November 30, 1964.[105] Another twelve states provided the basic five, but with substantial, even drastic, limitations on scope, duration, and availability of services. Over half of the plans made no provision for dental care; about half did not include drugs; and about one-fourth not only curtailed hospital care but eliminated anything else, even physician care.[106] The pattern resists easy generalization. Yet only two of the states providing all five services were poor or rural (Kentucky and West Virginia) while among the non-comprehensive states, over half were either poor, rural, or both.

Kerr-Mills did less than hoped to help the poor states or the medically needy within them. One of the main reasons for that outcome—as Senator McNamara had warned—was that many states were too poor or unwilling—after meeting other responsibilities—to put up the matching funds. Beyond that, there were some perversities or adverse consequences in the way the funding worked. Many states, both rich and poor, took advantage of the more generous matching to transfer Old Age recipients into the MAA program, thereby drawing down more federal dollars with the same number of bodies.[107] The enhanced matching was also used to pay for expensive facilities, such as hospitals and nursing homes—a tendency that began a persisting and pernicious imbalance between institutional and non-institutional care. Another popular money-saver with long-term consequences was to place elderly mental patients in nursing homes, where they could be covered under Kerr-Mills. These activities were of greatest benefit to the larger and more affluent states that, as a result, drew down a larger share of the federal matching funds. Poorer states that participated less got less. Those poorer states that did participate gained accordingly but, in some instances, lacked money to pay for their own Public Assistance programs. Among the perverse consequences of Kerr-Mills were to make some of the neediest even worse off and to bequeath to the future Medicaid program not only the traditions of public assistance and welfare medicine but unmet needs and institutional biases, some of which persist to this day.[108]

Medicaid

"Medicaid," as a program providing health care for categories of poor people has a long history beginning even before the voucher payments of 1950. One of the most important strands of this history has been the political role played by programs similar to Medicaid as either an alternative or a supplement to various social security based proposals for national health insurance. As an alternative to Wagner-Murray-Dingell in 1947 and again in 1949, Sen. Robert Taft (R., Ohio) had proposed a program of means tested federal matching funds for medical benefits for all categories of welfare recipients that was remarkably similar to the later Medicaid program.[109] At about the same time, Arthur Altmeyer, Wilbur Cohen, and other key Social Security policymakers were thinking of a Social Security financed hospital benefit for the elderly with the possibility of a later add-ons, such as a physician benefit and a program for the poor.[110] Cohen had already begun a related incremental strategy of adding voucher payments for health care to Public Assistance categories that led, fairly soon, to Kerr-Mills—adopted deliberately as an alternative to the Kennedy-Anderson bill, another version of national health insurance based on Social Security.

In the Kennedy administration, the campaign for health insurance began early in January 1961, with the King-Anderson bill, providing a hospital benefit for elderly Social Security beneficiaries. That effort failed for a number of reasons: lack of a decisive electoral mandate; the determined opposition of the AMA; a conservative Congress dominated by southern Democrats and the Kennedy administration's ineffectiveness in dealing with that body; and the opposition of Wilbur Mills and Robert Kerr.[111] Even after the assassination of President Kennedy[112] and the lop-sided electoral victory of Lyndon Johnson and the congressional Democrats in November 1964 there remained the obstacle of Wilbur Mills and uncertainty about what could move him.

The needs and the clamor for health insurance kept growing: more elderly, sharply rising medical costs, and lack of affordable insurance or health care. These needs got increased visibility through national advocacy groups[113] and the persistent and effective studies and investigations by the Senate and House special committees on the aging. State welfare commissioners, congressional delegations, and governors concerned about rising costs, increased welfare budgets, and local complaints were eager for relief and complained that Kerr-Mills needed expansion or replacement. Meanwhile, periodic reports on the progress of Kerr-Mills indicated that the program was not only failing to meets its objectives but getting bad press and becoming an embarrassment.[114]

Two themes tended to increase the visibility of Kerr-Mills, bestow upon it a kind of left-handed legitimacy, and accord it a larger role than it might otherwise have had. One was the argument that a revised and enlarged Kerr-Mills was an alternative to Medicare—an argument advanced repeatedly, at great length, and with compendious documentation by the AMA, once it got over its initial opposition to the program.[115] Of course, one danger with this argument is that health care advocates would begin demanding both, not one or the other, as they did in 1963 when political momentum grew for another try at Medicare.[116] Lyndon Johnson, newly inaugurated as president, did just that—endorsed both Medicare and expansion of Kerr-Mills in his health message to Congress in February, 1964.[117]

A second theme that emerged in the debates of 1963 was that a social security based Medicare, as it grew, might threaten the fiscal integrity of the Social Security program so that some kind of "firewall" needed to be built to stop legislators—in their kindly but imprudent benevolence—from bankrupting Social Security. One form of self-denial, originally suggested by Senator Jacob Javits in 1962 (R., NY) was to establish a "health insurance trust fund," similar to that created for Social Security.[118] The trust fund proposal was readily accepted, both by the Social Security Administration and by Wilbur Mills, but not seen by itself as sufficient.

According to Wilbur Cohen, this "firewall" concept was the moving cause for the Medicaid program. He recalls being asked by Wilbur Mills how to prevent Medicare from becoming the "entering wedge" for a nationwide "compulsory" system of health insurance for everyone. Of course, most of Cohen's colleagues would have been happy with such an evolution. Nevertheless, his recommendation was to cover key groups of the poor so that the incentive to expand Medicare would be lessened. According to Cohen, "Medicaid evolved from this problem and discussion."[119] He then went on to expand the state plan requirements, "taking into account the views of the State welfare directors."[120]

In the narrow sense of identifying one reason that moved Wilbur Mills to add a Medicaid title to the legislation, Cohen's account may be historically accurate, although it takes no notice of the fact that many health policy activists, as well as President Johnson, were already supporting a two-layer cake that would include both Medicare and Medicaid. It is also a narrow account of Mills' behavior—a person who seemed to think in comprehensive terms and have in mind multiple levels of concern and calculation. In any event, Mills' own account is different from that of Cohen's.

Unlike Lyndon Johnson, Wilbur Mills did not feel obligated to complete the policy agenda of the slain president. The election of Johnson in November 1964, he said, "made the major difference." As for Medicare, Johnson "had espoused it in the campaign, you know, and here he was elected by a two-to-one vote." As a result, Mills thought, the time had come to pass Medicare. Many others, he said, mentioning George Smathers (R., Fla.) and Russell Long (D., La.) were similarly affected by the election. He added, "I think we all realized the time had come for it."[121]

Then, "as they went into it," they realized that the pending legislation would take care of about 25% of the health care costs of the elderly. At that point, according to his account, Mills went to President Johnson and said, "If we pass your program, Mr. President, and the American people find out we're taking care of 25% of them, we're going to be the laughingstock of the country. We've misled them, they'll think, and it'll react seriously on us." According to Mills, Johnson replied, 'Well, do what you want to about it, then, and develop it as you want to develop it."[122]

As for the origins of Medicaid, a succinct statement by Mills is worth quoting in full:

> It became increasingly clear to me, however, as I studied the programs and consulted with many interested groups that a Medicare hospital insurance program for the aged alone was not sufficient to meet the many medical needs of aged, blind, and disabled or the mothers and children receiving aid for dependent children. With Wilbur Cohen's help, we developed what eventually became Medicaid (Title XIX) and Medicare. Then, with the support of John W. Byrnes, the ranking minority member on the Committee, we added voluntary coverage of physicians services in what became part B or supplementary medical insurance (SMI).[123]

In a later oral account, Mills spoke less about his own perspective and more of the work of the Ways and Means Committee as a whole. He emphasized that the three-part package was not just "pieced together" but intended as part of a long-term plan (whose?) and based upon a consensus reached after much deliberation and whittling away of differences. This version is more in keeping with Mills' style as chairman, which was to grind through the legislation with the Committee members, aim for inclusive legislation and a consensus that would ensure close to unanimous support, and report out only legislation assured of passage in the House. Nevertheless, Medicaid seems to have received almost no consideration in the Committees deliberations nor in floor debate in the House.

Finally, the origins of Medicaid remain obscure, except that discontent with Kerr-Mills and the role of the two Wilburs seem important. In the

debates over Medicare, the AMA's "Eldercare"—an expanded version
of Kerr-Mills—was one of the three alternatives being considered. At
the time, dissatisfaction with Kerr-Mills was widespread and the program, as it stood, was an embarrassment to Wilbur Mills and needed
fixing. Despite his fiscal conservatism, Mills was almost a healthcare
liberal when it came to the "downtrodden" and women and children.[124]
Wilbur Cohen had long supported a Medicaid option and was largely
responsible for nudging the Public Assistance program in that direction.
He was close to Mills and had been appointed assistant secretary for
health in the Johnson administration to serve as liaison and point man
for health legislation. In this role, he had already worked up a plan for
expanding Kerr-Mills to cover welfare recipients.[125] Finally, a Medicaid
option was important to Mills for the reason ascribed by Wilbur Cohen:
it would protect the Social Security on the left flank as the Byrne bill,[126]
with its Part B voluntary option financed by beneficiary premiums and
the federal treasury, protected the right flank. For these reasons, the
Medicaid options seems not so much an afterthought as a forethought
and an important part of the mosaic.

For most of its legislative history, Medicaid was a low profile item. A
legislative draftsman said that he could scarcely recall working on Medicaid and doubted that it took as much as an afternoon of their time.[127]
Despite a large amount of consensus, the Ways and Means Committee
approved the bill on a straight party-line vote, 17-8. In House and Senate
debates, Medicaid as such occasioned little controversy. Many welcomed
the extension and strengthening of Kerr-Mills. Some said the Medicaid
legislation didn't go far enough and disliked the vestiges of welfare, such
as means-tests. There was so little comment that Medicaid did, indeed,
seem like a casual add-on. After an uneventful conference, the House
passed the Social Security Amendments of 1965 on July 27 by a vote of
307-116. The Senate voted approval on July 28 by 70 to 24. President
Johnson flew to Independence, Missouri along with 47 guests for a signing ceremony in the presence of retired president, Harry S. Truman, and
200 other witnesses.

Throughout, attention was on Medicare, not Medicaid. Talk of a
"sleeping giant" came later. Almost no one foresaw the potential of
Medicaid or would have imagined that it would some day overtake
Medicare and become, after Social Security, the country's largest
entitlement program.[128]

Title XIX, the "Medicaid" title, does not use the term: its caption is "Grants to the States for Medical Assistance." Both the House and Senate committee reports specify Title XIX's purpose as extending and improving the Kerr-Mills program, which it does; but that phrasing—with whatever intent—leaves undisclosed some other purposes, such as seeking to rise above Medicaid's welfare heritage, progressively cover in more of the poor, and "mainstream" the medical care they would receive. In characteristic American style, Title XIX did not so much resolve tensions in advance and strongly ground a new program as to accept and ratify an existing situation, set some boundaries and rules, and leave it to future partisans to resolve the differences between less and more ambitious agendas.

Much of the legislation followed the Kerr-Mills (and Public Assistance) template in requiring a single state agency and a state plan with a list of requirements. As with Kerr-Mills, participation in the Medicaid program was entirely voluntary, but had to include all the Public Assistance categories: Aid to the Blind; Aid to Families with Dependent Children; and Aid to the Permanently and Totally Disabled (Sec. 1901). There were some strong incentives and a deadline for joining—Kerr-Mills voucher payments under these titles would cease after December 31, 1969 (1915(b)). An even more important inducement was the provision under Title XI, Sec. 1118 that states participating in the Medicaid program could use the more favorable match under Title XIX for their other categorical assistance plans. As with MAA under Kerr-Mills, there was an open-ended authorization balanced by categorical eligibility and means-testing.

A remarkable feature of the new act was the provisions intended to equalize and standardize eligibility requirements and the services offered. The Medicaid legislation continued the basic state plan requirements of the Social Security Act such a state-wideness, a merit system, and the right to a "fair hearing." Also required were (1902a(1-5))—provisions originally intended largely to counter political spoils and racial discrimination, but promotive also of equalization and accountability. Beyond these requirements, the Medicaid legislation had some important all-or-nothing provisions. Participation was still voluntary and states could largely determine eligibility and benefits, but if a state chose to participate, it had to make medical assistance available to all individuals "receiving assistance" under any state plans approved under OAA, AFDC, AB, APTD or Kerr-Mills (1902)(a)10). Also, if they covered the "medically indigent," they had to do so for all categories of aid and under comparable standards. Finally, the medical assistance for any group could not be less in "amount, duration, or score" than for any other group. (1902(a)(10)B).

At first impression, these provisions would seem to be an effort to bring Medicaid eligibility and assistance determinations up to more common and generous standards. In fact, their main thrust was to protect the categorically eligible *recipients* of public assistance—to ensure that the neediest came first, that the income and assets determinations for them be accurate and fair, and that they not be discriminated against with respect to the medical care and services they received. One notable expression of this objective was the requirement that eligibility determination and means testing at the state level be made by "the State or local agency administering the State plan approved under Title I or Title XVI..." (1902(a)(5)—in most instances, the state welfare department.—on grounds that this agency would be most expert and experienced. As further insurance, guidelines for reasonable determination would be prescribed by the Secretary.

One effect of these provisions, over time, was to add greatly to the layered complexity of the Medicaid program as state administrators struggled with additional categorical determinations and the meaning and application of "state wide" and "amount, duration, and scope" requirements. A laudable purpose of protecting the neediest also tied the Medicaid program even more tightly to the theory and practice of welfare administration.

In sharp contrast, "medical indigence," originally introduced by Kerr-Mills, received little attention in this legislation. States that provided assistance and/or services for the medically needy still had to meet categorical requirements, such as blind or disabled. All categories of need had to be covered. And the coverage had to be comparable for all those included, regardless of category. This was a significant effort at mainstreaming and the legislations seems to have been based upon a presumption—not unreasonable given the history of Kerr-Mills—that states would be moderate in taking up this option and set eligibility standards and income and assets tests close to those for Public Assistance recipients.[129]

In any event, subsequent developments revealed some perversities of categorical schemes. Efforts to protect the categorically eligible and reform eligibility determination and means-testing mitigated some of the abuses and anomalies. But poorer states declined or were slow to take up on the "medically indigent" option or raise the income levels for Public Assistance. As a result the poor in the poor states suffered doubly—from the low eligibility levels which prevented them from getting coverage and from the linking of their medical coverage to Public Assistance levels of income eligibility which meant that they would lose coverage when their income rose above the Public Assistance level,[130] even though they (or their family) continued to need Medical Assistance. In effect, and contrary to congressional intent, much less than intended was done to help the neediest and much more the less needy.

Under the statute, "medical assistance" was "payment of part or all of the cost" of a list of required and optional care and services. The five required care or services were 1) inpatient hospital, not including mental illness or tuberculosis, 2) outpatient hospital; 3) laboratory and X-ray; 4) skilled nursing home services for those over 21; 5) physicians' services. Notably absent from the required list were prescription drugs, dental care and dentures; eyeglasses and prosthetic devices; hearing aids; and physical therapy. These were included under a long list of "optional" services, ending with "any other medical care [or] remedial care recognized under State law, specified by the Secretary..." 1905(a)(15).

In retrospect, and especially considering the short history of Kerr-Mills, the coverage seems generous. Today, the omission of prescription drugs and prostheses seems harsh and unfeeling. But it is well to remember that getting all the states to participate *and* provide the required services was not an easy task. Moreover, almost any legitimate health care or service was eligible for matching, and with the more generous matching for poor states, an opportunity for rich and poor states to expand their programs. Time proved, in fact, that the Medicaid program was much more expandable than anticipated.

One notable inclusion in the list was a pared down version of the Long Amendment to cover "institutions for tuberculosis or mental diseases." (1905(a)(14). This provision was of particular concern to states with large public institutions, especially for the mentally ill. In the consideration of Kerr-Mills, Senator Russell Long (D., La.) offered an amendment to make tuberculosis and mental hospitals eligible for voucher payments. After much finagling, Long's amendment was passed by the Senate but dropped in conference, much to his chagrin. His amendment was eventually adopted as part of Medicaid, though restricted to those over 65, as it would have been under Kerr Mills. This anomaly, and others like it, were embedded in the Medicaid legislation, with important consequences for future paths of development.

Along with this extension of coverage went a remarkable subsection, (1902(a)(20), that requires States choosing this option to determine the "reasonable cost" of such institutional care; engage in "joint planning" and development of alternate methods of care; develop individual treatment plans with periodic review and determination of need for continuing institutionalization; and progress toward a "comprehensive mental health program," including utilization of community mental health centers, nursing homes and other alternatives" to public institutions, with descriptions of the staffing, standards of care, and plans for cooperation between public and private institutions.

This mental health provision—an oddity out of keeping with the rest of the act—was a manifestation of two enthusiasms within the Kennedy-Johnson administrations. One was a thrust toward deinstitutionalization and treatment of the mentally ill at the community level. The other was an emphasis upon comprehensive health planning as a way of rationalizing and improving care and to same money. It also anticipated the use of Medicaid matching as a means to reshape the health care delivery system, not just as a way of paying for services.

Various protections or restrictions were added—incorporating Kerr-Mills provisions, but also going beyond them—dealing with liens on property, age requirements above 65 or below 21, and residency or citizenship restrictions. Much attention was devoted to improving the accuracy and fairness of eligibility determinations and means testing. Medicaid recipients were sheltered in various ways from enrollment fees, premiums, deductibles, and co-pays. One addition of considerable future importance was permitting states to "buy in" to Medicaid by paying the enrollees Medicare premium deductibles, and co-pays (1902(a)(15).

Scant attention was given to quality of care. The merit system and the statewide, comparability, and amount, duration, and scope requirements addressed quality indirectly at a cost of some rigidity. A guarantee of freedom of choice of providers might help assure quality, but was not mentioned in the statute.[131] State plans had to designate a statewide authority responsible for maintaining standards for institutions caring for Medicaid patients; and plans for "comprehensive mental health programs" had to describe standards for institutional care. In only one instance, were standards of care directly addressed—for mental patients.

Cost containment received relatively little attention, at least explicitly— which is surprising, given the expansive potential of the program and Wilbur Mills' usual concerns about fiscal prudence and parsimony. One expectation was that state eligibility requirements and the expense of matching would hold participation down.[132] The requirement that medical services had to be comparable across categories was a kind of ratcheting up provision that would deter promiscuous coverage increments. Also, the stigma of "welfare" would discourage many potential applicants.[133] Beyond that, the Medicaid act required that hospitals be reimbursed on a "reasonable cost" basis and left methods of payment for physicians and other providers up to the states.[134]

One of the most remarkable paragraphs in the Medicaid statute appeared at the end of Sec. 1903, "Payment to States," set there almost as a parting homily. It is quoted in full:

> The Secretary shall not make payments under the preceding provisions of this section to a State unless the State makes a satisfactory showing that it is making efforts in the direction of broadening the scope of the care and services made available under the plan and in the direction of liberalizing the eligibility requirements for medical assistance, with a view toward furnishing by July 1, 1975, comprehensive care and services to substantially all individuals who meet the plan's eligibility standards with respect to income and resources, including services to enable such individuals to attain or retain independence or self care.

According to Wilbur Cohen, he "included this provision in the law because [he] was acutely aware of the inadequacies of the State medical assistance plans in the 1960's [and] knew that we had to start from where we were, but [his] hope was to broaden the program over a 10 year period." He added that "there was no opposition to this ambiguous and general provision in 1965."[135]

Section 1903(e) nicely illustrates both the promise and the peril of Wilbur Cohen's incremental strategy. Events quickly revealed that the time horizon as well as the enforcement methods were politically unrealistic and the Sec. 1903 mandate was postponed and then repealed. But eventually much of Wilbur Cohen's vision with respect to Medicaid was realized. How we got there and whether it was the best way to go remainsto be considered.

Notes

1. Pat McNamara (D., Mich.) one of the most influential members of the Senate Sub-Committee on Long Term Care, opposed Medicaid. Many state and local officials were cool to the legislation, fearing especially that it would involve them in conflicts with physicians in their own states. Wilbur J. Cohen, "Reflections on the Enactment of Medicare and Medicaid," *Health Care Financing Review*, 1985 Annual Supplement, 3-11, at 3.

2. Robert J. Myers, *Medicare* (Richard D. Irwin: Homewood, Ill., 1970), p. 267. 267.

3. Wilbur J. Cohen, "Reflections on the Enactment of Medicare and Medicaid, *loc. cit.*, 3.

4. Pat McNamara especially objected to the strategically important step of expanding Kerr-Mills, which he had opposed. Edward D. Berkowitz, *Mr. Social Security—The Life of Wilbur J. Cohen*. Lawrence, Kansas: University of Kansas Press, 1995, 360, n101.

5. Medicare Parts A and B, and Medicaid. The expression is often attributed to Wilbur J. Cohen, although "layer cake" metaphors were much in use in the health insurance debates of 1964.

6. For instance, rejection rates for the military draft ran as high as one-third because of bad health and lack of education in the poorer regions of the country. Cf. War-time Health and Education, Hearings before a Sub-committee of the Committee on Education and Labor, U.S. Senate, 78thth Congress, 1944-45.

7. During the war, both the American Medical Association and the American Hospital Association were gravely concerned about shortages of hospital beds and physicians and about the role of health care in the future. Cf. Daniel M. Fox, Health Policies, Health Politics—The British and American Experience, 1911-1965. Princeton, NJ: Princeton University Press, 1986.

8. World War II has been described as the first war in which science was decisive. The war rapidly accelerated scientific and technological progress in many fields, including medicine and biomedical science.

9. As chairman of the Board, Altmeyer was the administrative head of Social Security.

10. Altmeyer, *The Formative Years*, 94-95.

11. *Ibid.*, 94-95; Fox, *Health Policies, Health Politics*, 89-90.

12. *Ibid.*, 91.

13. Altmeyer, *The Formative Years*, 96.

14. Altmeyer failed to make clear whether President Roosevelt supported this step or not. More than once, the Social Security leadership acted on its own when such a step seemed justified by the occasion.

15. Senator Wagner gave a public radio address before the introduction of the bill, making clear that such issues were for the "State plans" and that nothing in the bill was intended to impose a "Federal strait-jacket." *Ibid,* 115-116.

16. Fox., *Health Policies, Health Politics,* 79 ff.

17. William Beveridge's report, *Social Insurance and Allied Services* was published toward the end of 1942. It was notable for the publicity given it in Great Britain, for its comprehensive approach to social insurance, and for associating the National Health Service with social insurance.

18. Altmeyer, *The Formative Years,* 143-144. The earlier report from the National Resources Planning Board was itself a spin-off from the original Social Security legislation. It was seen as an American version of the Beveridge Plan. The Social

Security Board built upon this report with more specific recommendations. As one part of a well-organized scheme, John G. Winant, a former chairman of the Social Security Board and, in 1942, ambassador to Great Britain, arranged for a visit by Sir William which coincided with Prime Minister Winston Churchill's address to a joint session of Congress. While he was in this country, Sir William met with prominent officials and discussed his plan (luncheon arranged by Altmeyer) with members of the Senate Finance Committee.

19.   *Ibid.,* 144.
20.   The earlier attempt was in 1939. The 1943 delegation was Arthur Altmeyer, Wilbur Cohen, and I. S. Falk. Edward D. Berkowitz, *Mr. Social Security,* 51.
21.   J. Joseph Huthmacher, *Senator Robert F. Wagner and the Rise of Urban Liberalism.* New York: Athenaeum, 1971, 292.
22.   *Ibid.,* 293.
23.   David Brody makes the point that Roosevelt's conservatism on domestic issues was more pronounced in wartime because he was usually ahead of the country in foreign policy and needed to retain the support of a conservative, isolationist Congress. In Brody's words, "he was willing to trade [a] scheduled increase in social security contributions for Senator Vanderberg's support in foreign policy." John Braeman, Robert H. Bremner and David Brody, *The New Deal* (Columbus, Ohio: Ohio University Press, 1975), vol. 2, 274.
24.   Huthmacher, *Senator Robert F. Wagner,* 293.
25.   This was done to avoid Senate Finance Committee jurisdiction. Senator Walter George (D., Ga.), who chaired Finance at that time, was opposed to WMD. Senator James Murray (D., Mont.) chaired Education and Labor, a more hospitable venue. *Ibid.,* 320.
26.   *Ibid.,* 321; Altmeyer, *The Formative Years,* 154.
27.   Huthmacher, *Senator Robert F. Wagner.* 321.
28.   Harry S. Truman, *Memoirs—Years of Trial and Hope.* New York, Doubleday, 1956, Vol. II, 17 ff.
29.   *Supra.,* footnote 6.
30.   Theodore R. Marmor, *The Politics of Medicare*, 2nd ed. New York: Aldine de-Gruyter, 2000, 6.
31.   President Truman had made the failure of the Republicans to provide health insurance part of his campaign against the 80th Congress. He also promised to work for passage of such a program if re-elected.
32.   House Democrats lost 28 seats, going from 263-171 to 235-199. In the Senate, they were reduced to a majority of two seats. With southern Democrats dominant in key committees, Democratic control was weak at best and non-existent on such issues as health and education.
33.   Robert M. Ball, interview by Judith Moore and David Smith, May 12, 2004
34.   There is some dispute about Oscar Ewing's role in developing this strategy, but both Wilbur Cohen and Robert Ball recalled that the group suggested this approach to Ewing and not the other way around. Robert Ball interview with Moore and Smith, and Wilbur Cohen, "Reflections on the Enactment of Medicare and Medicaid," 4.
35.   The 1939 Wagner bill would have vastly extended social security coverage and also included grants to the states to help care for the poor. The 1946 version, which was to implement President Truman's health message, pared down the bill to health insurance for social security contributors and their dependents, with grants-in-aid for state public health and child care programs. In the same year,

Senator Robert Taft proposed, as an alternative to W-M-D, federal grants-in-aid to assist the states in providing health care for means-tested low income families. This plan lacked the categorical restraints of the later Medicaid program, but otherwise largely anticipated that program. As early as 1945, twenty years before the eventual passage of Medicare/Medicaid, the essential elements were there, but not the necessary political consensus.

36. *Ibid.*
37. Fox, *Health Policies, Health Politics,* 152-153.
38. The Bingham Associates Fund of Boston was active in the field of hospital planning and helped initiate, in the early 1930s, the Tufts-New England Medical Center, a forerunner of later huge medical school-teaching hospital complexes. Anne R. Somers, *Hospital Regulation: The Dilemma of Public Policy.* Princeton, NJ: Princeton University, 1969, 133.
39. Cf. Thomas Parran, "Medical Services of the Future," *Yale Review*, Vol. 35(2) Mar. 1946, 385-390.
40. *Ibid.,* 394; also Stephen P. Strickland, *Politics, Science, and Dread Disease: A Short History of United States Medical Research Policy.* Cambridge, MA: Harvard University Press, 1972); and *Research and the Health of Americans.* Lexington, MA: Lexington Books, 1978.
41. Thomas Parran, "Medical Services of the Future," 394.
42. Fox, *Health Policies, Health Politics,* 130.
43. Physicians especially attacked the health stations (or clinics) as intruding upon the private practice of medicine. Congress was not enthusiastic about the categorical health grants and would underfund or earmark them. President Eisenhower disliked departures from traditional federalism and the Bureau of the Budget under Eisenhower discouraged project grants. David G. Smith, "Emerging Patterns of Federalism: The Case of Public Health," Arnold Blankenship and John Hess, *Administering Health Systems: Issues and Perspectives,* Englewood, NJ: Prentice Hall, 1971, 131-142 at 134 ff.
44. Strickland, *Science, Politics, and Dread Disease*; Richard Rettig, *Cancer Crusade.* Princeton, NJ: Princeton University Press, 1977 ; Elizabeth Drew, "The Health Syndicate," *Atlantic Monthly* 12/67.
45. To borrow from Robert and Rosemary Stevens.
46. Social Security Amendments of 1960, Title VI—Medical Services for the Aged, P.L. 86-778, September 13, 1960.
47. Fully twenty years before Charles E. Lindblom published his famous article on incrementalism, "The Science of Muddling Through" *Public Administration Review* 19, 1970, 79-99.
48. After World War II there was some veterans' provisions and re-conversion legislation with health-related titles, most of which terminated.
49. Staff and legislators referred to it as a "train." One author called it an "incremental engine." Berkowitz, *Mr. Social Security,* 76.
50. At the time, revenue bills were debated under a "closed rule" allowing no amendments from the floor except those moved by a member of the Ways and Means Committee. The Senate Finance Committee tended to defer to the House and to the Ways and Means Committee on Social Security legislation. Back then, the jurisdiction of the Ways and Means Committee was enormous, covering almost half of the work of the House and all of the Social Security titles.
51. Martha Derthick, *Policymaking for Social Security* (Washington, D.C.: Brookings Institution, 1979), 81.

52.   Harry S. Truman, *Memoirs—Years of Trial and Hope, op cit.,* 170-171.
53.   Altmeyer, *The Formative Years of Social Security,* 170.
54.   *Ibid.,* 171
55.   Ball, interview by Judith Moore and David Smith, May 12, 2004.
56.   Edwin E. Witte, *Social Security Perspectives—Essays by Edwin E. Witte,* Robert J. Lampman, ed. Madison, Wisc.: University of Wisconsin Press, 1962, 31, 37. The bill was silent or vague in many particulars. This was especially true for the finance provisions, which were left incomplete so the bill could go to health committees rather than Ways or Means or Finance. Even so, the bill was never endorsed by President Truman, nor did it reach the floor of either House or Senate. The Oscar Ewing bill and its successor, the Forand bill as well as King-Anderson all assumed primary jurisdiction of Ways and Means.
57.   Berkowitz, *Mr. Social Security,* 66.
58.   The Advisory Council was originally largely imposed upon the Social Security Administration by Senator Arthur H. Vandenberg as an alternative to some hostile hearings that he intended to conduct on the size of the Social Security reserve fund. The Council was meant to be a watchdog. The Social Security leadership soon co-opted it and succeeding Advisory Councils and were able to use them to advance their own programmatic objectives. Cf. Martha Derthick, *op. cit.,* 90-91 and Ch. IV, "Advisory Councils."
59.   *Ibid.,* 43-44.
60.   "The Social Security Act Amendments of 1950 (P.L. 734, 1950).
61.   Altmeyer, *The Formative Years.* 187.
62.   Disability insurance was not seriously considered by the Committee on Economic Security. It was proposed in the Wagner bill of 1943 and again in the Social Security Amendments of 1950. Unlike welfare assistance for the permanently and totally disabled, which was not strongly opposed, disability insurance raised difficult technical and policy issues—for instance, how to define the benefit so as to minimize moral hazard and what emphasis to put upon rehabilitation. It was also strenuously opposed by insurance companies, the AMA, and states-rights legislators and got, at best, lukewarm support from the Eisenhower administration. It passed in 1956 by a Senate vote of 47-45. One vote would have created a tie, with Richard Nixon, the vice president, as the tie-breaker. Cf. Berkowitz, *Mr. Social Security,* 64-77.
63.   *Ibid.,* 64 ff., 77 ff.
64.   Wilbur J. Cohen, "Reflections on the Enactment of Medicare and Medicaid," 3-4; Derthick, *Policy-making for Social Security,* 26-27.
65.   *Ibid,* 27.
66.   *Ibid.,* 27.
67.   *Ibid.,* 27.
68.   Robert Ball, interview by Judith Moore and David Smith, May 11, 2004; Martha Derthick, *Ibid.,* p. 27.
69.   At this time, the maximum federal match was $30 of the first $50 spent by a state for Old Age Assistance or Aid to the Blind. For Aid to Dependent Children, it was $16.50 for the first $27 a month spent for the first child with a lesser amount for each additional child. Stevens and Stevens, *Welfare Medicine in America,* 22.
70.   According to Robert Ball, this provision for cash payment was regarded as the "Magna Carta" or "Declaration of Independence" for the recipients. Their right "to waste their money the same way everyone else can." Interview by Moore and Smith, May 12, 2004.

71. Wilbur J. Cohen, "Reflections on the Enactment of Medicare and Medicaid," 9.
72. The Omnibus Budget Act of 1986 (SOBRA) went most of the way, 179-184 for pregnant women and children and the elderly and disabled. *Infra.*, 179-180.
73. Wilbur J. Cohen, "Reflections in the Enactment of Medicare and Medicaid." *Ibid.*. 9.
74. His plan, first proposed in 1949, would have incorporated a dollar increment ($6 for adults; $3 for children) based upon the *average* number of recipients receiving aid under the state plan. This formula would not only have funded medical assistance, it would have made large lump sums available to the states—much easier to work with than fluctuating numbers and individual accounts. *Ibid.*, p. 6.
75. With 37 states reporting. Estimates were difficult because state records were sparse and unreliable, with payments often buried or incorrectly classified. Cf. Ruth White, "Vendor Payments for Medical Assistance," *Social Security Bulletin,* 13 (6) June, 1950, 3-7.
76. This was a six-fold increase in less than ten years with one-fifth of the states not taking part and some that participated not reporting.
77. Note that this incrementalism was not the "salami slicing" sort, in which many slices would make a sandwich, but a series of marginal changes in a process or structure to create a new capability that left the original much the same.
78. There were a number of NIH initiatives, but these were primarily research and training and, except for NIMH programs, not seen as health care. Another exception, that was deflected, was Heart-Cancer-Stroke.
79. So at least do Robert and Rosemary Stevens argue. The AMA supported vendor payments as an alternative to national health insurance, though the political effects of this support are arguable.
80. Stevens and Stevens, *Welfare Medicine in America,* 10. With respect to domestic affairs, the fabulous fifties were a decade of prosperity and contentment for most people. This circumstance left Democrats searching for policy issues during the popular Eisenhower administration. Older Americans were one group that did not share equally in these good times and for whom health problems, medical care costs, and lack of insurance were increasingly troubling.
81. Members of the group were Wilbur Cohen (moving at this point to become dean of the School of Welfare at the University of Michigan); I.S. Falk, who had left the Social Security Administration and was then a consultant to the United Mine Workers; Nelson Cruikshank, head of the AFL-CIO Department of Social Security; and Robert Ball, the top Social Security official. Theodore R. Marmor, *The Politics of Medicare*, 24.
82. When the Forand bill was first introduced, Wilbur Mills refused to hold legislative hearings. A year later, when re-introduced, hearings were held, but the Committee rejected the bill by a vote of 8-17. 24.
83. Berkowitz, *Mr. Social Security,* Chapter 6, " Courting JFK, Expanding Social Security." Cohen had also worked with Kennedy on the Social Security Amendments of 1958.
84. The Committee was renewed as the Senate Special Committee on Aging in February 1961 and repeatedly renewed thereafter. It held hearings in Washington and at sites across the country and was especially influential in making the case for Medicare, helping develop policies adopted in the Social Security Amendments of 1972, and in exposing nursing home abuses—an investigation that led to the establishment of the HHS Inspector-General. Val J. Halamandaris, *Congressional Encyclopedia,* (1) 117-18. At one time, the Senate "sub-committee" had a mem-

bership of 12 and was a cross between a semi-permanent investigative committee and a bipartisan caucus on the aging.

85. "The Aged and Aging in the United States: A National Problem" Rpt. #1121, February 23, 1960, U.S. Congress, Senate, Subcommittee on Problems of the Aged and Aging of the Senate Committee on Labor and Public Welfare, 116.

86. *Ibid.,* 116. Sen. McNamara was strongly opposed to means-testing.

87. Mills was a fiscal conservative and concerned about the actuarial implications of any legislation that went through his committee. He was deeply committed to maintaining the fiscal solvency of the Social Security Trust Fund. Fully aware that a favorable report by his committee would usually assure passage in the House, he sought to exercise his enormous power moderately and responsibly: by striving for bipartisanship, inclusiveness, and near unanimity within his committee and, on principle, never reporting out a bill he thought unlikely to pass the House.

88. Mills kept his intentions secret. Without any previous notice or hearings, the bill was presented to the Ways and Means Committee and immediately approved. Sheri David, *With Dignity: The Search for Medicare and Medicaid* (Westport, Conn.: Greenwood Press, 1985), 37.

89. Harry F. Byrd was the chairman but was elderly, in poor health, and initiated little.

90. David, *With Dignity,* 37.

91. Richard Harris, *A Sacred Trust.* Baltimore, MD: Penguin Books, 1969, p. 111.

92. Wilbur Cohen was then at the University of Michigan and so could engage in such consulting. He was well known to both Kerr and Rader and during the 1950s had collaborated with them on various projects. Most recently he had worked closely with the Senator on the Social Security Amendments of 1958 and helped devise an equalization formula that increased the matching rate for poorer states. Berkowitz, *Mr. Social Security*, 125-126.

93. David, *With Dignity,* 47.

94. *Ibid.,* 40. Few in Congress thought the Forand bill would pass. The best hope seemed to be to attach it to the Kerr bill and then try in conference, but Forand never cleared the Senate Finance Committee.

95. The main objection was cost. *Ibid.,* 41,

96. *Ibid.,* 43.

97. *Ibid.,* 38.

98. Means and assets tests for OAA recipients were specifically required by law. According to Robert and Rosemary Stevens, the states, without exception, applied means tests for applicants in implementing their programs for the "medically indigent" under Medical Assistance for the Aging—in some instances, even harsher tests than for Public Assistance. Means tests were not just a federal requirement. States also used them for their own fiscal protection. Cf. *Welfare Medicine in America,* 30-31.

99. Richard Harris, *A Sacred Trust,* 114.

100. *Medical Assistance for the Aged—The Kerr-Mill Program, 1960-1963,"* Committee Print, U.S. Senate, Special Committee on Aging, October, 1968, 3.

101. *Performance of the States—Eighteen Months of Experience with the Medical Assistance for the Aged (Kerr-Mills) Program,* Committee Print, U.S. Senate, Special Committee on Aging, June 15, 1962, 13.

102. "Public Assistance: Number of Recipients and average payments, by Program and State," Table XIV, *Social Security Bulletin,* Vol. 28, December, 1965, 46-47.

103. *Ibid.*

104. *Medical Assistance for the Aged—The Kerr-Mills Program, 1960-1963,* 35.
105. The five major services were hospital, nursing home, practitioners, dental, and drugs. The five states were Indiana, Massachusetts, Minnesota, New York, and North Dakota. *Hearings before the Committee on Finance on HR 6675,* Part 1. U.S. Senate, Committee on Finance, 89th Congress, 1st Session, April 29, 30 and May 3-7, 163.
106. *Ibid.*
107. In 1963, transfers were estimated to account for about l/4 of all new enrollees in the MAA program. *Ibid.,* l4-15.
108. Over half of Kerr-Mills funds went for hospitals and nursing homes.
109. David, *With Dignity,.* 35.
110. Ball, interview by Moore and Smith, May 12, 2004.
111. Cf., David, *With Dignity,* esp., chs. 4, 6; and Gordon, *Dead on Arrival.*
112. November 22, 1963.
113. For example, the trade unions, public welfare associations, and advocates for the aged and for nursing home reform, etc.
114. Wilbur Mills, who eventually grew eager to mend his own program, recalls one Arkansas reporter referring to the program as "Cur-Mills." *Transcript, Wilbur Mills Oral History Interview II,* March 25, 1987, by Michael L. Gillette, Internet Copy, Lyndon B. Johnson Library., 38.
115. One representative, Joel Broyhill (R., Va.) proposed to Wilbur Mills that they "sweeten up" Kerr-Mills so that the elderly would neither need nor want Medicare—to which Mills responded that they should be getting people off Public Assistance, not adding to the program. David, *With Dignity.* 110-111. Robert Ball stated that the Social Security Administration was aware of the role of Kerr-Mills as a potential alternative to Medicaid, which was one reason they sought to keep improving the program in tandem with Social Security. Interview by Moore and Smith,, May 12, 2004.
116. Cf. statements by Arlin M. Adams, Secretary of Public Welfare, Commonwealth of Pennsylvania and by Evelyn M. Burns, for the National Consumers League, *Medical Care for the Aging, Part I* , Hearings on HR 3920, House of Representatives, Committee on Ways and Means, Nov. 18, 19, 20, 1963, 510 and 292.
117. David, *With Dignity,* 109.
118. *Ibid.,* 91.
119. Wilbur Cohen, Reflections on the enactment of Medicare and Medicaid, 3.
120. *Ibid.,* 3.
121. *Transcript, Wilbur Mills Oral History Interview II,* March 25, 1987, 1.
122. *Ibid.,* 1.
123. Wilbur D. Mills, "Building a Better Safety Net," in *20 Years of Medicare and Medicaid,* Health Care Financing Review, 1985 Supplement, 1.
124. *Transcript, Wilbur Mills Oral History, Interview II, loc. cit.,* 45. In 1943. for instance, Mills had sponsored the Mills-Ribicoff bill that would have provided $282 million in matching grants for maternal and child health services. *Ibid.,* p. 45. More immediately in point, he supported the Child Health Act, an option proposed by the administration for FY 1965, that extended Kerr-Mills to cover needy children.
125. Berkowitz, *Mr. Social Security,* 215.
126. Mills version on Medicare, Part B is interesting in this context. He was asked whether the Byrne amendment was done in concert with him. Mills responded, "Oh, I developed the whole thing in Committee. I mean, we did, with the help of the staff people, by my questions, and the questions of other members we devel-

oped the idea and then the program. Then I whispered in his ear, 'John [Byrne], I wish you'd offer a motion to include it.' 'I'll be glad to.' He did." One could speculate on what steps preceded this event.

127. Larry Filson, telephone interview by Smith, Nov. 4, 2002. However, there were previous drafts from HEW.

128. Robert J. Myers, the HEW actuary, predicted a figure of $3 billion for Title XIX, a much larger number than had been assumed. Senator Leverett Saltonstall (R., Mass.) warned that, despite the lack of discussion, Title XIX was a "sleeper" in the bill and within five years could "dwarf" Medicare. Both were wrong. Stevens and Stevens, *Welfare Medicine in America,* 108-109.

129. Note that the original concept was not that any definition of "needy" was acceptable but that another way of interpreting "needy" (or poverty status) was that medical expenses ate up income and assets and did or would reduce the individual to a "needy" state if the costs of medical care were not paid or reimbursed.

130. This was one expression of the so-called "notch effect," that plagued welfare programs and their recipients for many years. For the "medically needy" there is no "notch," so long as the recipient "spends down" to the "medically needy" income and asset levels.

131. Added by the Social Security Amendments of 1967.

132. Unlike other categorical programs, Medicaid required states to put up 40% of their match immediately and 100% by July 1, 1970.

133. Myers, *Medicare,* 267.

134. At the time, cost containment methods were in their infancy. Also, the Ways and Means Committee was basing its estimates on 1964 Kerr-Mills expenditures, and that led to a dramatic under-prediction of the federal share—$200-238 million for the first year. *Social Security Amendments of 1965*, U. S. Congress, lst Session, Ways and Mean Committee of the House of Representatives, HRpt 213, 75.

135. Wilbur Cohen, "Reflections on the Enactment of Medicare and Medicaid," 10.

3

Medicaid Implementation

The period from 1966 to 1980, roughly fifteen years, can be thought of as a first stage or era in the history of Medicaid, because state and federal officials were implementing the Medicaid program as originally designed: a state-driven system of categorical eligibility with traditional forms of service delivery and a claims (or voucher) method of payment. Amendments to the program were sought primarily to improve the original system rather than change its structure. Later, in the 1980s, expansion and adaptation of Medicaid got high priority and the program was transformed into its "modern" form. But early implementation of the program and the modest reforms sought in this first period were of a fee-for-service, claims-paying system that presumed traditional modes of service delivery.

The Medicaid program began with a hurried start in the last two years of the Johnson administration: writing regulations, developing and approving state plans, certifying providers, determining eligibility, enrolling recipients, paying claims, and reviewing reports and monitoring procedures. Following the initial implementation there was a lengthy period of growth in the Medicaid program matched by neglect or partial efforts at reform that left a legacy of uneven program and institutional development, problems in need of attention, and a mixed bag of tools with which to work. The bad news was that little visible progress was made during this first period. The good news was that the program reached a "take-off" position—with developing agendas for reform and some of the materials for achieving them.

Given the historic importance of Medicaid, one question is why more attention was not paid to the program in its early years. An obvious and important reason was the program's low visibility. It was more than an "afterthought" for national health policymakers but a high priority for no more than a handful within the administration, the Congress, or the welfare constituency. Moreover, leaders within Social Security or the Welfare Administration started with the presumption that it was mainly a state program—up to the states to run as they pleased so long as no federal laws or restrictions were violated.[1] State governors and administrators were, of course, a large and attentive group, but concerned primarily with getting matching funds from the program and with a variety of local concerns, not primarily with cost containment or systemic reforms. There were some noisome issues such as unexpected levels of utilization and cost increases, fraud and abuse and nursing home scandals. In time, each of these became highly visible and urgent topics of concern, but this was years in building, and Medicaid[2] costs did not become a widespread and politically "hot" issue until late in the 1970s.

The program was neglected because more important or more urgent issues pre-empted the agenda. The first decade—1966 to 1976—was a turbulent era, with attention centered upon civil rights, the Vietnam war, and "Watergate." In the Johnson administration, the domestic issues were civil rights, education, and poverty. After their passage, President Johnson mentioned Medicare once and Medicaid not at all.[3] Under the Nixon administration, the big domestic issues were the Family Assistance Plan ("welfare reform"), inflation and federalism, along with Watergate and the threat of impeachment.[4] A national health insurance proposal was developed primarily as a counter to a more sweeping Democratic plan. Medicaid figured mostly as an adjunct to the Family Assistance Plan or to the administration's National Health Insurance Partnership Act.[5]

Under the Carter administration, domestic politics was calmer, illustrating another point: that even when health care is on the agenda, Medicaid policy often depends upon strategies with respect to larger concerns such as national health insurance or Medicare. The major Medicaid issues were the merging of Medicare and Medicaid to form the Health Care Financing Administration (HCFA), the Child Health Assurance Program, fraud and abuse legislation, and increased support for Medicaid Management Information Systems (MMIS), all sought in large measure as preludes to national health insurance. Medicaid was not so much crowded out as dealt with piecemeal when it fit with larger strategies.

Political weakness also helps account for the absence of attention or of systemic reform. The Medicaid program lacked a strong or united constituency and was unable to mobilize support in its own behalf, so that controversial bills standing alone were almost certain to fail. Even incremental changes often required a vehicle or legislative "train" such as the Social Security amendments or, in later years, reconciliation bills.[6] Either alternative meant that Medicaid considerations were subordinate to some other major purpose, and amendments mostly restricted to the incremental and uncontroversial. More comprehensive reform would be addressed in staff reports and committee hearings, but no free-standing Medicaid bill was passed during this entire period.

Initial Implementation

A safe statement about Medicaid administration is that little is entirely new: programs have antecedents and tend to be grounded in previous experience and built upon institutions and traditions already in place. That is fortunate, since administrative routines, institutional memory, and agency expertise are important resources. Before Medicaid, there was Kerr-Mills, and before that, Public Assistance and the voucher payments. By 1965, forty states had participated in Kerr-Mills and all fifty of them in the federally subsidized Public Assistance program, so they were familiar with state plans, eligibility determinations, means testing, and other procedures and requirements. Both federal and state officials had been through the initial implementation of Kerr-Mills with its rituals of advance explanation, letters to the governors and state officials, publications and conferences, technical assistance, and advisory groups.[7] Kerr-Mills provided five years of antecedent experience with a program similar to Medicaid. During that time, staff from the Division of Medical Services and the Bureau of Family Services were in frequent communication with state welfare administrators and would regularly attend meetings of the American Public Welfare Association.[8] So there was a modest fund of experience, some trailblazing and creation of routines.

Previous experience confers advantages, but the situation with respect to the initial implementation of Medicaid was less desirable than this account suggests. For an item, the Kerr-Mills Medical Services staff was tiny, consisting of a physician, one or two additional professional staff, and administrative support, not sure whether they were a "division" or not. They were administratively located in the Bureau of Family Services that was, in turn, part of the Bureau of Public Assistance (later Welfare Administration) headed by Ellen Winston. She was a career civil servant and an aggressive administrator, but devoted to the cause of social work, not health care. She was also reputed to oppose growth in the Medical Services division.[9] Whatever the foundation for this opinion, there were three different directors during the five years of Kerr-Mills and the staff grew little and slowly even as the division later became an "administration" and then a "bureau." In 1965, there were 23 members in the central administration of whom only twelve or thirteen were professional staff and several of them fresh from college with no previous administrative or professionally related experience.[10] Of the eleven Health, Education, and Welfare (HEW) regions, only four had a Medicaid representative.[11] With the passage of Medicaid, 35 additional people were added, and with the 1967 amendments a few more; but as late as 1972, the Medicaid staff was just over 100, including regional positions.[12]

The Medicaid program had a short grace period—five months, from July 30, 1965 to January 1, 1966—before it was scheduled to start reviewing state plans. Of course, savvy officials were aware months in advance that something big in health care was coming and began planning for the event.[13] But there was a comfortable assumption that Medicaid would be largely an extension of Kerr-Mills, and a "state program" so that there was less anxiety than was appropriate. For Medicaid program there was nothing comparable to HIBAC[14] and the eleven months that Medicare had to pre-vet procedures and regulations with providers and beneficiary groups, identify glitches, negotiate differences, and smooth the transition to a fully operative system.

With a lack of time or expert staff, the Medicaid administration had, perforce, to be largely reactive rather than proactive—that is, take the business as it came in, get on top of the most urgent and immediate, and hope that, in the future, successful protocols could be developed. These constraints meant that most of the needed skills, administrative expertise, and lines of communication had to be developed on the job. Some like this kind of life and some do not; but a large part of the ultimate success of the state and federal Medicaid programs is attributable to their ability to attract and hold officials who accept and thrive under such conditions.[15]

An important and pressing need was to prepare for the submission and approval of state plans—important because of the central role of the state plan in Medicaid administration and immediately pressing because six states were already lined up to file before the official date of July 1, 1966, with sixteen others to follow before mid-year.[16] Moreover, these state plans would be different, requiring the interpretation of novel statutory requirements and language and their application to a much larger and rapidly changing universe of recipients and providers.

After the initial letters, publications, and conferences, the Division of Medical Services and the Bureau of Family Services continued to facilitate the state plan process in several ways. State letters went out frequently; Washington staff attended professional meetings, and state officials were frequently invited to Washington for informational sessions.[17] Over the telephone, federal officials answered questions about state plans, segregation, how to write requests for proposals (RFPs), contract with providers, and so forth. Technical assistance or more extensive conferences were dealt with by the regional offices or by sending a person or a delegation from Washington.[18] A crash course was developed to teach additional recruits how to review state plans.[19] Meanwhile, staff from the Bureau of Family Services and the Division of Medical Services worked on a definitive manual to guide their own staff and state officials.[20]

Little advance planning went into such concerns as cost containment or fraud and abuse, aside from seeking to enhance the Division's computer capabilities. This was an important step, although a long distance from developing the software and information flow needed to mount a credible effort either to contain costs or stem fraud and abuse.[21] These concerns received scant attention from the tiny Division staff, already spread thin. There was also a tendency to trust the states and to believe that the matching requirements would constrain utilization. Beyond that, the future was dimly perceived and little was known about what to expect or how to deal with program costs or with fraud and abuse. Upon reflection, it may have been better not to have known more since the puny efforts of the Medicaid administration would likely have been swept aside within months of their implementation.

Another omission was the lack of advance planning to deal with racial discrimination in Medicaid supported programs. It would have been preposterous for this miniscule, unformed agency to take on such a task—not least because neither Title XIX nor Title XVIII for that matter, mention the topic. Civil rights strategy was high-level politics at that time, not to be decided, so to speak, at the platoon level. And in the upshot, desegregation for Medicaid was mostly dependent upon what was decided first for Medicare.

Although not directly related to the early implementation of Medicaid, the history of these events is important for later developments, and a fuller account is given in an addendum at the end of this chapter. The campaign to desegregate community and public hospitals was a heroic effort and largely successful, but limited in scope. It dealt with the more blatant forms of discrimination such as denial of admission or segregated wards and did not cover Part B physician services or more subtle forms of discrimination[22] or effectively monitor compliance beyond the initial certifications. With a few exceptions, Medicaid policies and practices were largely determined by Medicare or HEW decisions or left to state plan administration—an outcome that avoided conflict but left much to existing local and private orderings of health care for racial minorities.

State Plans and "Supplement D"

Under the various titles of the Social Security Act, the state plan has been historically important as a way to achieve and sustain a balance between federal requirements and state initiatives or freedom of action. Among the purposes of the state plan have been to counter political spoils, assure statewide coverage and equal levels of service, and see to it that federal dollars are spent for approved purposes. The underlying notion was that state expenditures would not be matched if they were not spent according to an approved state plan or amendments thereto. What got approved was a matter of interpreting the statute and of argument and negotiation between state administrators and federal officials, with politicians involved as occasion permitted or demanded. In principle, withholding of funds could be used as a sanction, though almost never was. Like kinship or other inescapable unions, much depended in practice on mutual understandings, often unspoken, about how to play the game without breaking it up.

In the early stages of Medicaid implementation, reviewing and monitoring of state plans was important both for negotiating over content and to find out what the states were doing, which was difficult especially in the absence of developed data collection and reporting systems. In the new program, these state plans provided an opportunity to raise aspirations and start the Medicaid program on a better trajectory than Kerr-Mills. Under the Johnson administration—especially within those agencies involved in health services such as the Office of Economic Opportunity, the Public Health Service, and the Bureau of Family Services—there was a strong sense of mission about bringing health care to the poor and using the available options and alternatives creatively to that end. For that reason, reviewing state plans was more than routine—it was for some a strategically important activity, a matter of conscience, and of serving a cause.

This high aspiration on the part of some federal officials was often a long distance from where the states were at this point. Mostly, they started with the presumption that Medicaid would be like Kerr-Mills, only bigger. But Medicaid *was* different—more like dealing with a whole industry than traditional purchase of service. Though not politically realistic, there should have been at least a year of preparation, with program manuals, Q&A routines, and fully staffed technical assistance. But time was short, resources limited, and the initial presumption, even at the federal level was that program administration would be up to the states, guided and monitored by the state plan process.

As applied to Medicaid there were two important gaps or thin patches in this process: one the lack of expertise to develop an adequate state plan and the other a low level of aspiration in many states with respect to programmatic goals. *Supplement D,* issued on June 17, 1966, with additions to follow, was a manual dealing primarily with the state plan that addressed both these deficiencies and served over the next decade as a primary guide available both to federal and state officials.

Supplement D

The manual was, officially, one of many supplements and appendices issued as part of the Handbook of Public Assistance, which makes it seem more routine and innocuous than it was. It was prepared primarily by the Bureau of Family Services, with the participation of some members of the Medical Services and in consultation with congressional committee staffs.[23] As a manual, it did not itself have the force of law, but federal officials often treated it as "law" and it served as a framework or template for negotiation and the development of later regulations. It did two things imaginatively, though not always well. One was to provide a "nuts and bolts" guide for initial implementation of the Medicaid program. And the other was to preserve and begin the "embedding"[24] or institutionalization of a more generous vision for Medicaid.

Supplement D does an admirable job of laying out the general principles and specific details of initial implementation. Over 220 single-spaced pages are devoted to state plan requirements, setting forth in clear prose—not murky "bureaucratise"—what the law says and intends and how to apply it to administrative arrangements, eligibility requirements, and service delivery. Included with the exposition are "interpretations," "criteria of administration," recommended forms, and a series of appendices, with a 22-page "State Plan model," as a guide for state plan submission.

Beyond the "black letter" requirements, *Supplement D* states that state plans for Medicaid would be "substantially different" from existing state plans, though without spelling out what "substantially" meant. One difference lay in the attention paid to the state plan model, an elaborate document of 22 single-spaced pages addressing not just the form and bare requirements of the state plan—at a time when state plans were often one page or less—but laying out in detail all sorts of requirements with respect to eligibility determination, service provision, and administrative procedures directed at raising levels of state administrative performance.

Another major difference was Sec. 1903(e)—the mandate to liberalize eligibility, expand coverage, and provide "comprehensive care" to "substantially all" eligible individuals by July 1, 1975. This expansive and controversial addition—originally a Wilbur Cohen initiative—came at a time when notions like "comprehensive care," "regionalism," and "planning" were popular and often associated with an onward—or renewed—march toward national health insurance.[25] Some of the interpretive language in *Supplement D* that dealt with the state planning process was permeated with this persuasion. For instance, states were told that Title XIX was the "beginning of a new era in medical care for low income families," that the law "aims much higher than the mere paying of medical bills," and that states, in order to achieve its "high purpose" would need to "assume responsibility for planning and establishing systems of high quality medical care, comprehensive in scope and wide in coverage."[26] Much of this language was imperative; and the Secretary was ordered by law not to make payment to the states without a "satisfactory showing" of progress in this direction.[27]

Of course, "comprehensive care" was an aspiration and 1975 was almost a decade away. Immediately, the most pressing tasks were to get the Division of Medical Services organized and individual state plans approved and operative. Yet some within the embryonic Division as well as the Bureau of Family Services did see their mission as "getting health care for the poor" by expanding the category of "medically needy," exploring the available coverage options, and working toward "comprehensive care" for as many as could be legitimately included.[28] States were also eager for expansion and some, especially New York and California, moved ahead with a vigor that precipitated an early crisis.

This expansive vision was only one element of a broad effort to raise local aspirations and performance through state plans, with a variety of techniques and mandates that made much of the relatively small and cautious increments of federal authority added by the statute. One approach was to emphasize the authority to issue or endorse standards: for instance, standards for eligibility determination, for facilities, health care professionals, and medical services and remedial care.[29] Continuing education and increased participation of administrative and health care staff was encouraged and tied to higher levels of federal matching where appropriate. Ways of expediting and simplifying eligibility determination were mentioned along with promptings to interpret coverage broadly. In a few specialized areas, such as skilled nursing homes, mental health and tuberculosis hospitals, and children's services, *Supplement D* was quite prescriptive with staffing requirements, access and admissions criteria, consideration of less restrictive alternatives to inpatient placement, and mandates to collaborate with state health, vocational rehabilitation, and crippled children's programs and, as appropriate, the provision of and criteria for social services.[30]

An important source of potential conflict was between a strict interpretation of the law and the expansive agenda contemplated by Sec. 1903(e). In working with this problem, the authors of *Supplement D* made good use of four expository categories: 1) legal requirements; 2) administrative requirements; 3) criteria for administration; and 4) interpretation. In most instances, the law would be stated first, accurately and clearly, in plain language. This would be followed by administrative requirements explaining how the law was to be applied, but paying attention to places where he law was permissive and offering opportunities for expansive interpretation.[31] Usually, these administrative requirements would be followed by "criteria of administration," which set forth—often in lengthy and prescriptive detail—what should or could be done to comply with specific plan requirements. These criteria, it was explained, were not mandatory—it was just that their absence would be "questioned" in reviewing the state plans.[32] In other words, they were subject to discussion, bargaining, and give and take. The fourth category, "Interpretations," was sometimes just that, explanations of what was intended or expected, but often with brief "sermons," meant to point out the moral dimensions of choice and to inspire the states to seek the higher road that led toward "comprehensive care."

The importance given to liberalizing eligibility, expanding coverage, and moving toward comprehensive care is remarkable, especially considering the casual way in which Sec. 1903(e) was treated by Congress—as a worthy aspiration for the relatively distant future rather than as an urgent

mandate.[33] Ten years is a long time in the life of legislation—five elections away—so that it is plausible Congress saw Sec. 1903(e) that way.
It is true that Congress directed the secretary to withhold funds if a state
failed to "make a satisfactory showing of efforts" in the desired direction; but it did so without defining terms or specifying the circumstances
under which this death sentence would be invoked.[34]

Monitoring the States

As contemplated in *Supplement D*, the state plan would play a large
role in the implementation of Title XIX, a strategy that seemed necessary
and was thought to be possible. It was necessary, in an obvious way,
because of the broad effort to set a high trajectory for the implementation process and make a good start. It was necessary in a less obvious
way, because there wasn't time or resources to develop other means for
directing and monitoring the implementation process. In retrospect, the
agenda seems quixotic, but these were days in which small numbers of
career civil servants accomplished prodigies and there were reasons to
hope for success.

One source of optimism was the assumption, shared by Congress, the
administration, and most of the states, that Medicaid would be largely
a follow-on to Kerr-Mills and that the administration of the program
would (and could) be left largely to the states.[35] There was also the
comforting belief—supported by experience with Public Assistance and
Kerr-Mills—that the matching requirement would restrain state spending.[36] With good will on the part of state and federal officials, it seemed
not unreasonable to hope that most problems could be met on a case-
by-case basis and negotiated successfully especially with an auspicious
launching of the program.

In addition, there were some assets and favoring circumstances.
For an item, most of the state officials wanted the program to succeed.
Especially important in this respect were the state welfare directors
supported by their national organization, the American Public Welfare
Association. These directors lobbied for their own states to be sure, but
also wanted good things to happen nationally, were concerned about the
long-term success of the Medicaid program, and could and did intervene
with their state governments or with well placed representatives and/or
senators.[37] Another asset was the Welfare Administration and its Bureau
of Family Services.[38] During the first years of Medicaid implementation,
the Welfare Administration was headed by Ellen Winston, an aggressive
career civil servant, who took an active role in issuing program directives,

promoting conferences, and reaching out to state officials. The Medical Services Administration though small, was competent, enthusiastic, and hard working.[39] In the early years, moreover, there were funds for travel, conferencing, and bringing state directors to Washington.

Had the Medicaid program remained small like Kerr-Mills and moved at a similar pace, implementation might have been more even and effective. But the diversity, complexity, and dynamism of the new state programs were much underestimated. About a dozen states—mostly southern and/or rural—did not initially participate. Another dozen operated, at least initially, at about the level of the Kerr-Mills program.[40] The complexity and dynamism, as well as the explosive costs, came largely from another ten states—led by New York, California, Massachusetts, Michigan, and Pennsylvania—that were populous, politically powerful, and eager to take maximum advantage of the new program. This group was also the source of many of the early problems with implementation that severely taxed the new federal administration and revealed critical lack of staff, data collection, and monitoring capabilities.

Lack of staff tended to reduce activities to the essentials of coping with in-house administration, getting policies out, conducting site visits and reviewing state plans and amendments, meanwhile responding to or fending off administrative superiors, congressional inquiries or demands, and the prompting of various constituencies, such as state welfare directors, governors' offices, or advocacy groups.

One activity that suffered greatly was outreach to the states—in the form of technical assistance, partnering on projects, or helping to negotiate differences at a local level. Adequate regional staff would have helped, but only four out of eleven HEW regions had even a single designated Medicaid representative. Site visitations from Washington were an alternative, but expensive and prodigal of staff time.[41] As a result, an active federal presence was largely missing at the state and local level, except for the long-distance telephone and an occasional site visit. Given the "progressive" nature of the Medicaid agenda, this situation was particularly unfortunate since urging a higher level of aspiration and performance at a state or local level was likely to seem wrongheaded and fatuous without a thorough grasp of local circumstances. A further point is that, without local agents, the federal agency not only lacked an important resource for encouraging and guiding behavior but often did not know in a lively way what was going on at the state and local level.

Oversight of program activities suffered especially from a lack of information in the form of required reports and a flow of claims data suitable for analysis. The statute made provision for "such reports as the Secretary may from time to time require ..."[42] but "the Secretary" required none in the early days so that the staff had little to rely upon other than reviews of the state plans and amendments and some periodic updates. The other major source of periodic information was the Quarterly Reviews of expected and of actual expenditures.

By themselves, the Quarterly Reviews provided little help. Amounts were reported in aggregate numbers and with varying terminology. The data was "general and raw," and almost worthless for analysis or administrative control,[43] such as monitoring trends in utilization or identifying possible fraud and abuse. A number of federal and state Medicaid officials,[44] to their credit, soon grasped the important truth that moving from Kerr-Mills to Medicaid involved not just an incremental difference but was a systemic change opening up a huge technological and information gap that required a *system* for data gathering and information management with common definitions, reporting forms and requirements, payment edits and checks, and a capacity to synthesize and analyze data. In other words, a Medicaid information management system was needed.[45] So, what might seem to the outsider as a crankish fascination with technological gimmicks was, in fact, a vitally important prerequisite for tracking behavior and understanding what was going on in this humming, buzzing confusion of a dynamic and somewhat chaotic new program. To be sure, getting federal and state Medicaid management information systems up and running was a good decade away and, meanwhile, Medicaid officials at the federal and state level had to improvise.[46] But there was at least an understanding of the problem and of the direction that must be taken.

As noted, the state plan process, including initial approval, plan amendments, and some periodic reporting, was intended and did play a central role in implementing the Medicaid program. For various reasons, that process was less effective than hoped, though it should be said in advance that the state plan was and is vitally important in establishing a semi-contractual set of mutual obligations, allowing for change and renegotiation, and maintaining a tolerable and moving balance between a number of quasi-sovereign states and the federal government, and between particularism and the larger good.

Lack of time for advance preparation was one of the greatest problems—only five months to the January 1, 1966 deadline. One result was to cut short advance liaison with state officials; and another that the first installment of *Supplement D* was not issued until June 17, 1966, almost six months after the first state plan applications. In effect, this was setting the course after the runners had crossed the finish line. More specifically: six states applied in January, followed by California and New York in May—all of these before *Supplement D*. These were given provisional approval. Fourteen more applied in July 1966, also given provisional approval since they could not realistically have been expected to comply with *Supplement D* requirements in one month. In sum, 22 of the 37 states that joined within the first two years did so before the new state planning guidelines were in place.[47]

The number of states in this category of early joiners does not fully indicate their fiscal significance. Among this group, California and New York were 52% of the total Medicaid expenditures in the first year, even though California joined in March and New York not until May. Adding the next eight states accounted for 79% of the total first-year expenditures, while the remaining 27 states were only 21%. Of course, this distribution tended to become more equal over time. But the point remains that, initially, the state planning process was much less effective in reaching the more dynamic and fiscally important state programs.[48]

The top ten, sometimes referred to as "leadership" states—shared some significant characteristics.[49] Almost without exception, they had strong traditions of public health, social services, and/or public assistance. Several also paid out large sums for public hospitals and long-term care institutions, such as mental hospitals and nursing homes. With the exception of Oklahoma and Texas, most would be classified as "high tax effort" states. Although not in this category, Oklahoma had a strong public assistance program supported by an earmarked tax. Six of the ten applied with lengthy lists of optional services and with generous upper limits for the "medically indigent." In summary, most of these states had traditions of aid to the poor, were accustomed to pay for their preferences, and not likely to be apologetic about their expectations.

In the absence of a guide similar to *Supplement D*, the first states had little to rely upon other than the original letters from the secretary, memoranda from the Bureau of Family Services, and their own previous experience with Public Assistance and Kerr-Mills.[50] As a consequence, several of the twenty-two early joiners submitted brief state plans, five or six pages in length, with perfunctory "will comply" acknowledgements.[51] Federal officials complained that it was hard to tell what was going on with such states or to negotiate on the basis of such uninformative state plans.[52]

All of this early group were given provisional acceptances, making them subject to later review—which was hardly the same as an adequate review *ex ante*. At the later dates, programs were under way, authorizations and budgets approved, contracts in force and care-giving relationships established so that disruptions would be costly and painful. Also, the bargaining relationship would be different, with federal officials seeking to take away rather than to approve. By then, *Supplement D*, which guided the federal officials, might seem pretty irrelevant to the protean realities of a local Medicaid program.[53]

The first approach to oversight was both optimistic and ambitious. Under the Program Review and Evaluation Project (PREP), an initial state plan application included a site visit by a team of federal, regional, and state visitors. This was to be followed by periodic site visits and reports on progress toward implementation of the state plan, with remedial action plans and monitoring for compliance. Quarterly estimates and state plan amendments or exceptions to state interpretations or practices would provide further occasions for intervention and corrective action. Larger issues might require a Program Memorandum or a "Dear Director" letter, but the PREP process was important to give Medicaid officials a lively sense of what was going on and to get problem resolution close to the actual situation.

One difficulty with this ambitious approach was that site visits were prodigiously wasteful of limited professional resources. Initially, these visits were mostly staffed by people from the Washington area who would travel to local sites and meet with the state representatives and whatever staff might be available at a regional office. There was money for this activity, but it took time for travel and diverted energies from technical assistance and other oversight activities, including monitoring of compliance with remedial directives.[54] This pressure on administrative resources hastened the decentralization of amendment reviews and compliance monitoring to the regions which was beneficial to an extent, but made site reviews less useful for the Medicaid program as a whole and assigned to some regions tasks beyond their capacity to perform.[55] One positive result of this experience, though, was to raise a serious question about the merits of site visits versus paper reviews and lead to increasing awareness of the need for an MMIS both nationally and locally.[56]

In large measure, oversight of the states was by "exception," that is, by taking exception to a state plan, an amendment, or a reported activity or intention. States quickly learned how to turn this system to their advantage: by saying little or taking action first and then reporting it. As a result, state plans tended to be skimpy with important language deliberately obscured or buried in a sub-paragraph of an appendix. Reports were often similarly uninformative, sent late, or not sent at all. Some of the bolder state directors would simply take action and then put the proposal in the next plan amendment.[57] This kind of behavior left federal officials "flying blind," and tended to reduce them from prospective bargaining to retrospective wheedling.

In addition to lack of data or adequate reporting, there was an intimidation factor. As one former Medicaid official put it, "there was so few of us and so many of them," including state welfare directors, often well-connected at home and in Washington, with access to their own governors; the National Governors' Association; the American Public Welfare Association; and their individual congressional delegations and senators. He said that he would make bets with a colleague as to how long it would take for one of their denials to get from the state welfare director to the governor's office, then to the White House and the secretary and finally back to them. Maybe an hour, he guessed.[58] Small wonder that Medicaid officials often felt intimidated, beaten down and ineffectual—more so when Congress added its own critical appreciation of their efforts.

Medicaid people at the state level soon discovered that the federal officials lacked the will or even the power to do much about enforcement except to persuade, cajole, or bluff and, ultimately, trade a concession for a measure of compliance by the state. The only legal sanction was to withhold funds. In the parlance of the time, that was "dropping the atom bomb" and not likely to happen.

One official recalled his own attempt to find the state of New York "out of compliance," whereupon he was brought immediately before the deputy director and told that others would settle the matter.[59] That statement could mean various things. For instance, some state directors could not only stay administrative action but get changes in the interpretation of the law.[60] All of this is not to say that the early Medicaid administration was impotent. In some instances, the states were proactive and happy for a push from the federal agency which, in turn, enabled them to put pressure on their own governors or legislatures. With so much of the program as yet unformed, a handful of federal officials could often induce states to make concessions that would have been hard to exact at a later date. In that context, *Supplement D* and the state plan model articulated a coherent vision and set of principles from which to begin negotiations—though whether aiming so high was good or bad is hard to say. Certainly, it created a host of compliance problems and an almost hopeless task of monitoring implementation. Yet it also helped demonstrate the potential importance for Medicaid of the state plan and made palpable some of the most urgent and lasting needs of the program.

But much more in the way of commitment and resources was needed. One official who experienced those early years expressed his view that a huge federal-state program like Medicaid, with a large number of options permitted by law or regulation, couldn't be successful without strong analytical tools, technical assistance, consultation and follow-up, and periodic inspections. For that, he added, we lacked the people, the data and statistics, and a reporting system.[61]

Social Security Amendments of 1967

The Social Security Amendments of 1967 provided for an across-the-board 13% increase in Social Security payments, which was a major triumph for the Johnson administration. The statute also included a minor group of "Public Welfare and Health Amendments" that were changes in direction, if not significant retreats, from the Great Society. The welfare amendments established the "Work Incentive Program"—a work requirement for adult AFDC recipients; and the Medicaid amendments put significant limits on eligibility for the medically indigent.

This combination of bestowing and withholding reflected the troubled times.[62] The Great Society was still a work in progress[63] and 1967 was important as a run-up to another presidential election in 1968. But 1967 was a year of crisis—of deep political divisions and angry battles over civil rights, "poverty," and the Vietnam war. It was also a time of change—of increasing self-doubt among Great Society enthusiasts and of growing numbers and effectiveness of their opponents.

Under these circumstances, the Social Security Amendments of 1967 were of major political importance—as an overdue increase in the wage base combined with a substantial raise in benefits. In this larger picture, the Medicaid amendments were scarcely visible; nor would they have been possible except as part of a powerful legislative vehicle or "train" such as the Social Security Amendments. To continue the metaphor, they probably wouldn't have been included, even as one car of the train, without the nagging attention of Wilbur Mills.

Part of the background to this story was health care inflation, increasing steadily at a rate two times that of general consumer prices or cost of living. This was a topic of broad interest: in the private sector and for the government, at the federal, state, and local levels. There was intense concern about how to monitor, account for, and contain this inflation.[64] And the rise in Medicare and Medicaid costs was worrisome because of the huge increase on the demand side—millions of consumers with new and unlimited entitlements to health care.

One factor that made cost inflation in Medicaid disturbing, especially to the small cadre of people that monitored such developments, was the unexpected *rate* of increase in program expenditures. Prior to the Medicaid legislation, according to an often reported (but inaccurate) account,[65] Congress had been told by Wilbur Cohen that the additional first-year federal expense for Medicaid would be $238 million. The eventual figure, however, was over $1 billion, with a 20% increase expected for the following year and 12% or more per year thereafter. This development led to a supplemental appropriation for 1967 of $470 million, with a warning that "even this sum may be less than required"[66] and a Ways and Means Committee estimate that within three years federal expenditures for Medicaid, under existing law, would be as much as $3 billion a year.[67]

Who should tackle this problem, and how? The barely established Medicaid program lacked staff, data, reporting systems or proven techniques to mount a cost containment program. Elsewhere within the Johnson administration, there was little continuing interest in Medicaid, let alone Medicaid implementation. The salient health policy issue within HEW was hospital and health care cost inflation, some of this relevant to Medicare, but less so to Medicaid. The Gorham *Report to the President on Medical Care Prices*, for instance, recommended many ways to make health care generally more cost-effective, such as health planning, group practice, reimbursement methodology, drug formularies, alternate delivery systems, and so forth—none of it relevant to Medicaid in the near term.

The first step in addressing this pervasive and complex problem, so far as it pertained to Medicaid, came about in typical American fashion, as a panic response to a triggering event. The event was the passage and signing by Governor Nelson Rockefeller of the Social Welfare Act establishing a legislative basis for the New York Medicaid program. The most controversial feature of this law was the setting of an income eligibility level of $6000 per year for a family of four,[68] potentially making eight million people or 45% of the population of New York state eligible for Medicaid. Governor Rockefeller had calculated at the time that only about a fourth of those eligible would sign up, a figure that proved to be approximately correct.[69] Nevertheless, the $6000 income eligibility figure raised fears of public insolvency, and that "welfare medicine" would reduce the income of doctors in private practice, displace Medicare Part B, and "crowd out" employer-based insurance. In addition, some supporters of this legislation, most notably Dr. Samuel Bellin, who became the director of the New York City program, saw Medicaid in New York as an approach march to national health insurance.[70] There was a quick and negative response, especially from upstate New York, in the form of appeals to HEW to reject the New York state plan and of legislative proposals to cap this category is some way or other.[71]

Wilbur Mills felt moved, in 1966, to address this problem for reasons both personal and institutional. For him, a major reason for a Medicaid program was as a check to expansive social security schemes.[72] Moreover, he had assured the AMA that he would watch over the program to see that it did not get out of hand.[73] It seemed reasonably certain that is just what would happen if this particular hole were not plugged, especially because of the interaction of unlimited eligibility with full utilization of services and free choice of providers. With this concern in mind, he included in a 1966 committee report an estimate by Robert J. Myers, the HEW actuary, that the federal cost for Medicaid would soon rise to $3 billion a year "or even more without remedial steps."[74]

The bill he reported out of the Ways and Means Committee in October 1966 came too late for the Congress to take action that year. It addressed the problem in a gingerly fashion, taking only a few small steps. The report expressed the Committee's disapproval of state plans that "go well beyond ... the intent of Congress" and cautioned the states to avoid "unrealistic levels of income and resources in Title XIX eligibility" adding that it would continue to work toward "appropriate, objective, and equitable formulas" and that it "expects the Department" to obtain from the states and provide to the Committee "current information" on expenditures, income levels, numbers of recipients and types of services "promptly and periodically" so that "corrective measures" could be taken as needed.[75]

The formula eventually developed and included in the Social Security Amendments of 1967 was a limit of the medically needy category to

133% of the individual state's maximum AFDC payment level. The Senate version was 150%, and the final compromise was to begin at 150% in July, 1968 and phase down to 140% and then 133% by January 1, 1970. States could set any level they pleased, but federal matching would be available only for the specified levels.

The across-the-board limits may seem simplistic and arbitrary, but they were more crafted and elegant than they appear. This approach adopted a usable tool—one of the few available, given the level of information and the great range of state variation—to exert a calculated amount of braking on inflationary trends. It stayed clear of spending caps or limits on coverage and optional services and still achieved projected savings rising to 45% in four years. Contrary to what might be supposed, it was welcomed by both governors and legislators in most states, who said that they thought limits were desirable and that they would channel more dollars to the neediest states.[76] Many also approved a less obvious benefit, which was to encourage some of the laggard states to raise their AFDC levels of eligibility, and thereby qualify for a higher level of eligibility for the medically indigent as well as move toward more equal welfare benefits among all the states.[77]

Another important contribution of the 1967 Amendments was Early and Periodic Screening, Diagnostic, and Treatment (EPSDT) a program, like Medicaid, of obscure origins and uncertain mandate yet eventually of great importance. As to origins, EPSDT was descended primarily from Title V Crippled Children's Services and Maternal and Child Health block grant, which authorized small grants for screening, diagnosis, and treatment. The programs were not means-tested, but the authorization was skimpy. Under the Johnson administration—which was sympathetic to proposals extending health care—both the Children's Bureau and the Public Health Service sought to expand and consolidate efforts in this area. Another stimulus was a 1964 report entitled *One Third of a Nation: A Report on Young Men Unqualified for Military Service* which stated that one out of every two men called up for military service was unfit by reason of poor physical or mental conditions.[78] A 1966 program analysis developed within the HEW Office of the Secretary laid out details for a remedial program, including several options, one of which was an extension of the Crippled Children's Services to be supported by Title XIX, the Medicaid program.[79] This proposal became the basis for President Johnson's child health initiative, which in turn led to Wilbur Mills' inclusion of EPSDT as part of HR 5710, the Social Security Amendments of 1967.

In one respect, this legislation seemed like a suitably arranged marriage between child health—with its poor circumstances, but no means-test, and Medicaid, with its means-test but open-ended authorization. Later, there was much to be said for this union, but initially developing a viable relationship proved difficult. Much was left up to goodwill without deciding which partner—welfare or health—was in charge[80] to decide about eligibility, the appropriate course of treatment, and how to arbitrate differences and enforce responsibility, especially for treatment.[81] The final regulations took four and a half years to develop and the program limped along for twenty years. Nevertheless, EPSDT eventually became one of the most flexible and bounteous sources of funding of health care for children in poverty and almost, by itself, a separate entitlement.

The 1967 legislation took two related and important steps with respect to the nursing home industry. One was to recognize and define an "intermediate care facility" (ICF) and make this institution eligible for Medicaid funding. The second was to adopt the Moss Amendments with respect to these facilities, setting up a legislative basis for federal regulatory standards for nursing homes receiving Medicaid reimbursement. In these developments, two trends converged: one toward an easing of federal requirements so as to accommodate the nursing home industry; the other toward regulating that industry. Together, these developments illustrate again the programmatic weakness of Medicaid, especially when operating within the constraints of the federal system and dealing with a powerful industry.

The private nursing home industry began to develop rapidly with the Kerr-Mills legislation which authorized federal matching for voucher payments to private institutions providing nursing home care. By the time the Medicare/Medicaid legislation came along nursing homes were well-established institutions. They were also politically powerful since they were numerous, often with one or more in each state legislative district; individuals and families needed their services; and the nursing homes themselves depended, often heavily, upon public funds. They were too important to be ignored by the time the Medicare and Medicaid legislation was being implemented.

There was a curious kind of dependence of Medicaid upon Medicare in developments with respect to the nursing homes and the ICFs. In 1965-66, HEW and many within Congress would have preferred to ignore nursing homes entirely. For example, the administration's initial Medicare proposal provided for only 60 days of "extended care" benefits, which had to meet a high standard of care and was conditioned upon a hospital stay and hospital supervision. In the final legislation, the Medicare benefit of 60 days was extended to 100 in the hope of saving some money and possibly encouraging a number of nursing homes to upgrade their services.[82] Then, in developing the regulations and standards for participation, HEW introduced the concept of an "extended care facility." This facility also required a hospital stay and exacting standards of care that would have shut out most of the nursing home industry. The Medicaid legislation—largely ignored during these developments—provided for "skilled nursing home services," but without defining what these were. Quite soon, strong pressures developed within the Congress and from the states to create a broad nursing home benefit—not dependent upon a previous hospital stay or pervasively regulated—that would help care for the elderly, the mentally retarded, and other wards of the state and would support the nursing home industry itself. At the time, both HEW and the Ways and Means Committee were resolutely opposed to "custodial" care without a medical component, or to any such broad and undisciplined assault upon the federal fisc.[83] The compromise established another concept, the "intermediate care facility" (ICF), which has been aptly described as "a nursing home with just enough nursing to justify public support as a health care facility."[84] They were held to the life-safety and sanitary requirements for skilled nursing homes. Initially, they were ineligible for Medicaid payments, but could receive voucher payments under the public welfare cash assistance titles with matching funds based on the more generous Medicaid rates.[85]

An ironic twist was that the ICF compromise was made possible, in part, by backers of the Moss Amendments, who acceded to the ICFs in exchange for support of their Amendments.[86] These amendments received their name from Frank E. Moss (D., Utah), chairman of the Sub-committee on Long Term Care of the Senate Special Committee on Aging. Moss was a liberal Democrat, an environmentalist and consumer advocate, who was skillful in gaining national visibility for such causes. He began working with Senator John Kennedy to publicize issues relating to the elderly—especially health care and nursing home abuses—and helped build a consensus for the Medicare legislation that passed in 1965. Much of his concern about nursing home abuses grew out of a series of hearings begun in 1963. They not only covered this topic thoroughly, but gave it high visibility and helped initiate a reform movement that endured for decades.[87] In light of the lax administration of the ICF provision, it is ironic that it was associated with such a worthy campaign.

The Moss Amendments provided for the first time a statutory base for comprehensive regulation of the nursing home industry, including standards for custodial and medical care, staffing requirements for nursing services, licensing of nursing home administrators,[88] and authorization for HEW to withhold funds for institutions not in compliance.[89] First introduced in 1966 without success, these amendments were included in the omnibus Social Security legislation of 1967 and passed largely intact.

In retrospect, the Moss Amendments might be seen as grand, or even grandiose, in conception. They were important for setting high aspirations for the future. They were also, in one big step, getting deep into the regulation of health care, taking on a whole industry, and moving into an area that had been traditionally an affair of the states. In retrospect, this step might seem more valorous than prudent. Final regulations were published in 1970, after the nursing standards had been greatly weakened to accommodate the proprietary nursing homes. Little was settled, except to postpone the fight to another day. These Amendments and the approach they represented helped make "nursing home standards" one of the great symbols and rallying points—but whether they poured too much effort into this cause to the detriment of alternative approaches is

In addition to these major topics of eligibility restriction, EPSDT, the ICFs, and the Moss Amendments, the 1967 legislation also dealt with an assortment of small items, some of them important to individual Medicaid recipients and others matters of program administration. One in the latter category was the creation of a Medical Assistance Advisory Council (MAAC), intended in some measure to parallel the Heath Insurance Benefits Advisory Council for Medicare (HIBAC). No doubt, the Medicaid program could have benefited immensely from a preliminary year of preparation aided by a council similar to HIBAC, but the MAAC, coming as it did almost two years after the beginning of the Medicaid program proved to be largely useless, except as a source of occasional review and comment. It was discontinued by Sec. 287 of the Social Security Amendments of 1972 (P.L. 92-603).

Another administrative change of some significance was to extend the 75% matching ratio for physicians and health professionals working within the "single State agency" to support personnel working on Medicaid affairs within other health agencies. Also covered were services performed to help qualify other state agencies for participation in programs falling under the Social Security Act, including Medicare and Medicaid and child health.[90] This extended the reach of Medicaid and other health programs but it is notable that matching for general administrative expenses remained at 50% and no provision was made for increased administrative expenses incurred by the federal program.

Various steps were taken to bring Medicaid more fully into the mainstream of medical care and closer to the Medicare program. Effective July 1, 1969, states were required to extend free choice of qualified medical facilities and practitioners to Medicaid recipients—a measure which helped to mainstream Medicaid but also protected fee-for-service medicine from the encroachment of health plans and managed care. A related measure was to allow matching for direct payments to a recipient for doctors and dentists bills, which would make free choice a more robust option.

One Senate provision, dropped in conference, was interesting for the insight it affords into difficulties in securing claims data. This was an authorization for the General Accounting Office or HEW to perform audits of records and to *inspect premises* where services were performed "on a spot check basis or when there were indications of possible fraud."[91]

There were, in addition, a number of small, technical amendments indicating the need for constant tinkering with the Medicaid program as well as the usefulness of a legislative vehicle such as the social security amendments that permit both the adoption of whole new titles as well as minor and often precisely crafted specific changes, for instance: an adjustment in the way "maintenance of effort" would be measured; extending the SMI buy-in to the medically indigent and not just those receiving cash assistance; and allowing seven of fourteen services to substitute for the five specifically mandated by Medicaid.

Conclusion

As legislation, Medicaid was anything but a casual afterthought; it was the culmination of a lengthy development and of the strategic and tactical calculations of Wilbur Cohen and Wilbur Mills. The same cannot be said about the early stages of Medicaid's implementation, for which there was little advance planning, coordination, or staffing. In part that was because of the assumption that Medicaid would be, initially at least, much like Kerr-Mills, which was *true* for most states. For Congress and DHEW the main show was Medicare: negotiating regulations, desegregating and certifying hospitals, and preparing to enroll 19 million beneficiaries. As for implementation, Medicaid was not even an afterthought—other than by implication—except that whatever federal agency was responsible for the program had five months to get it up and running, with little additional staff or money.[92]

Although short of time and money, staff from the Division of Medical Services and the Bureau of Family Services fulfilled their primary responsibility of developing implementing policies and regulations, providing information and guidance to the states, and reviewing and approving state plans. The assistance was limited and most the initial approvals were provisional; but Supplement D and letters and memoranda served well to establish standards, procedures, and criteria for both federal and state officials in the early years.

During this initial period, Congress and the administration began some "marginal centralization,"[93] setting federal limits and introducing new options. Under the first heading, the 133% limits on optional eligibility proved to be a powerful brake on Medicaid expansion. The intermediate care facility (ICF) was a popular new option for the states. EPSDT and the nursing home standards, though more aspirations for the future than immediate prospects, were important for protecting the young and the elderly. All of these changes were significant markers, good for the future.

On the administrative side of implementation, lack of time and staff severely limited the amount of effort that could be devoted to outreach, technical assistance, and conferencing with state officials. One consequence was the loss of opportunities to raise aspirations, normalize criteria, and bargain for small concessions. In effect, the program began with a poor stance and lack of resources. It is impossible to calculate what may have been lost in this process, but much that could have been modified or challenged and put on notice was not.

On the other side of state plan activities, lack of effective methods, resources, or the infrastructure for monitoring compliance and claims-related behavior soon became obvious as critical deficiencies. Dealing with them was a huge and difficult project requiring new technology, effective reporting requirements, and the development of data bases. More staff and planning at this stage of initial implementation would not have made cost inflation and fraud and abuse go away. As with disease, crime, and disaster, though, these measures might have prevented some of the objectionable behavior involved or mitigated its effects and reduced its importance in the history of the Medicaid program.

Addendum

The Civil Rights Act of 1964 is essential background for understanding the posture of both Medicare and Medicaid with respect to racial discrimination. The civil rights movement, growing for a decade, erupted in the spring and summer of 1963 with bus boycotts, freedom rides, sit-ins, and protest marches. One part of the federal response was the Civil Rights Act of 1964 (P.L. 88-352). The act was vast in its reach, including voting rights, public accommodations, federal assistance programs, and public and private sector employment. Title VI dealt with grants, loans or contracts, "other than a contract of insurance or guarantee," and prohibited exclusion from, denial of benefits, or discrimination under any program receiving financial assistance (Sec. 601). Enforcement was by withdrawal of federal benefits, with the appropriate rules and regulations left up to the departments and agencies administering the specific programs.

Whatever one may say about the Civil Rights Act, it was a bold and risky venture, both in law and in politics. Much of the law to be applied was unsettled or yet to be made. Powerful voices in Congress were opposed and congressional oversight or appropriations committees could cripple enforcement. And massive non-compliance was a robust possibility.

The Civil Rights Act cut across almost every federal domestic program. Inevitably it would reorder priorities. It would also entail a huge mobilization of effort and detailing many already stressed federal officials to an intense and uncertain struggle. A venture into unknown territory, it would push people and institutions to their limits.

The Department of Health, Education, and Welfare (DHEW) would inevitably bear much of the brunt of this battle. The Department had fought the good fight against segregation for years; but there were also misgivings within the Department as to the size and timing of this effort and how it would affect individual programs. Health care was especially troublesome. To begin with, DHEW had a long-standing opposition to mixing health policy with desegregation efforts or a civil rights agenda.[94] At the time, much of the Department's staff and energies were engaged in desegregating education, where they already faced massive non-compliance and were neither prepared for or eager to take on another vast and intractable sector.

The misgivings were well founded. But the civil rights movement was a historic movement that could magnify small events into pivotal decisions and force choices that would otherwise be delayed—and such was the case with health care. One episode of that sort was the *Simkins* case, which held against racial discrimination by a Hill-Burton hospital.[95] This case figured prominently in the debates over the Civil Rights Act of 1964. Sen. Robert Byrd (D., W. Va.) asked DHEW for an opinion on the bearing of the decision on Title VI.[96] Both the secretary, Anthony Celebrezze, and high officials within HEW, including Wilbur Cohen, feared that the civil rights issue might derail the Medicare/Medicaid legislation and sought a way to contain this issue. The formula worked out—that was legal, seemed politically viable, and complied with the constitutional mandate—was that Part A (hospitals) had to desegregate but that Part B (physician services), which were voluntary and involved private insurance, did not. This separation helped avoid a direct confrontation with hundreds of Medicare physicians, but it was made with no consideration of a future Medicaid program and what it would mean for that program.

Despite this resolution in principle, both implementation and compliance in health care moved slowly, with an emphasis upon voluntary compliance and responsibility for desegregation activities largely devolved to the operating bureaus within the DHEW.[97] As part of the larger picture, compliance also lagged in education, job opportunities, and voting rights. A concurrent event, though, was a hardening of attitudes within the Johnson administration with respect to compliance. Meanwhile, the approach of July 1, 1966 forced action with the need to decide about desegregation in the Medicare program and organize for the task of reviewing the compliance in some 8,000 hospitals.

The revitalized campaign to desegregate the hospitals opened with a stern letter from the surgeon-general of the Public Health Service stating categorically that hospital participation in the Medicare program would require compliance with Title VI and enclosing a descriptive summary of the guidelines. Although direction would be centralized in the DHEW Office of Equal Health Opportunity, within the Public Health Service, the compliance efforts would engage broadly much of the staff, as this account illustrates:

> Secretary Gardner directed the temporary assignment of 750 people to the Office of Equal Health Opportunity from all areas of the DHEW bureaucracy. Robert Ball, Commissioner of Social Security, was instructed to provide some 10,000 square feet

and support for this operation. In a sleight of hand that would avoid dangerous delays in seeking supplementary appropriations, salaries and travel costs would be paid out of each employee's home agency budget. Each division chief would recruit a quota of volunteers to assist in the Medicare certification process. If there were not enough volunteers, staff were to be drafted.[98]

A part of this mobilization that is seldom mentioned was contingency planning against the possibility of widespread hospital and physician defiance, including mass refusal to provide health care services to African Americans, especially in the South—a worst-case scenario that could well have destroyed the Medicare and Medicaid programs before they were fully launched. Against this possibility, the Department developed a "Plan B." As one part of this plan, the U.S. Army would contribute troops and portable field hospitals. Wilbur Cohen, then the undersecretary, agreed to deliver 1,000 physician assistants. George Silver, deputy assistant secretary for health, supervised the training of nurse practitioners. Robert Ball, the Social Security administrator provided office space. Sargent Shriver, head of the Office of Economic Opportunity, pledged $10 million for expenses. Whether "Plan B" would have been effective or not, its existence makes the point that the desegregation campaign was in no way seen as a sure thing.[99]

The "volunteers" mentioned were part of an outreach effort to meet with local hospitals and government officials and help smooth the transition. They were also needed to do field investigations and verify compliance with the guidelines prior to certification. Mostly, they were government workers from the Social Security Administration and the Public Health Service, but they also included staff from the National Institutes of Health, the Food and Drug Administration, and the Indian Health Service as well as many veterans of the civil rights struggle.[100] Like other civil rights workers, their work sometimes involved danger, secret meetings at night, harassment, and arrests on trumped-up charges.

President Johnson described the campaign to desegregate the Medicare hospitals as, short of wartime, the greatest mobilization in American history. Although there were holdouts, the Medicare program began on schedule, with the Medicare hospitals desegregated—at least, in the terms laid out by the guidelines.[101] A number of the "volunteers" regarded this experience as the high point of their government careers. Surely, it was a glorious achievement in the annals of public service that, if not widely known, has at least been well recounted. Desegregation of the Medicare hospitals was vital for the future of Medicare and Medicaid, and possibly even for their survival.

With respect to Medicaid, though, it is important to be clear about what was and was not accomplished. Even though the legislative and administrative directives usually referred to "Medicare" hospitals, the ban on segregation definitely included Medicaid hospital patients and the successful initial campaign covered most of the acute care hospitals in the United States and its territories. Since Medicare and Medicaid patients would share these hospitals, this was a great step forward in providing access to care and "mainstreaming" health care for African-American Medicaid and other minority recipients.

At the same time, the main target of this initial effort was segregation in its more blatant forms—denial of admission or segregating wards—not racial discrimination in the more subtle forms it could take, such as use of non-racial categories to discriminate; shutting down or re-locating services heavily used by poor and/or black patients; granting staff privileges to those with desired admission or referral practices; and reducing hours of service or levels of amenity to discourage utilization.

A factor complicating the issue of pervasive discrimination was the DHEW interpretation that the Title VI ban did not apply to physicians, because of the voluntary nature of Medicare Part B, and a theory that physician care under Part B was an indemnity "contract of insurance" and therefore excluded.[102] Not clear, though, is why this theory should apply to Medicaid as well as Medicare. But there were practical reasons to avoid taking on most of the physicians in the country, not least of which was that Medicaid would lose the participation of physicians in the program soon and perhaps totally. In any event, this particular exemption has lasted, with the practical result that a whole category of non-institutional but pervasive discrimination remains largely untouched and unstudied.

With the exception of a few holdouts, desegregation of the community hospitals was a success, in part because of the potential leverage of Medicare and Medicaid dollars. Public hospitals and nursing homes were targeted for desegregation, in the next phase, and they illustrate how events can develop in the absence of such leverage. For the most part, mental hospitals were easily desegregated because their staffs and most of the public officials—including welfare directors, legislative leaders, and governors—were willing to have them desegregated. Some states actually staged mock battles with the "Feds" to show that they were being "forced" to do this. Also, these hospitals were public institutions and there was no question about "state action" so that the full force of the Fourteenth Amendment and the federal courts could be used, as they were in the most important federal court decision on mental health in American history.[103]

Nursing homes were a different story. Most were not "public" in the constitutional sense. Nor were Medicare or Medicaid revenues likely to provide much leverage.[104] They were small and numerous—frequently family affairs resembling a boarding house for the elderly—with their providers well connected locally and/or politically active themselves. The lurid scandals over the nursing home chains were still in the future; and timing was important. Nursing home payments were not scheduled to start until January 1, 1967, a full year after the hospitals and most providers. Before that, in July 1966, HEW published *Supplement D*, which, aside from making Title VI compliance part of the state plan, included a requirement that nursing homes meet the same conditions for participation as Medicare "extended care facilities,"[105] a provision that made no sense and raised storms of protest from the nursing home facilities. HEW backed down and later, in 1967, published an interim regulation that largely accepted existing state standards for nursing home certification. Meanwhile, HEW's desegregation campaign had crested; the "volunteers" had gone back to their offices; and federal officials were confronting increased hard core resistance in the South. As a result, the compliance achieved was largely on paper only. During 1966, more than 6000 nursing homes filed assurance and compliance forms with HEW, but little was done to determine the extent to which nursing home actions matched these statements.[106]

Beyond the phase of initial certification, the Medicaid program as such has had little connection with efforts to desegregate or eliminate racial discrimination. *Supplement D,* published in July, 1966, required state plans to contain "as a separate identifiable segment" a "Statement of Compliance and Methods of Administration," (or evidence of previous compliance) but with no effective provision for monitoring compliance. Medicaid officials would sometimes pass along data about service patterns; but no effort was made to collect this data systematically. Once the initial campaign was over, there was a movement away from active involvement in civil rights and a centralizing of desegregation efforts in the HEW Office of Civil Rights or the Department of Justice.[107] Thereafter, the strategy shifted more to law suits, with which the operating agencies had little to do, except as sometime and often reluctant sources of data and expertise or as parties joined in the suits. This proved, as one astute observer said, a regulatory process "overdesigned to fail."

In effect, relegating civil rights compliance to the state plan procedures was one more latter day concession to southern "states' rights" and its legacy of segregation. In a word, compliance was insufficiently institutionalized and got lost in the private orderings of health care provision and regulation. A charitable view would be that the government lacked the strength to do both: get the Medicare and Medicaid programs effectively implemented and take on the broader fight against racial discrimination in health care.

One result of this historic development has been that much of the effort to mitigate the effects of racial discrimination in health care for the poor has not been by conscious adaptation of Medicare or Medicaid policy but through the Civil Right Act, safety-net providers, and targeted subsidies. Such an approach had the advantage of "morsellizing" a politically difficult issue. Furthermore, until the 1990s Medicaid probably lacked the data and the infrastructure to make much headway against racial disparities.

Notes

1.   Robert Ball, interview by Moore and Smith, May 12, 2004.
2.   Initially, as with Kerr-Mills, participation in the program was uneven. By the end of 1968, for instance, 44 States were participating in the program, but four states (New York, California, Pennsylvania, and Massachusetts) accounted for 62% of the total expenditures. Much of the fraud and abuse was concentrated in these same states, *Medicare and Medicaid—Problems, Issues, and Alternatives.* Report of the Staff to the Committee on Finance, United States Senate, 91st Congress, 1st Session, February 1970, 244-245.
3.   Vaughn David Bornet, *The Presidency of Lyndon B. Johnson.* Lawrence, Kans.: University Press of Kansas, 1983, 222.
4.   *The Task Force on Medicaid and Related Programs* (McNerney Task Force) and the Social Security Amendments of 1972 were, in a sense, exceptions to this statement, but neither of these had a direct or immediate programmatic effect upon Medicaid, although they did lay a foundation for later reforms.
5.   President Nixon's strong preference for foreign policy is well known. An interesting personal note is that his *Memoirs* contain no reference to health policy, national health insurance, Medicare or Medicaid. *The Memoirs of Richard Nixon.* New York, Simon and Schuster, 1978.
6.   Until 1974, that vehicle was Social Security legislation, which often assured passage for incremental, non-controversial legislation. Later, it was the reconciliation process, but it was a decade before that became a powerful instrument of reform for Medicaid.
7.   *Medical Assistance for the Aged—The Kerr-Mills Program, 1960-1963.*
8.   J. Patrick McCarthy, telephone interview by Moore, March 10, 2004; Elmer Smith, a member of the early Division of Medical Services, describes himself and his colleagues as "constantly on the telephone" with one or another state official. Interview with Judith Moore and David Smith, May 26, 2004.

9. Stevens and Stevens, *Welfare Medicine in America.* 78. McCarthy describes her as "a smart woman," also "dedicated to cash assistance." Telephone interview by Smith September 7, 2004.

10. Stevens and Stevens, *ibid.*; McCarthy, interview by Moore, March 10, 2004.

11. John Spiegel, telephone interview by Smith, January 8, 2004.

12. Stevens and Stevens, *ibid.*; Howard Newman, interview by Moore and Smith, January 5, 2003. The contrast with Medicare is instructive. Medicaid staffed up hastily from a base of 23 (including clerical positions). When Medicare "went live," after a whole year of intensive preparation, the program had over 500 in place. The nascent Medicare program could also draw, to great advantage, upon the Social Security Administration's enormous stock of trained officials, administrative expertise and institutional memory, data and technical information.

13. McCarthy, telephone interview by Smith, September 7, 2004.

14. Health Insurance Benefits Advisory Council. See Judith M. Feder, *Medicare: The Politics of Federal Hospital Insurance.* Lexington, MA., D. C. Heath, 1977, 12-13.

15. An unfavorable comparison is sometimes made between the Social Security Administration—that fabled agency of incorruptibles who could take on any task and "do it right"—and the Public Assistance and Medicaid programs—collections of "social workers" that allegedly lacked administrative expertise and let their values get in the way of performance. It may well be that the Social Security Administration, along with the National Institutes of Health were, once upon a time, the best domestic agencies we have seen or are likely to see. It is also true that, for a time, the Bureau of Public Assistance recruited MSWs and that a number of Medicaid officials have been social workers. But, as Robert Ball has observed, the criteria of good administration vary according to the nature of the work. The Social Security Administration, in his view, successfully concentrated organizational resources, in-service training, and informational and computational capacity to make a huge number of individual, roughly identical decisions (about eligibility and benefits) accurately and promptly. For Medicaid, according to Ball, good administration is more a matter of employing a diffuse expertise to a variety of contextual decisions about complex situations—especially behavior mediated by political institutions. (Interview, *ibid*) With that distinction in mind, it may be good that the Medicaid program gets people of varied background who acquire much of their expertise on the job. It is also notable that many in the Medicaid program are "lifers" who spend their careers in Medicaid and related programs and that, despite fraud and abuse in the program, Medicaid officials have been remarkably less corruptible than those with whom they have had to deal.

16. *Intergovernmental Problems in Medicaid,* Advisory Commission on Intergovernmental Relations, Washington, D.C.: Government Printing Office, 1968, 19.

17. Dan Boyle, telephone interview by Moore, April 27, 2004.

18. In the early months, with Medicaid staff in only four regions, people were mostly sent from Washington, requiring large amounts of travel time, including weekends and "comp." time. This was expensive, but one advantage was that staff deployed in this fashion gained a comparative knowledge of states' experience. McCarthy, Telephone interview by David Smith, September 7, 2004.

19. One official recalls beginning his Medicaid career—just out of social work school—with a six week course in state plan assessment. Dan Boyle, telephone interview by Judity Moore, April 27, 2004.

20. *Handbook of Public Assistance, Supplement D, Medical Assistance Program* (Washington, D.C.: Social and Rehabilitation Service, 1966. Commonly known as "Supplement D."

21.   Computers were popular in those days, though it was still the punchcard era. Not only federal agencies but state administrations as well were computerizing services, even though they lacked the sophisticated data collection and software to do much with their information except to count and tabulate One official reported that they had no difficulty getting computers and setting up claims processing systems. For that matter, he said, that they were far more advanced than some of the private sector fiscal agents with whom they had contracts. At a time when his agency was using punch-card computers, one of their largest volume Medicaid fiscal agents still had individual "counters" sitting at long tables and running up and down stairs to check records. McCarthy, telephone interview by David Smith, September 7, 2004. Of course, computer capability was only the foundation—what was still needed was terminology (nosology), uniform reporting requirements, months of "clean" data, protocols, and software—not to mention, of course, an effective and politically acceptable method of assuring compliance.

22.   Such as use of non-racial categories to discriminate; shutting down or re-locating services heavily used by poor and/or black patients; granting privileges to those with desired admission or referral practices; and reducing hours of service or levels of amenity to discourage utilization. Cf. David B. Smith, *Health Care Divided: Race and Healing a Nation* (Ann Arbor, MI: University of Michigan Press, 1999), p. 145.

23.   McCarthy, telephone interview by David Smith, September 7, 2004; telephone interview with John Spiegel, January 8, 2004.

24.   A term borrowed from Smith, *Health Care Divided,* 323 esp.

25.   In 1963, the American Public Health Association officially endorsed the concept and called for implementing it through community health centers and "dynamic public health leadership." The concept itself is, of course, much older. Cf. *A Guide to Medical Care Administration,* Vol. I, p. 107 (American Public Health Association, 1965), 107.

26.   *Supplement D*, D-5130. 4, 5.

27.   1903(e), D-1100.

28.   John Spiegel, telephone interview by Smith, January 8, 2004.

29.   D-5130e, f, g; D-6420.

30.   Cf. D-2230; D-5141.d; D5141.l; D6330; D-7300; D-7500; D-7520.

31.   For example, the treatment of "categorical eligibility." Also, the "Long Amendment" (after Sen. Russell Long), establishing Medicaid eligibility for persons over 65 in mental health or tuberculosis hospitals.

32.   *Supplement D,* Appendix B, 1.

33.   Both the House and Senate Reports include this provision without comment as part of "Miscellaneous" arrangements. Wilbur Cohen commented at the time that no one objected to his proposal. Robert Myers noted later that the provision was "subject to different interpretations and ... may or may not be of great significance." Cohen, "Reflections on the Enactment of Medicare and Medicaid," 10; Myers, *Medicare*, 275.

34.   Reflecting on past experience with Public Assistance and a bitter and protracted confrontation with Gov. Davey of Ohio, Arthur Altmeyer concluded that the sanction of withholding funds "is so drastic that it can be invoked only in extreme situations." Altmeyer, *The Formative Years,* 77.

35.   This was true, for instance of Robert Ball, and of Dr. Francis Land, the first commissioner of the Medical Services Administration. Both House and Senate committee reports seem to share a like view. Also, Elmer Smith, interviewed by Moore and Smith, May 26, 2004.

36.   Smith, *ibid.* In fact, a number of the states *were* severely constrained by the matching requirement, even though the FMAP was especially generous for poor states.

37.   McCarthy, telephone interview by Smith, September 7, 2004.

38.   Some name changes: The Welfare Administration was created in 1962, and included the Bureau of Family Services, which succeeded the Bureau of Public Assistance.

39.   With the passage of Medicaid, an additional 35 positions were authorized. In August, 1967, the Medical Services Division was renamed the Medical Services Administration and given bureau status, with another small increment in staff. With such enormous responsibilities, the staff remained small, only reaching 100 in 1970. Although Ellen Winston had a reputation for assiduously seeking quality in the Welfare Administration, it was rumored that the Medicaid staff was deliberately kept small. Despite authorizations, for various reasons positions often remained unfilled for lengthy periods. Stevens and Stevens, *op cit.,* p. 78.

40.   *Intergovernmental Problems in Medicaid, op. cit.,* p. 27.

41.   Spiegel, telephone interview by Smith, Jan. 8, 2004; McCarthy, telephone interview by Smith, September 7, 2004.

42.   1902(a)(6).

43.   McCarthy, *Ibid.*

44.   Cf. statement by a state legislator in *Intergovernmental Problems in Medicaid, op. cit.,* p. 49. Among states with well-developed capabilities at the time were Michigan, Ohio, Texas, and Oklahoma.

45.   To assess this problem of data, Medicaid officials visited states and fiscal agents. Along with "shoe box" operations, they saw a few state operations that were advanced in computer technology and electronic data processing as well as some fiscal agents that were still processing claims by hand, lagging far behind the public sector in their EDP capabilities. One conclusion was that the fiscal agent wasn't likely to be a quick or universal "fix." Also, "mechanical' or electronic claims processing was still a long way from using data for administrative management and program analysis.

46.   Some interesting techniques of collecting data on fraud and abuse can be found in the Finance Committee studies and in the print, *Medicare and Medicaid—Problems, Issues, and Alternatives*, for example, getting IRS lists of physicians with more than $30 thousand annual income from Medicaid.

47.   *Intergovernmental Problems in Medicaid,* 19.

48.   *Ibid.,* Table A-2, 91.

49.   At the time, the top ten in Medicaid expenditures were, in rank order: New York, California, Massachusetts, Pennsylvania, Michigan, Illinois, Wisconsin, Texas, Minnesota, and Oklahoma. This ranking soon changed but, generally, there has continued to b e a marked difference between the top ten or twelve states and the rest of the country.

50.   Robert Baird, telephone interview by Moore and Smith, November 29, 2003.

51.   *Ibid.*

52.   McCarthy, telephone interview by Smith, September 7, 2004; Spiegel, telephone interview by Smith, September 8, 2004.

53.   Elmer Smith, interview by Judith Moore and David Smith, May 26, 2004.

54.   McCarthy, Elmer Smith, *Ibid.*

55.   McCarthy, *ibid.* Some regional offices were very active at the local level; in other instances, little of anything was done about monitoring corrective actions.

56.   Many made the point that MMIS was needed for management, but also to help define goals and measure progress toward them—which was good for program improvement, and to help defend the Medicaid program politically from its enemies as well as its friends.

57.   Lloyd Rader, the politically powerful and inventive Oklahoma State Welfare director developed a variant of this approach, which was to use state funds to pay for an innovation and, if it proved successful, to propose it for Medicaid funding. He got the same result later, but in a statesmanlike fashion.

58.   Elmer Smith, interview by Moore and Smith, May 26, 2004; William Toby, telephone interview by Smith, April 16, 2004.

59.   McCarthy, telephone interview by Smith, August 8, 2004.

60.   Reported especially of Lloyd Rader, who had close and good relations with Wilbur Mills, Robert Kerr, and Russell Long.

61.   Elmer Smith, interview by Moore and Smith, May 26, 2004.

62.   As indicated by elections in the previous November when the Democrats lost 47 seats in the House and three in the Senate.

63.   1967 was not as productive as 1966, but some important administration bills were passed, including major education and anti-poverty legislation, and a number of health related bills, among them the Medicare and Medicaid legislation in the Social Security Act of 1967.

64.   Cf. the "Gorman Report," *A Report to the President on Medical Care Prices*," Department of Health, Education, and Welfare, February, 1967; also Marmor, *The Politics of Medicare* (2d. ed.) 86 ff.

65.   The $238 million did not include institutional care (mental health and tuberculosis) for persons over 65 or the medically indigent (Ribicoff) children. Also, it did not count Kerr-Mills—which, though not technically Medicaid, was still an expenditure under Title XIX. Taking these into account produced a figure remarkably close to the actual numbers though fortuitously so, as Robert Myers points out, since New York and other late joiners drew down larger amounts than expected. None of these considerations prevented Sen. Williams from using the $238 million figure to attack Wilbur Cohen in committee hearings. Stevens and Stevens, 184.

66.   *Congressional Quarterly Almanac,* 1967, 199.

67.   Myers, *Medicare,* 285.

68.   New York history was important in explaining this number. New York had its own medical assistance program—in effect since 1929—under which the eligibility level had reached $5200 by 1963. Stevens and Stevens, *ibid.,* 163.

69.   *Ibid.,* 92.

70.   William Toby, telephone interview by Moore and Smith, April 16, 2004.

71.   It seems odd that the category of "medically needy" had no federal upper limit put upon income level, but such was the case. No limit was set under Kerr-Mills, which first established the category of "medically needy." One reason, also relevant for Medicaid, may have been the belief that the matching requirement would be an adequate restraint.

72.   *Supra,*

73.   Myers, interview by Moore and Smith, April 4, 2004.

74.   *Limitations on Federal Participation under Title XIX of the Social Security Act,* Rpt. No. 2224, Ways and Means Committee of the House of Representatives, 89th Congress, 2d Session, October 11, 1966, 2.

75.   *Ibid.,* 1, 3.

76.   *Intergovernmental Problems in Medicaid* ,pp. 34-35.

77. This would seem to have produced little effect.

78. Sara Rosenbaum, "Medical Necessity under the EPSDT Program: when is coverage required?" Washington, DC: School of Public Health and Health Services, George Washington University, 2002, 3.

79. Anne-Marie Foltz, *An Ounce of Prevention: Child Health Politics Under Medicaid.* Cambridge, MA: MIT Press, 1982, 22-23.

80. The Ways and Means Committee report would seem to make the Crippled Children's Program primary, stressing the objective of aggressive screening and early diagnosis, then adding that Medicaid would be modified in conformity with the Crippled Children's requirements The Committee Report also separated periodic screening, case-finding, and diagnosis from treatment. But how, then, decide who determines eligibility and who controls referrals, course of treatment, and responsibility for payment? *Social Security Amendments of 1967,* Report No. 744, U.S. Senate, 90th Congress, lst Session, 127; Foltz, *An Ounce of Prevention,* 27.

81. Note that *Supplement D* provides at some length for contracts between the two agencies—though with no provisions for settling disputes or enforcement and apparently with the presumption that the two agencies would cooperate.

82. Vladeck, *Unloving Care,* 50.

83. *Ibid.,* 63-64; Stevens and Stevens, 140.

84. Vladeck, *Unloving Care,* 63.

85. *Ibid.*

86. Jay Constantine, interview by Smith, January 19, 1988.

87. Val J. Halamandaris, *Profiles in Caring.* Washington, D.C.: Caring Publishing, 1991, 111 ff.

88. A companion bill introduced by Senator Edward Kennedy.

89. Vladeck, *Unloving Care,* 60; *Social Security Amendments of 1967*, 300 ff.

90. Vladeck, *Unloving Care,* 182.

91. *Social Security Amendments of 1967,* Report No. 744, 126.

92. With the passage of Title XIX, an additional 35 positions were authorized, bringing to 58 the number of persons in the Division of Medical Services. These people needed to be hired or re-assigned, which was not the same as having them on board. Many required training. Also, as Stevens and Stevens point out, these 58 persons were "expected to implement poorly drafted legislation, negotiate with powerful states, and administer a budget that was soon consuming a fifth of all federal expenses in medical care." *Welfare Medicine in America,* 78.

93. The term is from Frank J. Thompson, "The Faces of Devolution," in Frank J. Thompson and John J. DiIulio, Jr. eds., *Medicaid and Devolution: A View from the States.* Washington, D.C.: Brookings Institution, 1998, 14-55 @18.

94. Gordon, *Dead on Arrival,* 198.

95. *George Simkins v. Moses Cone Memorial Hospital,* 323F., 2d 959 (CB 41963), *cert. denied.*

96. Gordon, *Dead on Arrival.* 97; Also David B. Smith, *Health Care Divided: Race and Healing a Nation.* Ann Arbor, Mich.: University of Michigan Press, 1993, Ch. 3. The situation was complex. *Simkins* was an important event, but applied only to Hill-Burton hospitals and its narrow legal interpretation was that it excluded *future* Hill-Burton grants to segregated hospitals and the initial rule developed by HEW followed this distinction. As Title VI of the Civil Rights Act was being debated in Congress, the same Court of Appeals ruled in another case against racially motivated exclusions from hospitals staffs—another victory and a strong reason for legislation that would broaden the principle and rely less on case-by-case litigation.

97.   The Public Health Service had considerably better access to the states as well as extensive experience in dealing with state officials. The Social Security Administration lacked this kind of access and would be fully occupied with implementing the Medicare program on time. Smith, *Health Care Divided*, 129.

98.   George A. Silver, interview by Smith, May 19, 2004.

99.   Interviews with Silver on May 9, 2004 and with Philip H. Lee, May 5, 2004; also Smith, *Health Care Divided*, 180 ff.

100.   Another huge mobilization was getting 19 million Medicare beneficiaries enrolled on time. By July 1, 1966, 6,593 hospitals had received Title VI clearance; 327 were awaiting clearance; and about 300 others had not applied. A small number had applied but were defiant with respect to compliance.

101.   Smith, *Health Care Divided*, ch. 4.

102.   *Ibid.,* 161-164.

103.   *Wyatt v. Stickney; Partlow v. Stickney,* 344 F. Supp 373 (1972).

104.   Smith, *Divided Care*, 246-251; Vladeck, *Unloving Care*, 125 ff.

105.   Secs. D-9320; D-5141(K)(1).

106.   Smith, *Divided Care,* 160.

107.   *Ibid.,* 183.

4

Amending the Classical Model

In the spring of 1966, as the Medicaid program was being imple-mented, events in Washington and a number of individual states indicated that the program would need selective federal intervention and some amendments and reforms.[1] The Social Security Amendments of 1967 responded to these needs with a measured dose of federal intervention, the addition of preventive services for children, creation of a new category of ICFs, establishment of nursing home standards, and setting of limits on optional eligibility. These were instances of "marginal centralization,"[2] typical of this era in which federal control was exerted more to amend and/or reform the initial model than to restructure it or change its status as an entitlement.

The first eight years of this fifteen-year period was a time of divided government, which made systemic change in domestic programs difficult. Medicaid policy was also overshadowed and largely determined by de-velopments in other realms of social and health policy such as the Family Assistance Plan (FAP) and efforts to enact some version of national health insurance. Nevertheless, there were important changes in the Medicaid program with long-term impact—such as extending institutional ben-efits to the mentally retarded and mentally ill; "federalizing" the adult categories of aged, blind, and disabled; extending Medicaid coverage to the disabled; and getting serious about MMIS, cost containment, and the development of alternative delivery systems.

Most of the health policy legislation during this period of divided government was the work of a Democratic majority in Congress, some-times with an assist from the administration. There was less presidential leadership in health policy or health insurance than in other areas—such as economic policy or foreign affairs—and much of the administration's health policy was defensive or responsive, dictated largely by a need to counter a Democratic proposal rather than by an independent policy preference within the Nixon or Ford administrations. In point of time, though, some of the Nixon initiatives began earlier, while the Democratic Congress was still gathering materials and developing a consensus, so the narrative begins with that administration.

The Nixon-Ford Administration—1969-1976

The situation of the Nixon administration early in 1969 was not enviable. Richard Nixon won only 43% of the popular vote, the lowest percentage since Woodrow Wilson in 1912. He was the only president since Franklin Pierce in 1853 to begin his first term with both houses of Congress controlled by the opposition party. In the election, the Democrats suffered losses in the House (four seats) and in the Senate (five seats), but they had healthy working majorities[3] in both houses—and, much in point, firm control of the committees, especially Ways and Means in the House and Finance in the Senate. Moreover, racial appeals during the campaign had contributed to this reduced majority, so that the new administration began with a legacy of bad feelings.[4]

Richard Nixon's attitudes toward policy and the presidency were important. He much preferred foreign policy to domestic and once said that the country "could be run domestically without a President" so long as there was a competent cabinet.[5] In domestic policy, he hoped to delegate much and concentrate on a few major tasks, such as reforming welfare, structuring a New Federalism, and re-organizing the executive branch. He had little interest in social or health policy except as they intruded themselves or offered an opportunity for political gain. One expression of these attitudes was his decision not to take on the Great Society frontally but to modify and reinterpret programs.[6] The Family Assistance Program (FAP), for example, was desirable in part because it would not get the president bogged down in welfare "politics as usual." It was also a way to "dish the Whigs," that is, go the Democrats one better. He largely avoided health policy, except when driven to provide an administration alternative—as with his national insurance proposal—or saw a low-risk political gain to be made, as with his support of HMOs or his nursing home initiative. Overall, this may have been a good strategy for avoiding politically damaging defeats, but it ceded much ground to the Democratic Congress that controlled the details of health and social policy.

To these observations should be added that the Nixon administration confronted unfavorable economic conditions. The country was going through a spell of "stagflation"—a relatively stagnant economy with persistent inflation—much of the latter associated with the Vietnam war. Added to this was health care inflation, increasing pretty steadily at 9% to 12% a year, roughly twice the rate of general inflation, with hospital costs rising three to four times as rapidly. To complicate this problem, the experts differed as to the most important causes of health care inflation and what to do about them.[7]

The McNerney Task Force

The Task Force on Medicaid and Related Programs,[8] commonly referred to as the "McNerney Task Force" or "commission," was an oddity for an administration that sought largely to avoid health policy and assigned a low priority to Medicaid issues. A large body of twenty-seven distinguished members from private and public life, the Task Force was co-chaired initially by Walter McNerney, president of the Blue Cross Association and John Veneman, undersecretary of the Department of Health, Education, and Welfare (DHEW). It had a first-class staff headed by Arthur Hess, deputy commissioner of the Social Security Administration. They were charged by Robert Finch, then secretary of HEW to "deal immediately with the crisis in Medicaid"[9] and in so doing to consider recommendations within the existing law as well as new legislation that might be required. Seldom noticed, Medicaid suddenly had a commission that outweighed and almost outnumbered the program itself. Therein lies something of a tale, important for interpreting the Report.

Health care inflation and how to deal with it were salient topics in 1969 even though there was, as yet, little of an agenda for action.[10] At the time, DHEW had a cohort of talented and energetic new political appointees,[11] some with an itch to try new ideas and make a difference in social and health policy. A catalytic event was the bankruptcy of the New Mexico Medicaid program, seen as a warning of possible troubles with other state programs. Not knowing what to do, a departmental task force seemed like a good idea, although considerable effort was made to insure a commission that would not simply "bless this mess" but seek a way to restructure Medicaid and change it from an "old style social worker program."[12]

The final report was a solid document of 130 pages, containing over seventy major recommendations and more than fifty minor ones. It did not purport to be an exhaustive review of the Medicaid program, yet it remains to this day the most comprehensive review the program has ever had.[13] The report stated that it made "no prescription for a new

health care delivery system" and that such a quest would be "witless."[14]
Nevertheless, it proposed as a first major step changing Medicaid into
a program with a nationally uniform minimum level of health benefits
financed 100% by the federal government. Coverage would be extended
first to all those eligible under the Family Assistance Plan, then under
consideration by the administration. Others, such as single individuals,
childless couples, and migrant workers would be phased in over time.
With Medicaid currently covering only one-third of the poor and near
poor, the objective would be eventually to reach most of the remaining
two-thirds.[15]   States would continue to receive federal matching for
supplementary benefits and for individuals not covered under the plan,
but would be required to maintain their current levels of effort and to
move toward comprehensive care, covering in all needy and medically
needy, until all persons at or below the poverty level would have at least
the "Federal benefit package."[16]

This proposal would at least treat Medicaid more like an entitlement, as
a rightful benefit. It would also help greatly to equalize medical benefits
by establishing a federal "floor." Among less obvious improvements
would be to sever the "welfare" link, largely ridding the program of
demeaning means and assets tests and of the stigma attached to public
assistance, which were important barriers to access. Last, but not least,
the scheme would cover many of the working poor, an important objective for Republicans.

A second major theme was restructuring Medicaid to meet the rising
expectations of increased numbers of recipients as well as to curb unsustainable health care cost inflation. To create such enormous demand
would be, as the report put it, "like pouring new wine in old casks—some
of which are leaking."[17] Rather than price controls or traditional regulative approaches, the Task Force proposed a restructuring of the program
that would realign incentives, so that insurers, managers, providers, and
"consumers" would share risk and each have incentives to limit the use of
health care resources. Little was said about the microeconomics of such
an approach except that HMOs and "vouchers" were mentioned and much
was made of consumer education in how to use and not abuse the system.
Also recommended was a 5% set-aside and permitting the secretary to
modify the federal match by 5%-10% to encourage alternate delivery
systems that were better, more efficient, or more comprehensive.

In keeping with these conceptions, the Medicaid agency should no
longer be a "passive monitor" but become a "leader" and an active mentor.

Under this new dispensation, the state plan would be not just a "prospectus for gaining entry" but more of a performance contract to be "reviewed periodically for progress toward conformity with goals."[18] A prime objective would be to use Medicaid's purchasing power to make health services more available to the needy, improve their quality, and contain costs.[19] Within these parameters, though, leadership would be exercised cooperatively, by providing model standards, systems, and procedures, especially in such areas as eligibility determination, claims payment and utilization review—with active guidance, technical assistance, financial support for innovative projects, and help in developing resources, training personnel, and improving administrative functions.

When these recommendations were made, little was known about health care inflation, especially why it increased so much more rapidly than other costs. Even less was known about methods of cost containment, which at that time amounted largely to price regulation (fee schedules), rate regulation, or pre-payment—none of them particularly effective. All sorts of nostrums were being touted and tried, such as regional planning, incentive reimbursement, and prospective budgeting—none proven and some quite burdensome. From this perspective, advocating non-regulative approaches such as "incentive realignment" and consumer education was imaginative and sensible.

The Task Force encouraged HMOs and other payment schemes that would "align incentives"—put insurers, providers, and consumers on the same side in controlling costs. Notable in this prescription, in contrast to later HMO and managed care enthusiasts, is how little faith was put in competition or the "market." Competition, in their view, was good because it offered choice, both to consumers and providers.[20] But the "market" (which was not mentioned), is clearly imperfect and the system needed to be managed (with a light touch), and for that they advocated a mixed strategy of regulation, structuring incentives, and improving state administration.

Little was heard of the McNerney Task Force, which was too bad. In their notion of aligning incentives (without the ideology of "markets" and myths about competition) and their emphasis upon improving state performance through leadership and mentoring (rather than regulations and policy memos) they articulated an alternate approach that could have added a useful corrective to the course of Medicaid evolution over the next two decades. It is an instructive paradox that one of the few valuable proposals for restructuring Medicaid came from a Republican administration and that because of divided government and the political temper of the times, the Democratic Congress was not interested.

The McNerney Task Force was a small initiative, of note mostly to Medicaid specialists and in the wistful category of "what might have been." More generally, the Nixon administration's health policy during the first two years was to continue programs but to emphasize cost containment by supporting alternate delivery systems, construction grants that encouraged ambulatory and non-institutional care, increasing the numbers of trained health professionals,[21] and (for Medicaid), emphasizing administrative action and budget reductions to cut Medicaid expenditures and other payments to the states.[22]

There were no important Social Security amendments during the first years of the Nixon administration, since the major initiative was held up while the disposition of the Family Assistance Plan was being debated. But one minor act deserves comment: Public Law 91-56.[23] This legislation began life as HR 5833, a bill to suspend import duties on manufacturers' shoe lathes. To this was added a rider, at Senator Russell Long's initiative, to lower the federal matching percentage for the medically indigent, which would have saved over $300 million in FY 1969 but severely penalized the more generous Medicaid programs. Senate liberals were able to take much of the sting from this provision by requiring that the secretary would have to approve the reductions. In addition, states could not use the savings to increase payments to providers, and would have to maintain the same level of overall state spending, keep the five basic services, and put in place a program to restrain utilization and costs.[24]

Along the legislative way, the bill picked up enough riders to qualify it as a second "Christmas Tree" tax act. One of these additional provisions, another compromise, postponed the 1903(e) "comprehensive services" deadline from 1975 to 1977 as an alternative to repealing it outright, and stipulated that states would not be required to take steps to achieve this goal before July 1, 1971.

During the consideration of the bill, Senator Long cited data and testimony from staff investigations that revealed, in his words, "widespread abuse and fraud, as well as lax administration." He expressed concern over costs,[25] pointing out that Medicaid expenditures had been growing three times as fast as the number of recipients. And he promised a "thorough reappraisal of both Medicare and Medicaid" during the present Congress.

On the administrative side, Dr. Francis Land, the first commissioner of the Medical Services Administration,[26] observed that the Medicaid program had been created with little attention to cost estimation or the need for professional personnel to do this work.[27] He resigned that summer, as the McNerney Task Force was beginning its work. In the same hearings, John Veneman, the new undersecretary of HEW, put much of the blame for Medicaid's "administrative problems" on the failure of either the federal or state governments" to provide the kind and number of professional staff needed.[28]

Some good news about divided government is that Congress and the executive branch often come at problems from different perspectives and compete in trying to push ahead. That may also be bad news, particularly in the sense that they perceive different realities and may, between them, be unable to see or collaborate on some of the simpler and more effective remedies—such as staffing Medicaid adequately.

The Social Security Amendments of 1972

The Social Security Amendments of 1972 were, from one perspective, business as usual; they were, from another, a grand episode in the annals of legislation. Ostensibly, they were a next installment in the annual amendments of the Social Security Act. They were remarkable in that only a small part of the statute dealt with Social Security as such, while ninety pages were taken up with major and minor amendments of Medicare and Medicaid and another twenty with establishing Supplemental Security Income, which transformed the Public Assistance program with important long-term consequences for Medicaid. Moreover, the final legislation was passed after its most important original purpose—welfare reform—was dropped, providing yet another illustration of the staying power of the American welfare tradition.

The story begins with the Family Assistance Plan (FAP), introduced to the public by the Nathan Task Force on Public Welfare and sent to Congress with a presidential address on August 8, 1969.[29] Richard Nixon had promised welfare reform during his campaign and it was a burning issue at the time, with governors complaining about budget pressures and citizens scandalized by tales of welfare "cheaters" and successive generations raised on welfare. The story of how it developed within the administration is complex and interesting, but suffice it to say that it was considerably more than traditional "welfare reform": introducing America to a family-centered social policy with a guaranteed annual income and tied in with "New Federalism" and a strategy of revenue sharing.[30] In essence, FAP treated public assistance much like social security, with a guaranteed minimum income for families with dependent children at or below a federally established poverty line, whether or not the head of the household was employed or unemployed. States would be obligated to continue one-half of their previous support, to which the federal government would add 10%. This amount would be paid out in cash to the beneficiary— essentially a demo-grant, and much like a "guaranteed annual wage" that trade unions and some economists had long sought.[31]

FAP had some distinct political as well as policy advantages. It would do away with much of the existing "welfare bureaucracy" and the demeaning means and assets testing. It would devolve most of the administration to the states. Like Social Security, it would give people the right to waste their money as they chose. And it would make it easier to support the working poor without the incentive to split up families so as to stay on welfare.

A significant side benefit of this initiative was to stimulate a proposed revision of Medicaid along the lines suggested by the McNerney Task Force, at least for the AFDC population and the working poor. This was the initial impetus of the Family Health Insurance Program (FHIP), which would essentially insure families with dependent children under a federal program but with a sliding scale of premium contributions up to an income cut-off of $5000 for a family of four. As Robert and Rosemary Stevens observed, this was a novel instance of backing into national health insurance and, at the same time, relating premium support to the private market.[32]

Part of the background for Title II of the Social Security Amendments—which dealt with Medicare and Medicaid reforms—was the trilogy of cost inflation, lax administration, and fraud and abuse. To a considerable extent, these factors worked together, which was one reason for a comprehensive and systemic approach. Fraud and abuse were highly visible at this time—whether because they were only then being discovered or people were learning how to exploit the system, or both. Concern about fraud and abuse lent both a moral and a practical urgency to the need for reform.

Aside from their scope and particularity, the Medicare and Medicaid amendments were remarkable because they were largely the work of a small group of committee staff working over several years with whatever outside aid they could recruit from the Congressional Research Service and from within the DHEW. The story begins in December, 1966 when Senator Russell Long hired Jay Constantine to be a "watchdog" for the Medicare and Medicaid programs.[33] With the confidence of Russell Long, who was both the Democratic whip and chairman of the Senate Finance Committee, and that committee's broad jurisdiction, Constantine was strategically placed for the role. He was good at spotting able people and associating them with his causes—including, for example, Sheila Burke, William Fullerton, James Mongan, and Karen Nelson, all of whom distinguished themselves as health policy committee staffers. Especially important, under the Nixon administration, was the ability of this group to "network" with the CRS, the GAO, and a small number of health activists within the DHEW.

A small group of congressional staff, led by Constantine in the Senate and Fullerton in the House, and a scattering of people in DHEW and the CRS began working toward a general report on Medicare and Medicaid even as the 1967 Amendments were being developed.[34] They were not without expertise and understanding, but they lacked data, descriptive material, and testimony. Much of this had to be developed or gotten, with difficulty and imagination. In this respect, the 1970 report is notable as an illustration of the data that was obtainable and what could and was substituted in the absence of existing data bases: HEW audits of state plans; lists of physicians earning more than $25,000/year from Medicaid; Blue Cross fee schedules; and IRS information on nursing home sales. They also conducted site visits; with Constantine walking the wards of nursing homes to see for himself what the accommodations and patient stays were like.

Many of the changes recommended in the Senate Finance staff report were included in the Social Security legislation of 1970 (HR 17550), which passed the House, but was defeated in the Senate because of objections to the welfare proposals. The amendments were re-introduced next year and again passed the House, but this time were bottled up in the Senate Finance Committee—again over the welfare amendments. In 1972, the bill passed in both the House and the Senate, but the welfare part was dropped by the conference committee, after which the amendments passed unanimously in the Senate and by a vote of 305-1 in the House.

Relatively little happened to Medicaid during this two-year exercise in *immobilisme*, except for the creation of a new institutional category, the intermediate care facility for the mentally retarded (ICF/MR), which passed on December 28, 1971.[35] A well planned "rifle-shot," this bit of legislation was added as a final paragraph to a Social Security bill to establish a cash benefit for burial expenses. The amendment was offered by Sen. Henry Bellmon (R., Okla.) at the behest of Lloyd Rader, the welfare "czar" of Oklahoma, who had pioneered public institutions for the mentally retarded in his state and saw Medicaid funding as an important and appropriate source of support.[36] The legislation specifically excluded institutions for tuberculosis and for "mental diseases," but this early inclusion of mental retardation in the ICF category, as well as the continuing exclusion of mental illness, was important for the ways in which care and treatment evolved for both these categories. In the 1972 Amendments, Congress extended Medicaid coverage to include inpatient psychiatric hospital services for mentally ill persons under 21 years of age. Taken together, these two provisions significantly lightened the fiscal pressure on the states and shaped the development of therapy for the mentally retarded as well as the mentally ill.

From a historical perspective, the most important contribution of the 1972 Amendments to the Medicaid program was to establish the Supplemental Security Income program which more or less "federalized" the adult welfare categories of the aged, blind, and disabled. Title XVI, (Supplemental Security Income for the Aged, Blind, and Disabled) established for the first time a nationwide cash assistance program[37] with uniform income and asset tests, which was a big step forward. The level was set low, considerably below the Federal Poverty Level, with the expectation that states could and would supplement SSI allowances. Moreover, enrollment was not automatic: people had to come forward and submit to an eligibility determination, so that only about one-half of the potentially eligible enrolled.[38] Still, it was important in increasing eligibility for the aged, blind, and disabled.

As a general matter, under Title 1902(A)(10), states were obliged to provide Medicaid coverage for SSI recipients, but with various exceptions. The most important of these was Sec. 209(b) of the Amendments which provided in clear but analytically difficult language (1) that no state should be required to provide assistance to any aged, blind, or disabled person if that assistance was not required as of January 1, 1972;[39] but (2) that any such person should be "deemed" eligible if otherwise qualified as medically needy. In plain language, this was a loophole created for states that did not wish to be tied to the SSI definitions or levels of income eligibility but might still wish to cover the medically indigent.

The moving cause for this particular amendment was, again, Lloyd Rader of Oklahoma, who had a supplementary program for the aged, blind, and disabled and wished to keep control of it and administer it without being required to expand it drastically.[40] States also had the option of making supplementary payments and, as an incident of such payments, to extend Medicaid eligibility and optional services. As one result, what started out as an exercise in uniformity became, for some ten or eleven states an open road to yet greater variety (Sec. 209(b)).

Two points should be made before considering the Medicare and Medicaid amendments more generally. One is that their relevance to Medicaid was slight. The main thrust of the health related amendments was cost containment and, within that, the emphasis was upon approaches more suitable for Medicare. Also, it is worth recollecting how little was known then about the dynamics of cost inflation and what would work to contain it. Regulatory approaches were in fashion, though not so much proven as waiting to be tested. From a contemporary perspective, the 1972 Amendments revealed a faith in regulation along with a willingness to try whatever might work.

A major purpose of the new legislation was to encourage research into methods of cost containment, including alternate delivery systems. To that end, Sec. 222 established a broad authority for "the Secretary" to support "experiments and demonstration projects" aimed at developing a "prospective payment system" and other changes in payments systems that would lead to "efficiency and economy" of health services without "adversely affecting the quality of such services." For such projects, the Secretary was authorized to waive compliance with the usual restrictions of Titles V, XVIII, and XIX insofar as "such requirements relate to methods of payment..." (*e.g.,* statewideness, comparability, freedom of choice). Additional costs above what would "otherwise be reimbursed or paid" under these titles were to be "borne by the Secretary."

On its face, this broad authorization would seem evenhanded as between Medicare and Medicaid. It was not. Sec. 222 was well designed, as history has proven, to develop technically sophisticated and replicable national innovations—such as the Prospective Payment System of 1983 and the Medicaid Fee Schedule of 1990—but not so easily adaptable for institutional innovation in fifty different jurisdictions. Funding was also important. The statute provided that the trust funds for hospital and supplementary medical insurance could be tapped for Medicare projects, while like projects for Medicaid or Title V came from funds appropriated for these titles or from the secretary, an important difference. There were other reasons for the slow and halting progress in Medicaid program development; but lack of well-directed financial support was a major one.

Cost containment as such was supported with new authority and a new agency, including the extension of utilization review obligations, Sec. 1122 limits on hospital capital construction, cost and charge limits for hospitals and physicians' services, and establishment of Professional Standards Review Organizations (PSROs). These were all strategies developed primarily with respect to Medicare, but then extended to Medicaid, without much regard to their aptness for this latter use.

Both the PSROs (Sec. 249F) and the Sec. 1122 limits (Sec. 221) were ways to get at hospital costs without involving the government in direct price fixing. The PSROs were an imaginative program, supported by health care liberals and conservatives alike, to involve large and broadly representative groups of physicians in efforts at peer review based on their own professionally developed standards of health care and medical necessity. The Sec. 1122 limits sought to put some teeth into regional planning by withholding Medicare/Medicaid and Title V payments for capital invested in facilities not approved by state and regional planning agencies. Whatever their potential for Medicaid—which is doubt-ful—little was ever done to make them effective and they served largely to demonstrate the weakness of these regulative approaches.

The new legislation recognized HMOs but supported them with re-strained enthusiasm. For Medicare HMOs, it authorized payment (Sec. 226) in either of two forms: 1) actual allowable costs for new HMOs; or 2) for established HMOs, the average adjusted per capita costs (AAPCC) for a particular area, allowing a portion of the HMO's savings to be retained. These were formulas reflecting the wariness of the Senate Finance Com-mittee and likely to produce little, if any, savings. For Medicaid, managed care was recognized essentially by allowing waivers of statewideness and comparability in order to provide more comprehensive services. Nothing was said about encouraging these new entities. For that matter, the Senate Finance Committee turned down a House proposal for a 25% increase in the federal match for state contracts with HMOs or other comprehensive health care facilities.[41] The legislation specified that the payments could not be higher than the existing per capita Medicare payments in that area.[42] This was a rather chilly reception and one indicating that HMOs were not then well regarded as cost-saving devices.

Cost saving was also sought more directly, through regulation. For hospital and physician payments, states could develop their own versions of reasonable costs (subject to the secretary's approval) or of prevailing charges but the federal government would not match costs or charges in excess of Medicare limits.[43] For SNFs and ICFs a cap of a 5% annual increase in per diem costs was set for federal reimbursement. In addition, states were required to impose income related monthly premiums for the medically indigent and could require nominal co-payments and deductibles for the medically indigent as well as for optional services for them and for cash assistance recipients.

The thrust toward cost containment came with some strong inducements—both positive and negative—for the states to develop and apply utilization review and cost containment methodologies of their own. One such inducement was an enhanced federal match of 90% for the development and 75% for the operation of "mechanized" claims processing and information retrieval systems (Sec. 235). A 90% match was also included for developing mandatory "cost determination" systems in state-owned general hospitals (Sec. 235). Hospitals or SNFs providing Medicaid services were required to have in place systems for utilization review equal or superior to Medicare requirements (Sec. 237).[44] As for negative incentives, Medicaid payments for inpatient stays beyond a set number of days in hospitals (including TB hospitals), nursing homes, or ICFs[45] would be reduced by one-third unless an adequate system of utilization review was put in place (Sec. 207).

A major purpose of the Medicaid provisions in the 1972 Amendments was to raise the levels of state aspiration. This was approached in a variety of ways. One already mentioned was to subsidize state claims processing and management information systems: a prerequisite for cost containment but also for program evaluation and planning and to combat fraud and abuse. Another was the emphasis upon certification and inspection of SNFs and nursing homes, with full federal financing of these activities. Federal leadership in attacking fraud was important to contain costs but equally important for maintaining program integrity, essential to the ultimate survival of the Medicaid program. Most ambitious, but least successful of these activities were the Professional Standards Review Organizations (PSROs).

The PSROs grew out of earlier HEW experiments[46] and an AMA proposal—largely a response to concerns about more drastic forms of regulation—that physicians should take a larger role in developing standards of care and in implementing utilization review and quality assurance within health care institutions. It was, unfortunately, an idea born out of time. As passed, it quickly foundered because of a lack of adequate design or funding for the, unpaid demands upon physicians' time, issues of malpractice liability, and an unresolved conflict between the development of state wide standards and local utilization review decisions. Yet in conception it addressed a vital need for a way to bring a steady professional impulse toward quality improvement and standards of appropriate care into practitioners' individual decisions. A decade later, they were reborn in a different form as Peer Review Organizations (PROs)[47] which provides some testimony to their lasting importance as an underlying concept.

Dismay and anger over fraud and related abuse was one of the most powerful emotive forces driving the Medicare and Medicaid reforms and it provoked strong measures, some aimed at the actual offenses and others at unsavory activities that gave rise to them. Fraudulent acts, knowing false statements or misrepresentations, and kickbacks and referral rebates were made federal crimes with penalties up to $10,000 and one year in prison (Sec. 242). Included in this provision were persons fraudulently seeking benefits for themselves or a third party—in other words the individual beneficiary or recipient and, as well, a relative, friend, or representative. Also notable were penalties of $2000 and/or six months in prison for anyone making false statements or misrepresentations with respect "to conditions or operations" of hospitals, SNFs, ICFs, or home health agencies in the course of their certification or re-certification.

Suspect acts that often led to fraud or misrepresentation were addressed. "Factoring" was not subjected to criminal penalties, but Sec. 236 prohibited "reassignment of claims" and denied payment for them. A similar kind of provision required that ICFs disclose the identify of owners, partners, and directors (Sec. 236), which would help identify institutions at risk for substandard care or fraudulent resale and the parties and relationships that create the risk. [48]

As noted, the 1972 Amendments were more about Medicare than Medicaid and, with respect to the latter, dealt more with cost containments and improving state programs than with administration. There were other initiatives that did not fall readily into one of these categories but were of continuing importance for Medicaid. One of the most important dealt with a new entry, the "skilled nursing facility" (SNF), which supplanted both the Medicare "extended care facility" and the Medicaid "skilled nursing home." Pushed mainly by the Senate Finance Committee, it was a needed change and has endured. For Medicare, it established a more workable post-hospital step-down facility.[49] For Medicaid it provided care of a reliably higher quality than the "skilled nursing home" and, more clearly separated the SNF and "skilled nursing care" from the more institutional care in nursing homes or ICFs.

The SNF was one instance in which the Medicare and Medicaid programs were brought more closely together. By law, certification of a SNF for Medicare was automatic certification for Medicaid (249A). Standards of care were the same (Sec. 246). But reimbursement was not. One of the concerns of the Senate Finance Committee was that nursing homes and facilities were not paid enough to meet their costs. It was agreed that these costs should be reimbursed. At the time, the cost reimbursement process, in fully developed complexity, would have been difficult and onerous to impose on 50 states, so the provision was modified to require the states—by July 1, 1976—to develop "cost-finding methods approved by the Secretary" for reimbursement on a "reasonable cost related basis" (Sec. 249). The formula probably had no determinate legal meaning, but it served pragmatic needs. The Senate Report made clear that the Medicare cost reimbursement methodology was acceptable, but not required. It also deplored the "arbitrary rate setting currently in effect in some States" and encouraged states to experiment."[50]

Although the 1972 legislation was highly prescriptive and added a number of provisions that the states later denounced as "unfunded mandates," there were several in which requirements were eased. One such was "maintenance of effort," redolent of categorical welfare programs. The House wished to keep it for the five mandatory services; but the Senate prevailed in its determination to eliminate the stipulation entirely. Aside from the consideration that devising a way of measuring and enforcing maintenance of effort for health services had proved difficult and unsatisfactory, the Finance Committee was concerned about the effects of this requirement on contemporary efforts by the states to cope with a fiscal crises and that maintenance of effort requirements, generally, tended to function "as a barrier to orderly development and operation of the state programs" (Sec. 245).

A second concession was to repeal the Sec. 1903(e) "comprehensive care" requirement. In 1969, the July 1, 1975 deadline had been postponed two years until 1977. The requirement—by then not much more than an exhortation—was repealed in 1972, according to the Finance Committee

Report, because states were being forced to cut back on other programs or drop Medicaid entirely.[51] At the same time, the new "waiver" authority for Medicaid was coupled with a requirement that the agency involved must intend to provide "care and services in addition" to those already available in the geographic areas involved (Sec. 230), thus preserving a vestige of the "comprehensive care" aspiration.

Additional services were added, some as optional and others mandated. Most important, Medicaid coverage was extended to inpatient psychiatric hospital services for mentally ill Medicaid recipients under 21 years of age (Sec. 299B). For recipients over 65 and already in a TB hospital or an institution for mental diseases (IMD), services of inpatient hospitals, SNFs, and ICFs were also made eligible for coverage.

Along with the carrots went some sticks, in the form of sanctions for various categories of abuse or non-compliance. Previously noted (*supra*, 77) was the 1/3 reduction in payments for hospitals, SNFs and ICFs when inpatient lengths-of-stay were exceeded and states failed to have in place systems for reviewing institutional admissions and utilization (Sec.237). Family planning services received similar treatment: a 90% matching rate[52] with the proviso that the AFDC match would be reduced by 1% each year that the state failed to inform adults receiving AFDC funding of the availability of such services (Sec. 299E). For EPSDT programs, another 1% reduction in AFDC funds would be made if a state (1) failed to inform adults in AFDC about the screening services; (2) failed to provide or arrange for such services; (3) or failed to provide or arrange for treatment (Sec. 299F).

Among administrative details should be noted the demise of the Medical Assistance Advisory Council, which was terminated, effective October 30, 1972 (Sec. 287). Along with this change the Health Insurance Benefits Advisory Council (HIBAC) was directed to advise on general policy for both Medicare and Medicaid.[53] An "Inspector General for Health Affairs," which had been proposed in the staff report of 1970 and passed by the Senate in 1970, failed to survive in 1972, but was important as a precedent for the eventual creation of an inspector general for HEW in 1976.

The Finance Committee staff report of 1970 and the Medicare /Medicaid amendments that followed from it in 1972 were extraordinary achievements. The Sec. 222 R&D and waiver authorities supported work that led eventually to the hospital Prospective Payment System and the Medicare Fee Schedule. State fraud and abuse units and information management systems developed largely from the 1972 Amendments. Even the PSRO initiative helped sustain a movement toward utilization review and quality improvement that thrives today. The SNF was an important and lasting contribution. The statute is also full of small "fixes: elimination of irksome requirements, incremental extensions of eligibility and coverage, commonsense cost-savers, and occasional sanctions. Not least, the amendments expressed a bipartisan earnestness about making the Medicare and Medicaid programs work properly that stands as both an inspiration and a sad comment upon our own partisan era.

With that said, it is important to realize that the 1972 Amendments were aimed at making these programs work according to their original design rather than restructuring them—for instance, with community-based waivers or encouraging Medicaid managed care. These were directions taken in another era, but that is the point—that the 1972 Amendments belonged to an era, one in which FFS medicine and cost-reimbursement were taken as norms.

A major purpose of the statute was to improve state performance by building up infrastructure and encouraging remedial activities: the 90% match for implementing management information systems, the subsidies for state fraud units, payment for nursing home inspections, training of state inspectors, and PSRO expenses. These were subsides and painless. The other approach, for cost containment and mandated services, was to deny payment or impose penalties. One trouble with this two-pronged approach was that much of the pay-off from the institution building and performance improvement was some time in the future, as much as a decade away. By contrast, denial of payments, sanctions and penalties could be quick and often effective,[54] but, for Medicaid, they acted indirectly upon the provider and immediately upon the states—which made them angry, resentful of federal paternalism, and sometimes effectively resistant. Initially, this was not a big problem, in part because Medicaid was still a relatively insignificant operation, but over time, as this opposition led to increased mandates and organized and self-conscious opposition from the states, it became a divisive and serious matter.

Related Developments

After 1972, little happened during the Nixon-Ford administrations that related to Medicaid, except for implementation of the 1972 Amendments and some major initiatives that affected Medicaid indirectly. Health policy continued to be important. Both the Congress and the administration developed national health insurance proposals. Much attention continued to be directed toward public health, neighborhood and migrant health centers, the health professions, HMO legislation, and drug regulation. Two court decisions, *Roe v. Wade* (1973) and *Wyatt v. Stickney* (1971) had major impacts upon health policy.[55] There were also a few developments important for Medicaid.

The Nixon administration made some important changes in Medicaid administration: some serious recruitment went on, and the Medical Services Administration got more involved in state activities and the delivery of health services. Dr. Francis Land, who served as the first Commissioner of the Medical Services Administration from August 1967 to July 1969, was a physician who helped keep peace with the AMA but viewed Medicaid as a "state system," for them to run as they pleased, short of causing a scandal. Howard Newman, who succeeded him and served from December 1969 to August 1974 recruited a number of able and dedicated people and actively encouraged policy development and involvement with state affairs and with service delivery.[56] During this period, the MSA became more active at the regional and state levels, especially with implementation and enforcement related to EPSDT, nursing home standards, and fraud and abuse.[57] Staff authorizations grew along with increased responsibilities: by 1972 to 206 in Washington and 150 in the regional offices—by way of comparison, about half the number in Medi-Cal, the California Medicaid program.[58] Although still under the Social and Rehabilitation Service, the Medical Services Administration had become, by 1973, more of a "health" agency, staffed for much more than passive approval and monitoring of state plans to include rulemaking, enforcement responsibility, and a small program planning and evaluation capability of its own with publications, survey information, and program recommendations.[59]

Whatever additional resources and capabilities the MSA may have acquired, implementation of the 1972 Amendments largely employed them. First, the statute laid on a host of regulations to be developed and written with policies and often standards required for each of them. In addition, Medicaid shared in several new programs, such as SNF certification, PSRO implementation, and participation in President Nixon's nursing home initiative. Policies, definitions, data and technology were required for detection and referral of fraud and abuse cases. Protocols were needed for violations of the EPSDT regulation, finally published more than two years late. These were mostly new activities, added to other priorities such as strengthening regional offices, technical assistance, enforcement and participating in the President's nursing home initiative.

Part of the background for these efforts was the Nixon-Ford Economic Stabilization Program (ESP) which lasted from mid-1971 until 1974. Faced with "stagflation," a recession in 1970, a mounting deficit and a weakening dollar abroad, President Nixon initiated the ESP on August 15, 1971 with a ninety-day general freeze of wages and prices. This was followed by Phase II, a more selective and long-term approach. Under Phase II, hospitals and physicians appealed for and got a separate system of price controls more responsive to the special characteristics of the health care industry. This experience was important for learning about the political and technical difficulties of combating health care costs; and one legacy of ESP was a healthy skepticism about the effectiveness of regulation for controlling costs.[60] Also under ESP, the Nixon Administration made a determined effort to cut back on government expenditures, which were seen as an important driver of both inflation and the deficit. In 1972, Medicaid was so overshadowed by Medicare that it escaped attention. By 1973, though, Medicaid was included, with an emphasis upon implementation of the 1972 Amendments, administrative efficiency, combating fraud, eliminating inappropriate utilization, and reducing expenditures for optional services.[61]

Renewed quests for national health insurance were a staple of health policy during the Nixon-Ford administration. These efforts were important for Medicaid largely in diverting attention from the program. Initially, the Nixon administration had no intention of offering a national health insurance proposal, but in 1971, various initiatives were being pushed, including the Kennedy-Griffiths Health Security Act, which was a single-payer proposal similar to the earlier Wagner-Murray-Dingell bill, that would essentially have made Medicare coverage universal. There were alternatives, including an AMA "Medicredit" plan and a "National Health Care Act," proposed by the Health Insurance Association of America, that would set federal standards for insurance companies, but the Health Security Act was the lead proposal and Democrats, including Wilbur Mills, thought it would pass. Not wishing to veto a popular initiative and aware of the difficulty of beating a likely winner with nothing, President Nixon put forward his National Health Insurance Partnership in a health message to Congress in February 1972. His plan would have insured workers and their families with an employer mandate, continued Medicare for the aged, blind, and disabled, and covered low-income families with children through a new Family Health Insurance Plan—which had been an earlier health care addition to the Family Assistance Plan.[62] Both of these initiatives failed, but the episode illustrated the typical roles assigned to Medicaid when attention centers on national health insurance: a residual or supplement, but otherwise largely ignored or slated to be absorbed—with the paradox that Medicaid fares poorly when attention turns to national health insurance.

One by-product of the national health insurance initiatives was an additional prominence for HMOs, that led eventually to the HMO Act of 1973. Support for HMOs came largely from Nixon appointees, especially Californians who had local experience with managed care plans. They saw these alternatives as a way to get better health care for less and to dispense with cost-reimbursement and much of its attendant regulations.[63] HMOs were acknowledged in the 1972 Amendments as alternate payment methods for Medicare and Medicaid, but without encouraging their further development.[64] Still, they had been strongly endorsed by the McNerney Task Force and by the Ways and Means Committee in 1970.[65] Moreover, HMOs were innovative, called for little additional money, and aligned incentives in a better way without upsetting organizational structures drastically.[66] One option presented to President Nixon would have followed the McNerney report and combined HMOs with a proposal for 800 new neighborhood health centers as a way to reach the poor not covered by HMOs. The president preferred the HMO proposal standing alone as less controversial and as a way to showcase HMOs more effectively.[67]

Accounts differ about what happened, along the legislative journey to the HMO Act of 1973, but there may be a cautionary note worthy of attention. Some within the HEW and Congress were clearly policy conservatives who distrusted new-fangled gadgets and preferred to stick with Medicare, Medicaid, and health policy as they knew it. But much of the difference seemed not about HMOs as such but what kind of HMOs to back, what were the downside risks, and how to guard against them.[68]

In any event, the HMO Act of 1973 emphasized protectiveness to an extent that it seemed designed to discourage HMOs and required two later acts to get a workable statute. In none of these enactments was anything much said about Medicaid. But the point is that a federal HMO program was begun although, like many initiatives of the 1970s, it was almost dormant until the 1980s, when circumstances made HMOs more useful and attractive.

The "Watergate" episode and the impeachment crisis led to several important changes in national politics and, derivatively, in health policy. The term "Watergate" is commonly used as shorthand for a complex series of events brought on partly by the "Watergate" break-in of June 17, 1972 and the following "cover-up", but also by a developing impasse in the relations between the White House and the Congress.[69] These began an unfolding crisis that lasted over a year, beyond President Nixon's resignation on August 9, 1974 and well into the Ford administration (1974-76), diverting attention and postponing and/or hampering new policy initiatives.

Except for increased efforts to contain costs, few legislative initiatives dealt with Medicaid and those that did failed to pass. Two exceptions to this statement were the HMO Amendments of 1976 and creation of the Office of the Inspector General for HEW,[70] both of which came about at the end of the ninety-third Congress. A huge and ill-conceived initiative with marginal relevance to Medicaid was the National Health Planning and Resources Development Act of 1974,[71] otherwise known as the "Roy-Rogers Act," that brought out the worst in both health planning and resource development. Another attempt at national health insurance failed and early in 1975, President Ford imposed a one-year moratorium on any health proposals that would require new federal spending.[72] In keeping with a broad effort to contain health care costs, he proposed in 1976 a health block grant that would have rolled together Medicaid and all the categorical federal health services grants to the states into one $10 billion health services grant with a $500 million annual cap on increases.[73] For a Democratic Congress, wiping out so many carefully tended categorical grants for so many constituency groups in an election year scarcely seemed worth consideration. The bill was not reported, nor were hearings ever held.

An enduring legacy of the Nixon-Ford era were two institutional changes with great future impact on policy-making for both Medicare and Medicaid. Some of the impetus for these changes came from the Watergate turmoil and some from developments within the Congress. Whatever the source, these changes lasted and, when exploited with imagination and boldness, helped engineer major structural changes in the Medicaid program.

The Budget and Impoundment Act of 1974, as the name suggests, was largely a response to Watergate and to aggregations of presidential power. One aim was to build up a congressional budget capability to counter that of the presidency. Another was to keep Congress honest and on a fiscally sound path. A provision that addressed this particular concern was the budget reconciliation process—which required that the House and the Senate first agree on a budget resolution, setting categorical limits for the future budget, and then proceed, if needed, to a budget reconciliation, for which the authorizing and tax writing committees of each house would make the necessary changes in programs and expenditures to reach the targets already set. A related measure was the creation of the Congressional Budget Office, to supply Congress with the kind of expertise and policy options available to the president. To that end, CBO produces option papers for the Congress. It also develops five-year forecasts of the costs of proposed legislation and, upon request, "scores" proposals against projected "baselines."[74]

A more significant development was revision of the committee system within the House. More of a movement than an event, it was done by committee action, the Democratic caucus, and House resolutions over a period of years from 1971 to 1974. Among the objectives were realignment of committee jurisdiction and getting rid of odd scraps of jurisdiction, curbing seniority, and assuring some rights and perquisites to sub-committees and to the minority. One change in 1974 especially important for Medicaid was to strip much of the jurisdiction of the Ways and Means Committee, leaving it essentially with tax-related authority over unemployment compensation, social security, and health. Other health matters were assigned to the Committee on Interstate and Foreign Commerce. That meant—a significant change—that Medicare was divided between the two committees and Medicaid went to Interstate and Foreign Commerce. Other important changes were to triple the committee professional staffs, assuring the minority one-third of that staff, and to require the establishment of sub-committees, with rights and assigned jurisdiction of their own.[75] They were also given subpoena power and no longer had to depend upon individual House resolutions. Together, these changes amounted to a considerable shifting of power from the established committee barons. This vestment of power in the sub-committees created much more opportunity for "iron triangles" to form and for advocacy groups to be effective in pursuing specific categorical interests. Medicaid lost access to the powerful Ways and Means Committee—where it was usually ignored anyway—but gained access to a health sub-committee where it would at least receive some attention.

An obscure and bizarre incident related to the restructuring of the Ways and Means Committee. Wilbur Mills, at times described as more powerful than the president, was stopped at 2:00 a.m. on the morning of October 9, 1974 for speeding along the Tidal Basin, near the Thomas Jefferson Memorial. With him was an "exotic" dancer with the stage name of Fannie Fox, also known as "The Argentine Firecracker." She jumped out of the car and into the Basin, from which she was "rescued" by a patrolman. Mills survived this particular scandal and was re-elected in November, but his fortunes turned for the worse after he appeared on a Boston stage to congratulate Ms. Fox on her dancing. Next week, the Democratic caucus stripped Ways and Means of its control over Democratic committee assignments and enlarged the Committee from twenty-five to thirty-seven members. Meanwhile, Mills entered the Bethesda Naval Hospital. Shortly thereafter, he resigned his chairmanship and issued a statement saying that he was being treated for alcoholism. One account indicated that his performance as chairman had been deteriorating for some time and that his behavior was at times arbitrary and unreasonable.[76] It was also true that House members were increasingly of the view that the Ways and Means Committee was too powerful. Still, Fannie Fox could have been the opportunity, if not the reason, for the changes, illustrating the role of chance in the affairs of state.

The Carter Administration—1977-1980

The Carter administration saw another futile quest for national health insurance, in which Medicaid was to have been incorporated into whatever legislation finally passed. None did. Yet there were a number of important initiatives including child health assurance, hospital cost containment, the fraud and abuse program, the creation of the Health Care Financing Administration, patient protection legislation, and a mental health systems act. Some of these were seen as prerequisites for or elements of national health insurance. Several of the most important owed much to the previous administration and even more to the Congress. But they stood on their own merits and made important contributions to future policy developments in the Medicaid program.

President Jimmy Carter took office in January 1977 in the aftermath of Watergate with Democrats firmly in control of both houses of Congress. But it was a weak presidency, elected by a margin of 2% of the popular vote and without a strong mandate. In addition, the new president was inexperienced in national politics and made serious mistakes: not planning his transition adequately, alienating the Congress, and taking on too much in the first months of his administration.[77] President Carter also believed, rightly it would seem, that his administration was not prepared to push for national health insurance early on,[78] and held off full support until 1979, by which time much of the administration's limited political capital had been spent and a raging inflation, driven by energy and oil prices, made national health insurance seem neither prudent nor possible.

Unified government, with Democratic control of both the presidency and the Congress, did not bring added strength in health policy. Many in Congress, after Watergate and the Nixon-Ford administrations, shared the view that the balance between the presidency and the Congress needed to be redressed in favor of the latter. Another factor was the effects of congressional reorganization upon health policy. The Ways and Means Committee had been restructured and much of its jurisdiction ceded to Interstate and Foreign Commerce, within which the Health Sub-committee—loaded with health care liberals and with a staff of its own—generated new proposals and would often seek to go the president one better on administration initiatives.

The Senate waited until 1977 to restructure its committees and was more moderate in the changes made. One result—especially relevant for health policy—was that the Finance Committee remained as before, with its health jurisdiction intact and Russell Long (La.) as chairman and Herman Talmadge (Ga.) as the health sub-committee chairman. This was one power center. Edward Kennedy was the leading health care liberal in the Senate and a passionate advocate for national health insurance. But his power base was the Health and Scientific Affairs Sub-committee of the Labor and Human Resources Committee and he had little clout with Senate Finance. Yet on most health issues he had the confidence of organized labor, the Lasker Foundation, and other powerful national health constituencies and could negotiate from a position of great strength with the administration.

For President Carter, the situation created by this redistribution of power in the House and Senate was awkward, especially when seeking to lead on health issues: afraid of losing his Democratic base if he did not press for national health insurance, but unable to negotiate successfully with the major power centers for concessions he needed to pass such a bill and still remain politically viable. Even so, this changed environment was not all bad for Medicaid policy—several good initiatives developed in part because of a weak presidency and failed attempts at national health insurance.

Child Health Assurance Program

When first proposed by the Carter administration, the bill was entitled "Child Health *Assessment* Program" and appeared to be, as the title implied, a more effective version of EPSDT. At the same time, it was part of a larger agenda of covering the uninsured and progressing toward national health insurance. Ultimately, the Carter administration's CHAP initiative failed, but it was a token of things to come as well as another cautionary tale.

An important part of the background for this episode was the situation in Congress, with Democratic health care liberals pressing strongly for a comprehensive array of health service grants, such as mental health, migrant worker and community health centers, family planning, nurse training, and the National Health Service Corps. These had all been part of the Great Society agenda and Democrats supported them as a way of building infrastructure for national health insurance. They also had strong bipartisan support within the Congress. But this approach to health care was seen by both the Nixon and Ford administrations as contrary to the "New Federalism" initiative and President Ford defeated a 1974 reauthorization of these health grants with a "pocket" veto. In 1975, with a strong bipartisan effort, Congress passed the reauthorization, overriding a Ford veto for the first time.[79]

CHAP was not part of this original group of health service grants. It was introduced in the first months of the Carter administration as part of a further extension of health service grants, with a modest initial price tag of $180 million.[80] On its face, it was a larger and more effective version of EPSDT extending preventive health care to poor children not covered by Medicaid. In his April message to Congress, President Carter lamented that EPSDT reached only two million of the 12 million children eligible for Medicaid and that of the two million, only half received treatment for the conditions diagnosed.[81] CHAP would raise the federal match to 75% for screening and treatment and increase federal payments for administrative costs associated with the program. Eligibility would have been extended to an additional 700,000 children under six years of age who had a father living in the house. Children generally would continue to receive care for six months after a family's eligibility had been terminated; and all children under CHAP were to be immunized against childhood diseases.[82]

Several policy objectives came together in CHAP. One was a long-standing concern within HEW over the ineffectiveness of the EPSDT penalty and the administrative burdens associated with its implementation.[83] The Children's Defense Fund was pushing for a revision of EPSDT that would expand coverage to more children and had gained some allies within the Department.[84] The Carter administration was looking for a major health initiative and, in addition, had national health insurance in mind.

Within HEW concern was initially with fixing the EPSDT penalty rather than with program expansion. When seen as an opportunity for program expansion, the modest proposal becomes more interesting, both in its latent potential and as a precedent for the future. A major purpose of CHAP was to expand coverage, explicitly to 700,000 children under six years of age with a father living in the house. Not to be missed is that this modification moved beyond traditional welfare categories and by incremental steps could be extended to cover all children living in poverty independently of the existing categorical welfare eligibility. Along with prevention, came strong emphasis upon treatment by comprehensive care providers capable of follow-up on conditions diagnosed by EPSDT examinations. Moreover, President Carter proposed this bill along with his Hospital Cost Containment Act as a "crucial first step," leaving unclear whether the "first step" was toward more coverage for children or a step onward to national health insurance.

Either way, some members of the House Commerce Committee chose the more expansive interpretation. The chairman's bill (HR 6706) for instance, retained the "child health assessment" language, but stressed coverage. HR 7474, introduced by John Moss (D., Calif.) and Richard Ottinger (D., NY) emphasized primarily coverage—to include pre-natal services and children up to twenty-one years of age. Rep. Ottinger spoke frankly of this extension as "getting ready for national health insurance," and recommended a 90% match for diagnosis with 100% for treatment. He called for aggressive outreach and a system of "coupons" so children could go to any qualified provider and get their services. He added that his program might cost more, say, $500 million as opposed to the administration's $180 to $200 million.[85]

Although bills were reported out in both the House and the Senate, CHAP was a low priority item in 1977 and neither bill reached the floor.[86] In 1978, a modified and enlarged version of the president's proposal passed the House, but was blocked in the Senate by a procedural maneuver. CHAP was passed again by the House in 1979 (HR 4962), this time with "assurance"[87] in the title and with many of the accumulated changes desired by health policy liberals. It was again defeated in the Senate. The initiative died in 1980. Among the reasons given for its failure were that it would duplicate coverage included in a pending national health insurance proposal[88] and that it would be too costly for poorer states.[89] In addition, the House bill had picked up some anti-abortion amendments which the Senate opposed.[90] Still, it was a defeat that carried with it seeds of future victories. Especially to be noted are the broadened eligibility and mandated coverage of pregnant women and of children to the age of 18 (with 21 optional). Also important was overriding state public assistance limits with floors tied to the Federal Poverty Level. A third key feature was to make Medicaid services generally available to "assessment" children, *i.e.,* under EPSDT. Together, these would have created a great potential for expansion of Medicare eligibility and coverage. In this respect, the developing alliance between health care liberals on the health sub-committee of Interstate and Foreign Commerce and advocacy groups such as the Children's Defense Fund was of historic significance. They had an agenda, skill and energy, and political support that could be mobilized; but they needed a better vehicle for their legislation. That would come about under the conservative Reagan administration.

Health Care Financing Administration

Like other events that have overtaken the Medicaid program, the establishment of the Health Care Financing Administration (HCFA) was an instance in which external imperatives impinged upon the Medicaid program with little thought given to the administrative and programmatic consequences or even the expectations giving rise to these mandates. It was not so much that the idea of uniting Medicare and Medicaid was wrong in itself, but that it involved unreal expectations, was done hastily with little concern for administrative detail or organizational culture, and then followed by years of neglect—or worse—of Medicaid.

The first push toward combining the Medicare and Medicaid administrations within one agency came not from the Carter administration but from the Congress, specifically the Talmadge Sub-committee on Health of the Senate Finance Committee. At the time, the sub-committee was working on a Medicare/Medicaid Administrative and Reimbursement Reform Act[91] that included a number of changes in the administration of the two programs. Fraud and abuse was then a salient issue, with current incidents involving nursing home and hospital practices. As they probed these activities, the committee staff became concerned about the lack of shared information and the differences in awareness and capabilities as between the Medicare and Medicaid programs, especially in relation to fraud and abuse. As one step, they recommended a partial unification, with emphasis upon several shared activities to foster the dissemination of information and data as well as to leaven both agencies with different points of view.

Behind the sub-committee's efforts was a conviction that health care financing should be an instrument for shaping health policy and health care delivery. Unification would make that tool more effective. It would also make people aware of health care financing as an activity and keep control of it out of the wrong hands.[92] All of this meant that the new agency should be a relatively independent unit and, especially, not under the jurisdiction of the Social and Rehabilitation Services or the assistant secretary for health. Another advantage, not particularly discussed at the time, would be to increase the separation between Medicaid and Public Assistance.

As conceived by the Health Sub-committee, the united agency was intended to administer the Medicare and Medicaid programs somewhat reformed though much as these programs were conceived at that time, not as way-stations on the road to national health insurance. Therefore, the calculations started with a presumption that Medicare would remain a centralized, unitary system and Medicaid a federal one, largely responsive to the states. Taking this fundamental structural difference as a constraint, the sub-committee version specified the three activities of research and statistics, data processing, and program integrity as initial areas for coordination. These were activities that lent themselves to agency wide collaboration and exchange of information. They were the most necessary for moving ahead with cost containment, quality improvement, and monitoring fraud and abuse.[93] And this plan seemed achievable without too much disruption of existing program activities and personnel.

Although the Talmadge sub-committee proposals seemed reasonable and feasible, they got lost in the disorder of the incoming Carter Administration. The result was a near fatal disaster for the Medicaid program, providing an instructive lesson about the perils of reorganization schemes and demonstrating why going slow and even consulting the Congress about such ventures may be a good thing.

Joseph A. Califano, Jr. took over his post as secretary of HEW full of energy and eager to get things accomplished. He was not new to government, having served as a domestic affairs staff assistant to President Johnson, but he had little experience with health policy. High on his list of priorities was reorganizing HEW to get administrative control over all the major agencies[94] and to promote greater economy and efficiency. This was, for Califano, both a personal challenge and a way of advancing President Carter's strong interest in re-inventing government. The notion of moving Medicare out of Social Security and Medicaid out of the Social and Rehabilitation Service fit with these objectives and seemed, initially, the most important reason for this step. As he got more involved with national health insurance he also realized that demonstrating an ability to slow health care cost inflation and curb fraud and abuse would be essential for winning congressional appropriations for added health services and, beyond that, for national health insurance.[95]

The secretary's view of reorganization was that, like a battlefield amputation, it should be done quickly with as little warning as possible. Therefore, he decided to operate under executive authority without seeking new legislation. He conferred closely with a small number of political appointees and senior civil servants and showed the final plan only to the president, the vice president, and two top aides. To prevent premature disclosure, he had the plan printed for distribution secretly across the Potomac in the Department of Defense where he had served in earlier years. He also chose not to inform Congress, saying that it was "impossible to debate issues of turf" with all those "special interest groups." When announced, a few within Congress grumbled, but Jody Powell, speaking for the administration, said that President Carter considered it a "superb example" of the kind of economy and efficiency measures the president had promised during his campaign.[96]

This approach toward Medicare and Medicaid was drastic and procrustean rather than selective and incremental. Medicare and Medicaid were to be united "to the maximum degree the law permitted." In expounding his plan, Califano would—according to report—pound a fist and clench his hands to show how the programs had to be "smushed together."[97] Medicaid was to be physically moved to Baltimore, along Security Boulevard, and merged with Medicare down to the office level.[98] It was a tall order. The first HCFA administrator, Robert Derzon, proved insufficiently ruthless in executing it and was fired. Both Medicare and Medicaid lost good people in the move and suffered in other ways; but Medicaid could least afford the losses. Medicare came through the merger much as before—an intact agency and much the dominant partner, while Medicaid lost much of its institutional memory and expertise, had little influence over such central activities as program development, operations, R&D, and data collection, and felt despised and inferior in an organizational culture dominated by elitists that did not respect their professional qualifications or comprehend a state-oriented point of view.[99]

On the lighter side, there was discussion about what to call the new agency. One suggestion was "Federal Bureau of Insurance," another was the "Central Insurance Agency." The eventual choice, "Health Care Financing Administration," was descriptive of the agency's putative role under national health insurance; but the acronym, "HCFA" would inevitably be rendered as "Hick-vah," which lacked euphony. But "Medicare and Medicaid Agency" (MAMA) was worse. So, "HCFA" it remained, which was also descriptive in the sense that Medicaid largely disappeared except as an attachment to HCFA's functional units and did not re-emerge as a bureau until 1990. In 2001, the agency was re-named as "Center for Medicare and Medicaid Services" with a handy acronym of "CMS," in which Medicaid again disappeared.

Fraud and Abuse

Fraud and abuse legislation was another initiative in the Clinton administration that gained momentum from its association with national health insurance, in this instance because of the seeming unfairness—and probable futility—of asking the citizenry to support major new expense for health insurance with fraud and abuse siphoning off large amounts of tax dollars. Program integrity was also important to bolster public confidence that such programs could be viable. In addition to these pragmatic concerns, many in Congress and the administration shared strong views about a public trust and protecting fiscal integrity and were deeply outraged by what they saw as cheating and outright theft. From a superficial perspective, the fraud and abuse legislation of 1977 was an impromptu event, put together hastily for the advent of national health insurance, but it had deep roots in the past as well as strong, independent grounds for contemporary support.

By 1977, there was a long and rich history of fraud and abuse in the health care programs serving the poor and elderly. Prior to Medicare and Medicaid, nursing homes were a fertile source of horror stories not just about fires, poisonings, gang visits and bed sores but also kickbacks, extortion, and real estate swindles. Legislative hearings about these scandals supported nursing home reform and provided strong impetus for the original Medicare/Medicaid legislation and thereafter.[100] Fraud and abuse in Medicaid took some time to reach critical mass, but by 1968 they were already a subject of lawsuits, indictments, and investigations at the state level, and major factors in giving rise to both the McNerney Task Force and the Senate staff report of 1970.

Another important precursor of fraud and abuse legislation was the development of management information systems. These were generally seen within HEW and in many of the states as important not only for the prompt and accurate payment of claims but to screen claims for indications of possible fraud and abuse, develop provider profiles, help identify and diagnose sources of trouble, and build data bases useful for program analysis and planning. The Social Security Amendments of 1972—following the Finance Committee staff report of 1970 and the McNerney task force—encouraged the development of state Medicaid managed information systems (MMIS) and provided enhanced matching rates of 90% for developing such systems and 75% for operating them. Along with the enhanced match, HEW was to supply technical assistance and develop a model MMIS. Meanwhile, a number of states had realized the importance of such systems for their own use,[101] and had begun acquiring them by contracting with Blue Cross/Blue Shield or with private consultants such as H. Ross Perot of Electronic Data Systems—so in this respect, the fraud and abuse legislation built upon well established trends.[102]

The Medicare/Medicaid Anti-Fraud and Abuse Amendments (to the Social Security Act) (PL 95-142) passed Congress on October 13, 1977 by a vote of 402-5 in the House and by a voice vote in the Senate. It was based largely on the earlier anti-fraud legislation in the 1972 Amendments, with some important assists and amendments over the intervening years. One important event was a 1975 investigation by the L. H. Fountain (D., NC) Sub-committee on Intergovernmental Relations and Human Resources of the Government Operations Committee. Among the Committee's conclusions was that the administrative measures taken by HEW to contain and reduce fraud were inadequate. The Committee introduced a bill that would establish an inspector general within HEW appointed by the President and reporting only to the secretary.[103] This initiative received an assist from a Moss sub-committee[104] investigation showing that the Medicaid program and nursing home patients were losing over $1.8 billion a year to fraud and abuse, which was over 10% of a $15 billion dollar program. Responding to this opportunity, the Senate added some amendments, including most of the fraud and abuse provisions of a Finance Health Sub-Committee bill dealing comprehensively with Medicare and Medicaid.[105] This part of the bill was stripped and the inspector general legislation passed standing alone in 1976. When the House passed a fraud and abuse bill the next year, the Senate bill was added to it and became the main basis for the final legislation.

In broad outline, the statute established and defined a number of illegal acts, including defrauding the government and offenses such as kickbacks, bribes and rebates, requiring contributions as a condition of admission to a heath care institution, and "willful and repeated" violations of a participation agreement. A number of misdemeanors (under the 1972 Amendments) became felonies with penalties increased from $10,000 and one year in prison to $25,000 and five years in prison. A wider range of penalties was established: requiring suspension of physicians or other practitioners for a criminal offense related to the Medicare or Medicaid programs; allowing states to suspend Medicaid recipients convicted of defrauding the program; and making a violation of a participation agreement a misdemeanor.

Criminal offenses would be referred for prosecution to the attorney general of the United States. The House Ways and Means Committee had originally sought to have a special section established within the Criminal Division of the Department of Justice and dedicated to the prosecution of Medicare and Medicaid offenses. This met with strenuous objection by Griffin Bell, the attorney general, and was dropped. But anxiety about the diligence and capability of the Department of Justice to deal with Medicare/Medicaid fraud and abuse found expression in a provision of the act requiring the HEW inspector general to report annually to the Congress on cases referred to the Department of Justice and their disposition, including the inspector general's own recommendations about how the DOJ's performance could be improved (Sec. 204(a)).

The "abuse" part of the legislation was left largely up to the PSROs, whose assigned responsibility was to review for medical necessity and appropriateness. In general, these institutions were weak and faltering and important mostly for hospital activities. Still, the legislation took several steps that were significant for Medicaid, in principle or as precedents for future action. One provision was to make PSRO decisions conclusive, not merely advisory, for determining payment.[106] Specifically relevant to Medicaid was the extension of the PSRO's scope of activities to include review of "shared health facilities," defined so as to get at the so-called "Medicaid mills" (Sec. 5(b)2). PSROs were required, within two years of reaching operational status, to undertake the review of ambulatory facilities (Sec. 5(c)(1)). If and when a PSRO decided to move on such facilities as SNFs, ICFs, and ambulatory care services, the statute required that an amendment (in scope of activities) be submitted to the "Social Security Agency" and the proposal forwarded to the governors for comment before going to the secretary of HEW for approval (Sec. 5(c)2).

Fraud and abuse in Medicare/Medicaid shared with some types of commercial fraud—for instance, in banking and the stock market—the need to discover, understand, and be able to document what was going on in dark and secret places, what was happening systemically, and the relations between the two. Getting information was, therefore, an important feature of the statute, with a dual emphasis upon probing into private, hidden areas as well as collecting and systematizing an enormous amount of data.

Disclosure requirements—important for identifying potential sources of fraud—were broad in their sweep, covering Medicare/Medicaid, Title V "Maternal and Child Health" and Title XX social services and moving beyond owners and direct providers to include HMOs and clinical laboratories, contractors and sub-contractors, carriers and fiscal agents, mortgage holders, and indirect financial relations (Sec. 3). Providers had to disclose the names of owners, partners, directors, and officers (if a corporation) and any managing employees who had been convicted of defrauding either a federal or state health program. As a next step, "any disclosing entity" could be required by the secretary or the "single State agency" to provide "full and complete information as to their significant business transactions" between the provider and a contractor or wholly-owned sub-contractor over the last five years" (Sec. 3(a)1, amending Sec 1124(b,c)). Compliance with these requirements was made a condition of initial or continuing participation in, or certification for, Medicare/Medicaid, Maternal and Child Health, or Title XX social services.

Reaching broadly and deeply these provisions were relatively self-enforcing—that is, the provider either complied or faced discontinuation in the program. In fact, they seemed attractive enough to the comptroller-general that he, either from quickened desire or status consciousness, sought and got for his office an authorization to subpoena information needed to review federal health programs and seek compliance through the federal courts.[107]

One step that was important, even critical, for MMIS and fighting fraud and abuse, as well as for state and federal health programs more generally, was to require the secretary, with appropriate consultation, to establish uniform systems for reporting utilization of services. This involved costs, charges, and volume, both in the aggregate and broken out by services provided, functional activities, and categories of patient and provider. Capital accounts and discharge data were also important. Strong emphasis was upon *uniformity*—providing data that could be part of an intelligible body of information, usable for planning, comparing effectiveness and efficiency of activities, and communicating across many data-using entities (Sec. 19).

Efforts to upgrade state efforts emphasized suasion and encouragement, in part because past efforts met with little success and considerable resentment. Enhanced matching of 75% continued as before, but with requirements for qualifying eased and simplified. Past penalty assessments were waived with the new concentration upon remediation rather than punitive measures. Independent state anti-fraud units were encouraged, though not required, with a 90% match through FY 1980 for establishing them. And state initiatives to develop new, more effective attacks on fraud and abuse were given some cachet by making them eligible for funding under Sec. 222 of the Social Security Amendments of 1972.

For some perspective on this legislation, it is useful to recall the broad approach to "fraud and abuse" in the statute. As noted, "abuse" was to have been largely dealt with by the PSROs and through encouraging provider restraint and self-policing. Along with HMOs, they were touted as a last chance for provider freedom and self-government. It could be argued that this noble experiment was never really tried.[108] In any event, it failed to achieve the aims sought. One result was an imbalance—a statute with a truly formidable set of criminal penalties,[109] but lacking effective intermediate remedies and techniques short of hauling miscreants into court and sending them to prison—measures so harsh, expensive, and unpopular that they were seldom used.

These reflections help explain why the fraud and abuse legislation was sometimes seen as less than helpful. State Medicaid officials generally acknowledged the need for such measures and applauded federal leadership in supporting MMIS, though they would have preferred a more gradual development and more technical assistance.[110] They also said that less emphasis was needed on fraud and more on provider education and adaptation of PSROs to state needs,[111] since Medicaid officials and their providers had to live together in the same state. As usual, there was complaint that the legislation took inadequate account of interstate variation: those already far along and those with years to go. As one result, laggards got the greatest benefit from the enhanced matching while proactive states gained less and "suffered" for their virtue.[112] Some states lacked data or were not far enough along to implement more sophisticated modules, such as SURS,[113] and often had to scramble, pay large premiums to entrepreneurial software consultants, and stood to gain much less from MMIS than the more advanced states. In various ways, the statute was well designed to support federal prosecutions, but of little present help to many states in combating either fraud or abuse.

Boren Amendment

The so-called Boren Amendment of 1980-81 was, historically, two amendments—one in 1980 and a second in 1981. It began its career with Sec. 249 of the 1972 Amendments, a provision that was intended to give states a modicum of freedom in setting rates for SNFs and ICFs. Sec. 249 was almost repealed in 1977, but survived, as amended, to become an important protection for hospitals and sometimes for patients, as well as a major source of litigation and vexation for governors and state Medicaid directors.

The original purpose of Sec. 249 was to enable the states to get away—but not too far from—Medicare cost reimbursement, which could be both cumbersome and costly (*supra,* 109). But even the "cost-related" requirement was objectionable to some, especially Lloyd Rader, the Oklahoma welfare director, who paid his nursing facilities a statewide negotiated rate. Largely through his efforts, implementation of Sec. 249 was delayed until 1976, with a final compliance date set for 1978. In 1977, Rader enlisted the help of Sen. Henry Bellmon (R., Okla.), who was well placed on the Finance Committee to get Sec. 249 repealed. His amendment passed both houses, but was dropped in conference. In January 1979, the same amendment was introduced by Sen. David Boren (D., Okla.). By then, various additional groups had come to the table, including the nonprofit nursing home industry, the National Citizens' Coalition for Nursing Home Reform, and the National Governors' Association, with the result that the original simple repeal became a rather complex and troublesome paragraph embedded in OBRA 1980.[114]

The operative language is quoted at length because parts of it are often cited. Also, the text gives a lively sense for how productive of litigation the provisions might be. For SNFs and ICFs, states could

> use rates (determined in accordance with *methods and standards* developed by the State) which the State *finds* and makes *assurances satisfactory to the Secretary* are *reasonable and adequate* to meet the *costs* which must be incurred by *efficiently and economically* operated facilities in order to provide care and services in conformity with applicable State and Federal laws, regulations, and *quality and safety* standards... (ital. added).

The Boren Amendment has been cited as an example of well-intentioned language that can miscarry, especially when parsed by lawyers. The italics are used to suggest briefly some points of attack hospital attorneys were able to use to good effect. For instance, what "methods and standards" of rate-setting pass muster? What kind of a "finding" must the state agency make? Are the rates "reasonable and adequate?" What is "efficient and economical" operation? and how are these criteria established and applied? Are federal and state quality and safety standards met? And in doing so, what costs must be incurred? In addition to all of this, federal courts have held that they owe no special deference to state regulatory agencies in these matters and have often determined *de novo* what constitutes compliance with the Boren Amendment, and what are reasonable rates and methods of rate determination.[115]

In 1981, the Boren Amendment was greatly extended, primarily at the instance of Rep. Henry A. Waxman, the increasingly influential chairman of the Health and Environment Sub-committee of the House Interstate and Foreign Commerce Committee. As an early example of Henry Waxman's ability to swim against the tide, this amendment was part of the notorious and huge OBRA of 1981 that drastically slashed domestic programs and sought to cap the Medicaid entitlement. One part of the Waxman amendment was simply to insert the word "hospital" in front of SNFs and ICFs.[116] The other, especially important for Medicaid, was to provide that reimbursement had to "take into account the situation of hospitals that serve a disproportionate number of low income patients with special needs" and add that "individuals eligible for Medical Assistance [must] have reasonable access (taking into account geographic location and reasonable travel time) to inpatient hospital services of adequate quality" (Sec. 2173).

The Sec. 249, "reasonably cost-related" requirement had traveled some distance from a modest amendment designed to ease SNF and ICF reimbursement methodology to a provision aimed mostly at protecting hospitals and subsidizing inpatient care for Medicaid recipients. It took roughly a decade for the Boren Amendments to develop full momentum and for the DSH scandals to emerge in mature and florid growth. At a minimum, this evolution helps to illustrate the hazards of incremental fixes applied to the regulatory process.

Related Developments

In 1976-77, there was another attempt to amend Federal HMO policy that had some importance for Medicaid, mostly by keeping the HMO initiative alive and by introducing the notion, once again, that HMOs might be an attractive option for Medicare and Medicaid. In part, this renewal of interest came from the push for national health insurance as well as concern about rising health care costs, both in the public and private sectors. It also stemmed from an awareness that the HMO Act of 1973 needed additional repair and that the amendments of 1976 had not sufficed. The new legislation was a hard sell, in part because of provider opposition, but also the eruption of scandals in managed care and the reluctance within Congress to move from experiment to subsidized development.[117]   Supporters of the legislation were able to get about half of what they had sought. That half amounted to a three year, $163 million re-authorization for federal grants and loans, with some easing of administrative requirements, increased individual amounts and better structuring of grants and of loan guarantees, and more reporting requirements and closer monitoring. In brief summary, the 1976 amendments helped make federally qualified HMOs administratively feasible and the 1978 amendments provided funding for a modest number to become operational

The good news was that the HMO movement stayed alive, to become an important option for both Medicare and Medicaid at a later date. HMOs also received a substantial amount of attention, including a general restructuring of the program and the creation of a specially designated central office of Health Maintenance Organization Services (HMOS) within the Department. The administration backed HMOs with some enthusiasm but a low level of priority. In April 1978, though, the Senate Permanent Sub-Committee on Investigations reported on its four year investigation of prepaid health plans in the California Medi-Cal program[118] and revived bad memories from the past, confirming in many what they already thought about HMOs. This was followed by complaints of HEW laxness in nursing home enforcement, providing more indications that a go-slow policy might be wise. The administration's Medicare and Medicaid initiatives were dropped in the ultimate legislation, although Medicaid enrollments in HMOs received recognition of a sort: enrollment practices were limited to methods approved by the secretary.[119]

The Mental Health Systems Act (PL 96-398) was a late Carter administration initiative that had little direct or immediate significance for Medicaid, not least because it was repealed before it could be implemented by the incoming Reagan administration. It was, nevertheless, path breaking and precedent setting legislation, built upon the work of a highly successful presidential commission, and took a large step in the concept of mental health therapy as well as pioneering a new version of "de-institutionalization" that has become important for Medicaid programs dealing with disabilities.[120]

The origins of this new approach lay in a tardy and painful recognitions that a large proportion of the mentally ill were "chronic"—they were not going to get well. This was counter to a previous optimism that saw the main task as early therapeutic intervention to get mental patients back in the community before they severed primary ties and became "institutionalized", that is, psychologically resigned to an institutional status. In the later view, "aftercare" was even more critical: to enable the chronically ill to function in the local community, with newer and less debilitating psychotropic drugs and access to community based services that would help with employment, housing, and socialization.[121] But this approach meant reaching far beyond the earlier community mental health centers to develop a broad array of community based services, coordinate those services, and create a system that would make the dollars follow the individual being served.

These considerations help explain the importance of the "systems" emphasis: getting public and private, state and local services to work together. A new array of categorical grants would be available for the chronically and severely ill, as well as for social services, preventive initiatives, and administrative expenses. These grants, which would go primarily to existing or new community mental health centers (CMHCs) to support primarily services for the chronically ill, the elderly, and severely disturbed children. In this manner, the CMHCs and the powerful NIMH constituencies would be engaged. But much of the new funding would be targeted to specific priorities and distributed by the states operating under approved state mental health plans—a strategy that recognized the need for an "intermediate sovereign" to coordinate mental health services and support. States would have great freedom to oversee, prioritize, and manage the mental health "systems," but only if they stayed within broad federal guidelines and the overall purpose of coordinated and community based service delivery. They would also have to provide job security for institutional mental health workers displaced by the shift toward community care—a frank recognition of the politics of mental health at the state level.

The Mental Health Systems Act stands out especially because it was one of the few attempts to address comprehensively the problems of community based health care delivery within the federal system. Based as it was upon new therapeutic insights and possibilities as well as a realistic assessment of the politics of mental health, it was an important experiment—which, unfortunately, was never implemented.

Since 1980, much has changed in mental health policy and in attitudes toward persons with disabilities and the resources available to help them, so that the details of the MHSA are of little immediate relevance. But it is an important reminder of a central problem that continues: of how to "go to scale"—implement a therapeutic model that sustains individuals with disabilities in the community, that is comprehensive and truly state-wide, and that can be effectively monitored and maintained.

Conclusion

Surviving and growing, were important accomplishments during the Medicaid's first fifteen years. A welfare-based, categorical program was successfully implemented, lived through an initial crisis, was joined by all the states but Arizona, established viable and cooperative federal-state relations, and grew steadily (except for 1978) reaching a total of 22 million by 1980.[122]

Program integrity was vital for the credibility of Medicaid and a number of measures strengthened Medicaid's institutional foundations. Most essential were the fraud and abuse and MMIS initiatives which combated these evils directly and helped improve administration, planning, and program development. The PSROs and the establishment of a DHHS inspector-general also strengthened program integrity. Related developments were penalties for laxness in enforcing hospital utilization limits, in determinations of Medicaid eligibility, and failures to implement EPSDT requirements. As with enforcement generally, some of these measures were less than successful; but they demonstrated a seriousness of purpose and were, over time, improved with constructive modifications.

New benefits and service delivery changes addressed the needs of separate populations: children, the elderly, and those with specific disabilities. EPSDT, an early initiative, added preventive health care and early intervention for children. The ICF and the ICF/MR were service delivery innovations that had important and lasting effects. Inpatient psychiatric services were authorized for Medicaid recipients under 21 and the IMD exclusion lifted for those over 65 years of age. Though initially small in impact, these changes were precedents for incremental additions to existing benefits and extending them to new populations.

During all this time, Medicaid expenditures grew at a brisk pace, averaging more than 30% in the first five years and 18% over the next ten,[123] a rate that gained for Medicaid increased visibility both nationally and locally and changed views about the program from tolerant indifference to anxious concern. Even so, relatively little systematic attention was given to cost containment for the program except to apply methods devised for Medicare to Medicaid and retain existing AFDC categorical and income limitations. But it was important to learn what does not work, and one legacy of this period was a growing consensus that regulative approaches that seemed plausible for Medicare do not work well for a health care system as decentralized as Medicaid, with its "large numbers of independent professionals and institutions [and] apparently infinite capacities for adaptation."[124]

This period in Medicaid development revealed some of the undesirable characteristics of untended incremental growth, among them a tendency to follow and deepen existing channels and to grow excessively in areas where resistance was low or attraction high. One consequence of the continued linkage of categorical eligibility with welfare cash payments, for instance, was to perpetuate interstate variations and even heighten them when fiscal pressures led states to hold down or lower welfare eligibility levels. With the additional effects of optional Medicaid populations and benefits, these variations and their administrative permutations grew apace, adding to the inequities and layered complexity of the Medicaid program.[125]

Unchecked incrementalism also contributed to the growth of long-term care and the "institutional bias" of Medicaid by paying for nursing home care[126] and extending coverage to near substitutes such as the ICFs and the ICF/MRs. In the absence of Medicare coverage or community-based alternatives, the Medicaid match made such institutional placements attractive—at least to Medicaid directors and relatives of the impoverished elderly and of those with various mental and other disabilities who would otherwise be without care or dependent on relatives or other unpaid caretakers. By 1980, Medicaid spending for nursing homes and other long-term care institutions had risen to $11.5 billion or 42% of total Medicaid expenditures, much of that for inappropriate placements,[127] which seemed both wasteful and a poor deployment of resources.

The situation was complicated in 1972 by SSI, which "federalized" income support for the adult welfare categories of aged, blind, and disabled. Soon these populations were enrolling in Medicaid at a percentage rate of increase twice that for AFDC recipients. Since many in these adult categories were chronically and/or severely ill, suffered from one or more disabilities, and often required institutionalization, they were more expensive than the AFDC children and their parents. A consequence was that expenses for adults and the disabled began to rise as a proportion of total Medicaid budgets and those under AFDC to decline so that by 1980, roughly 70% of Medicaid expenditures were for the aged, blind, and disabled that were, numerically, only 28% of the number enrolled in Medicaid while 30% of the money was going for AFDC recipients that were 64% of the total number of Medicaid recipients.[128]

A perverse consequence of this squeeze on AFCD eligibility was that it tended to be most onerous for poor and rural states, including several with large minority populations.[129] In that respect, the Medicaid program was being deflected from one of its prime objectives of supporting health care for the neediest. Also, a huge amount of money was being poured into a less productive and inappropriate use for institutional care.

Such developments were systemic and raised questions about the future of the whole program. Despite Medicaid's wide acceptance and strong growth, trends and asymmetries such as those described made the case—for some, at least—that incrementalism, even with some well-directed "marginal centralization," was not enough. The program had design flaws and needed "restructuring," of the entitlement as such, a retrofitting of a new part, or some measures in between.

In looking toward the future, the contributions of this first stage of development should not be slighted. Over fifteen years, the Medicaid program got well established, gaining in acceptance and credibility. Some major initiatives such as EPSDT, MMIS and fraud and abuse, and the nursing home standards increased the federal stake in the program, upgraded state efforts, and got some urgent needs addressed. They also cleared the policy agenda for later efforts. As to those, most of them—

Medicaid managed care, home and community based services, a major child health initiative—were live options, being seriously considered, in 1980. OBRA '80, passed under the Carter administration, was the first reconciliation bill extensively used for program amendments, another precedent for the future.

For good and for ill, Medicaid is a program in which the future develops from the past, much like an organic growth. The period from 1966 to 1980 can be seen as creating both the need and many of the materials for a restructuring of the Medicaid program. That restructuring combined familiar elements from the past, but the ways that was done were at times new and surprising.

Notes

1.   For a sampling of such events, see Stevens and Stevens, *Welfare Medicine in America,* Ch. 6, "The Beginnings of Disillusion."
2.   Thompson and DiIulio, *Medicaid and Devolution* 18-19.
3.   In the House, 243-192; and in the Senate, 58-42.
4.   A "southern strategy" adopted by Richard Nixon and by George Wallace, in his Independent Party candidacy, which won five states and 46 electoral votes. *Congressional Quarterly Almanac* (1969), pp. 1200-1201.
5.   A. James Reichley, *Conservatives in an Age of Change* (Washington, D.C.: Brookings Institution, 1981), 59.
6.   Daniel Patrick Moynihan, who for a time served as President Nixon's main advisor on social policy, argued strongly for this approach. *Ibid.,* 70-72; Nixon admired Disraeli and once said to Moynihan that "Tory men and liberal politics are what have changed the world." *Ibid.,* 72.
7.   Michael Zubkoff (ed.) *Health: A Victim or Cause of Inflation.* New York, Milbank Memorial Fund, 1976, 12-13.
8.   *Report of the Task Force on Medicaid and Related Programs*, Department of Health, Education, and Welfare (Washington, D.C.: Government Printing Office, 1970).
9.   Stevens and Stevens, *Welfare Medicine in America,* 217.
10.   One law (P.L. 91-56) passed that year allowed states to: 1) cut back on optional services, so long as they did not reduce cash payments; and 2) put in place a plan to reduce utilization. They could not use the reductions to increase payments to providers. *Congressional Quarterly Almanac* (1969), 201; HEW also acted administratively to put a curb on payments to physicians and eliminated the cost-plus factor for hospitals. *Ibid.,* 867.
11.   One price for divided government was partisan differences between Congress and the administration, increasing the need for political appointees in the agencies. The Nixon administration created a large number of new political appointees, some of them partisan and others reflecting private sector approaches to problems.
12.   Lawrence S. Lewin, interview by Moore and Smith, November 7, 2002. Fred Malek took charge of the staffing. He was a political appointee, then in HEW, who later became personnel director for the Nixon administration largely because of his "loyalist" sympathies and hard-headed approach to decisions.
13.   In 1983, the HCFA Office of Research and Demonstrations began a series of Medicaid program evaluation projects, initially dealing with OBRA '81 program

changes. This initiative expanded in various ways, including a survey of the states that produced a compendious list of suggested reforms that were forwarded to William Roper, then the administrator of HCFA, but went no further. Although these evaluations were voluminous and of good quality, they were not aimed at overall assessment and reform.

14. *Report of the Task Force on Medicaid,* 3.
15. *Ibid.,* p. 18.
16. *Ibid.,* p. 17.
17. *Ibid.,* p. 106.
18. *Ibid.,* p. 68.
19. *Ibid.,* p. 64.
20. *Ibid.,* p. 3.
21. There were general shortages of health personnel and facilities and of physicians and hospitals in rural areas. There was also the erroneous view that a good way to lower health care costs was to "break the manpower bottleneck" by increasing the number of physicians. Cf. Rashi Fein, *The Doctor Shortage: An Economic Diagnosis.* Washington, D.C.: Brookings Institution, 1967, esp. Ch. 1.
22. For instance, the new Medicare regulations limited doctors' payments to 75% of prevailing charges and eliminated the 2% "cost plus" payments for hospitals (1.5% for the for-profits). The first Nixon budget proposed cumulative cuts of almost $500 million for Medicaid (as compared with $65 million for Medicare) to be gotten by reductions in Medicaid outlays and in payments to the states. *Congressional Quarterly Almanac,* 1969, 989.
23. A bill "To continue until the close of June 30, 1972 the suspension of duty on certain copying shoe lathes" P.L. 91-56 (1969).
24. *Congressional Quarterly Almanac,* 1969, p. 201; also Stevens and Stevens, *Welfare Medicine in America,* 145 ff.
25. *Ibid.,* 202, 205.
26. He served in this position from November 1966 to July 25, 1968. He was followed by Howard Newman, who was more alert to Medicaid problems.
27. *Ibid,* 385.
28. *Ibid.,* 385.
29. Reichley, *Conservatives in an Age of Change,* 132-140.
30. Reichley provides a good summary account of its origins and basic outlines.
31. The notion of a family grant (rather than categorical eligibility) had two important lines of descent—one from the "Guaranteed Annual Wage," advocated by trade unions and liberal Democrats, and the other from the "negative income tax," supported by free-market economists such as Milton Friedman. "Family Assistance Plan" as a title had some political cover and better resonance.
32. Stevens and Stevens, *Welfare Medicine in America,* 235-236.
33. Jay Constantine, interview by Edward D. Berkowitz, August 24, 1995. CMS Oral History Interview.
34. Constantine, interview by Moore and Smith, August 1, 1903.
35. PL 29-223.
36. Michael Fogerty and Charles Brodt, interview by Moore and Smith, August 11, 2003.
37. The same was also true in the Family Assistance Plan.
38. Sheila R. Zedlewski and Jack A. Meyer, *Toward Ending Poverty Among the Elderly and Disabled Through SSI Reform.* Washington, D.C.: Urban Institute, 1989).
39. In other words, states could follow their own eligibility criteria so long as they weren't more restrictive than those the state had in effect on January 1, 1972.

40. Interview with Fogerty and Brodt, August 11, 2003.
41. The Finance Committee reasoned that if HMOs were indeed more economical, the states should not need a subsidy to use them. Stevens and Stevens, *Welfare Medicine in America,* 346n65.
42. *Ibid.,* n66.
43. Secs. 224, 232.
44. ICFs were required to have an independent professional review of placements and of care for Medicaid patients.
45. 60 days for hospitals, ICFs and nursing homes and 90 days for IMDs. The nursing home limits were never implemented. Constantine, telephone interview by Smith, October 18. 2004.
46. Experimental Medical Care Review Organizations (EMCROs) were sponsored in a number of areas across the U.S. and cited in the Senate Report as "prototype organizations ... [providing the Committee) convincing evidence that peer review can—and should be—implemented on an operational, rather than merely experimental basis." *Social Security Amendments of 1972,* 257-258.
47. Tax Equity and Fiscal Responsibility Act of 1982 (TEFRA), P.L. 97-248, Pt. III, Subtitle (C), now referred to as Quality Improvement Organizations, though specific titles vary by state.
48. already applied to skilled nursing homes.
49. The ECF was especially troublesome because of payment disallowances. *Social Security Amendments of 1972,* 58-59.
50. *Ibid.,* pp. 287-288; Vladeck, *Unloving Care,* 68.
51. The argument may seem weak, since the "comprehensive care" requirement wasn't being enforced and the state of the economy required cutbacks independently of the 1903(e) requirement. At the same time, states differed greatly in their tax efforts and how seriously they took this obligation, so that 1903(e) did tend to bear more heavily on the states making conscientious efforts.
52. It was 90% because a previous rate of 75% had failed to provide enough stimulus.
53. It was reconstituted to become a 19-member panel, appointed by and to meet at the call of the secretary (but not less than once a year) to advise on both Medicare and Medicaid.
54. One veteran state Medicaid director remarked on how hard they worked to avoid federal disallowances because of their impact upon credibility, morale, and program administration. Michael Fogarty, Interview by Moore and Smith, August 11, 2003.
55. *Roe v. Wade,* 410 U.S.113 (1973) held that a woman's Fourteenth Amendment right to "privacy" protected her freedom to choose an abortion. *Wyatt v. Stickney* and a companion case, *Partlow v. Stickney* 324 Fed. Supp. 781 (1971) dealt with both the mentally ill and mentally retarded in public institutions and held them entitled to appropriate treatment and least restrictive alternatives. The decision led to an administered decree that was not finally terminated until 2003.
56. When Newman arrived, the headquarters staff was sixty persons, thirty-five of whom were support, plus a small regional staff. Forty more were authorized to help implement the 1972 Amendments, though the net gain is hard to assess because of staff turnover during those troubled times. As for the forty-person increase, that was an authorization, not actual staff. As one former staff person put it, "You've got your forty positions. Now, go fill them!" Joseph Manes, interview by Smith, October 29, 2002.

57. Stevens and Stevens, *Welfare Medicine in America,* ch. 12; Howard Newman, interview by Moore and Smith, January 15, 2003; Joseph Manes, interview by Smith, October 29, 2000.

58. Stevens and Stevens, *Welfare Medicine in America,* 243, 239.

59. *Ibid.,* pp. 240, 254n8, n9.

60. David G. Smith, *Paying for Medicare—The Politics of Reform.* New York: Aldine deGruyter, 1992, 133-134.

61. *Special Analyses: Budget of the United States for FY 1974* (Washington, DC, GPO, 1973), 151. According to a former budget official, one reason for the emphasis upon fraud and abuse and implementation of the 1972 Amendments was that they knew so little, reliably, about aggregate spending for health care. He recalls using the state estimates minus 3% as a rough way to calculate aggregate expenditures. Lynn Etheredge, telephone interview by Smith, October 19, 2004.

62. Stated in this summary fashion, the administration's proposal seems slap-dash. That was not the case. It and the later Comprehensive Health Insurance Plan (CHIP) of the Ford Administration depended upon a precise articulation of different insurance plans, multiple simulations, and careful explication. Many Democrats as well as Republicans believe it may well have been the best chance for a workable and politically acceptable scheme of NHI the country ever had. On the proposals generally, see *Congressional Quarterly Almanac, 1971* pp. 541-554; and 1974, pp 386-393. See also, Peter D. Fox, "Options for National Health Insurance: An Overview," *Policy Analysis,* 3(1)1977, 1-24.

63. Joseph L. Falkson, *HMOs and the Politics of Health System Reform.* (Chicago, Ill., American Hospital Association, 1980, 25 ff.

64. *Ibid.,* 95. Much as an apothecary might treat poison, they were regarded as seldom curative and, in any event, to be dispensed in small doses. By then disturbing reports were coming in from California, Illinois, and elsewhere about bad experiences with "prepaid health plans." Constantine, telephone interview by Smith, October 10, 2004.

65. Falkson, *HMOs and the Politics of Health System Reform,* 94.

66. *Ibid.,* p. 93; also Lawrence D. Brown, *Politics of Health Care Organization: HMOs as Federal Policy.* Washington, D.C.: Brookings Institution, 1983, 222.

67. Falkson, *HMOs and the Politics of Health System Reform,* 57 ff.

68. Cf., "Medicare-Medicaid Health Maintenance Organizations (HMOs), CCR No. 5, Staff Report on HR 1, Senate Finance Committee, 92d Congress, 1st session, March 8, 1972; also Falkson, *HMOs and the Politics of Health System Reform,* 134 ff.; and Brown, *Politics of Health Care Organizations,* 278 ff.

69. Cf. Reichley, *Conservatives in an Age of Change,* Ch. 12; Richard P. Nathan, *The Plot That Failed: Nixon and the Administrative Presidency.* New York: John Wiley & Sons, 1975.

70. This passed as Title II of PL 94-505, an attachment to a bill transferring a parcel of federal land on a military reservation to the Shriners' Hospital for Crippled Children in Colorado.

71. PL 93-641, known as the "Roy-Rogers" bill because of its sponsors, Reps. William Roy (R., Kans.) and Paul Rogers (D., Fla.).

72. *Congressional Quarterly Almanac.* 1975, p. 635.

73. With a promise that no state would get less than it did in FY 1976. *Ibid.,* 1976, 11-A.

74. Projected program costs without new legislation. Over time, the CBO developed an enviable reputation for competence and impartiality. It has also helped on many occasions to moderate some of the "liars' contests" that develop over budgets

and deficits and change them into more measured discussions about believable numbers.

75. For instance, to elect their own chairpersons and control their staff, budget, and procedures.

76. William Fullerton, telephone interview by Moore and Smith, January 29, 2003.

77. He failed to anticipate the difficulties of melding his campaign supporters with the new appointees who would run the government. He failed to respect (and seemed largely unaware) of the courtesies and dispensations expected by the Congress. He inherited a faltering economy along with a number of domestic problems left unresolved by the previous administration. Also, he took on too much too early, including executive branch reorganization, urban and welfare reform, energy policy, hospital cost containment, taxation, and social security. By August, 1977 all of his major initiatives had stalled, with the exception of executive branch re-organization. Burton Kaufman, "Jimmy Carter" in *Encyclopedia of the American Presidency.* New York: Simon and Schuster, 1994, Vol. 1, 173-179.

78. Cf., Joseph A. Califano, Jr. *Governing America.* New York: Simon and Schuster, 1981, 104 ff.

79. *Congressional Quarterly Almanac,* 1975, 591.

80. HR 4976, Health Services Extension Act.

81. Existing federal matching levels would have been raised 25% up to totals of 95% for treatment and from 50% to 75% for outreach and follow-up. A bonus of 25% for administrative costs could be added for "reasonable" performance, with 20% reduction for states that failed to meet a minimum standard.

82. Childhood immunization was a Carter administration priority. In April 1977 a crash program was announced to immunize 90% of American children by 1979. *Congressional Quarterly Almanac* (1975), 495.

83. Which were quite considerable. See Foltz, *An Ounce of Prevention,* 65-75. It would be an understatement to say that federal officials were eager to get out of this business. The penalty was repealed by OBRA '81, Sec. 2181(a)(1).

84. *Ibid.,* 72-73.

85. *Child Health Assessment Act,* Hearings before the Subcommittee on Health and the Environment of the Committee on Interstate and Foreign Commerce, House of Representatives, Ninety-Fifth Congress, 1st Session, August 8, 9, 1977 (Washington, D.C.: GPO, 1977), 35.

86. *Congressional Quarterly Almanac,* 1979, 499.

87. The initials stayed the same but the name was changed to "Child Health *Assurance* Program" (italics added).

88. Constantine, interview by Moore and Smith, January 8, 2003.

89. One fear was that CHAP might put pressure on the poorer states to raise their Public Assistance eligibility levels; also that it might strongly encourage the general movement toward more government-supported health care. Constantine, *Ibid.*

90. The "Hyde Amendment" first passed in 1976, applied to appropriations. HR 4962 (the version that passed the House) was the first time anti-abortion legislation was applied to Medicaid legislation as such.

91. Hearings before the Subcommittee on Health of the Committee on Finance, U. S. Senate, 95th Congress, 1st Session, on S. l470, 1977.

92. For instance, *not* under either the Social and Rehabilitation Services or the Assistant Secretary for Health.

93. Constantine, interview by Berkowitz, August 24, 1995. *loc. cit.*

94. Califano, *Governing America,* 44-45.

95. *Ibid.,* 157-158.

96. *Ibid.,* 44.

97. Fullerton, telephone interview by Moore and Smith, March 26, 2003.

98. Leonard Schaeffer, interview by Berkowitz, August 17, 1994, CMS Oral History Series.

99. Richard Heim was a notable exception.

100. Nursing home abuses helped make the case for programs that would protect the aged, under both Medicare and Medicaid. The many investigative hearings by the Senate Special Committee on the Aging and the House Select Committee on Aging were at least as much for visibility and raising consciousness as they were for investigation.

101. Like the federal officials, state Medicaid authorities wanted to contain fraud and abuse. Reliable data were also needed for planning and budgeting as well as to make the case for agency policies with advocacy groups or state legislators. William Hickman, interview by Moore and Smith, March 26, 2003.

102. Not all of this process went smoothly. To get the enhanced match required approval of an Advance Planning Document by the SRS, after which the state would, in most cases, contract with a software consultant which might be Blue Cross/Blue Shield, H. Ross Perot's EDS, or any of a small group of less well-known competitors. Not surprisingly, the firms in this business tended to be entrepreneurial and unscrupulous and the state and federal agencies to be inexperienced and lacking firm-specific data. Under these circumstances, there was much activity directed toward rigging the bidding process, including industrial espionage, bribery, and intimidation, with a small number, led by EDS, emerging as victors. Eventually the states learned more about contracting and did more for themselves. But the episode was ironic, with a federal-state program dedicated to curbing fraud and other dishonest practices but giving rise to much of both. Cf. *Medicaid Management Information Systems (MMIS),* Hearings before the Permanent Sub-committee on Investigations of the Committee on Government Operations, U.S. Senate, 94th Congress, 2d Session, 1976 (Washington, D.C.: GPO, 1977). esp. 161 ff.

103. *Congressional Quarterly Almanac* (1976), pp. 563-564.

104. Frank E. Moss (D, Utah), Long-term Care Sub-committee of the Senate Special Committee on Aging.

105. "Medicare-Medicaid Administrative and Reimbursement Reform" (S 3205).

106. Conditioned upon a determination by the secretary that the PSRO was competent to review the particular activity.

107. (Sec. 1125). One staff member described the comptroller-general's state of mind as "subpoena envy."

108. Constantine, for instance, claims that they were never properly funded. Interview by Moore and Smith, January 8, 2003.

109. As an historical aside, Constantine said that they drew upon the Civil War False Claims Act of 1863, aimed at contractors who were selling the government sawdust as gunpowder. Ultimately, the "false claims" approach became a major tool in fighting fraud upon the government, but was not especially powerful until after the 1986 amendments (PL 99-562), which allowed triple damages, facilitated *qui tam* suits, and provided "whistle blower" protection.

110. Robert Baird, interview by Moore and Smith, November 19, 2003.

111. Richard Heim, telephone interview by Moore and Smith, January 15, 2003. Directors often preferred to deal informally with fraud and not acknowledge it publicly; also, a major anti-fraud campaign, for instance, against the nursing home industry, would rock many boats. Education could be a way of smoothing over problems, for good or ill.

112.   Richard Heim, who had been a Medicaid director in New Mexico (and later director of the Medicaid Bureau, 1978-79) made the point that they missed out on the most advantageous match because they had already developed their system. They also had a huge backlog of claims for which they got only a 50% match. Altogether, a poor state lost a lot of money because it had been proactive. Interview by Moore and Smith, January 15, 2003.

113.   SURS was the "Survey and Utilization Review System," especially important for creating profiles, tracking utilization, and flagging suspect behavior. Cf. *Medicaid Management Information Systems (MMIS)* 158, ff. esp. statement by Harold F. Weinberg.

114.   PL 96-449, Sec. 962(a); Fogarty and Brodt, interview by Moore and Smith.

115.   Cf. Gerard Anderson and William Scanlon, "Medicaid Payment Policy and the Boren Amendment," in Rowland, *et al.* (eds.) *Medicaid Financing Crisis,* 87-88.

116.   PL 97-35, Sec. 2173.

117.   Cf. Falkson, *HMOs and the Politics of Health System Reform,* 184-186; also, *Prepaid Health Plans* Hearings before the Permanent Subcommittee on Investigations of the Committee on Government Operations, U. S. Senate, 94th Congress, 1st Session, 1975.

118.   Brown, *Politics and Health Care Organizations,* 373-375.

119.   PL 95-559, Sec. 14.

120.   Cf. Chris Koyanagi and Howard H. Goldman, "The Quiet Success of the National Plan for the Chronically Mentally Ill," *Hospital and Community Psychiatry,* 42(9), 1991. 899-905.

121.   Ruth Knee, interview by Smith, March 3, 2003; as one program official put it, the mentally ill should have, at a minimum, "a job, a house, and a date on Saturday night." Frank Sullivan, interviewed by Smith, April 16, 2003.

122.   The decline in 1978 (of 720,000) was primarily the result of reduced AFDC enrollment. *Health Care Financing Review,* Vol. 4(2), 1983, p. 169.

123.   *Medicaid Source Book: Background Data and Analysis* (Washington, D.C.: Government Printing Office, 1993), 81. (The Yellow Book).

124.   Stephen M. Davidson, *Medicaid Decisions: A Systematic Analysis of the Cost Problem.* Cambridge, Mass.: Ballinger Publishing Co., 1961, 51.

125.   Thomas C. W. Joe, Judith Meltzer, and Peter Yu, "Arbitrary Access to Care: The Case for Reforming Medicaid," *Health Affairs,* Vol. 4 (1) 1985, 59-74, at 69. According to these authors, fiscal pressures led some states, especially the poorer ones, to hold down AFDC rates, thereby constraining Medicaid costs but also making the disparity between these two Medicaid populations even greater. *Ibid.,* 71.

126.   An important factor contributing to overutilization of nursing homes was the absence of Medicaid support for alternatives, such as home and community based services and institutional placements for the mentally ill. Another element was states' discretion with respect to income and asset requirements. The 133% limits of 1967 applied to the AFDC population, not the elderly. The federal government imposed a 300% limit in 1973 (P.L. 92-233, Sec. 13(a)(3)) the effect of which was to limit eligibility to 300% of an SSI rate for a "nursing home only" group. This provided an alternative to the "medically needy" spend down, but did not eliminate it. Some states use both. With special thanks to Andy Schneider.

127.   *Health Care Financing Review,* 4(2) 1983, 168. Also, testimony by Bruce Vladeck, "Medicare Community Care Act of 1980," Hearings, Subcommittee on Health and the Environment of the Committee on Interstate and Foreign Commerce, U.S.

Congress, House of Representatives, 96th Congress, second session, on HR 6194, 1980. 195-207.

128.   *Health Care Financing Review,* Vol. 3(3), 1982, 123-124.

129.   Thomas C. W. Joe *et al.,* "Arbitrary Access to Care: The Case for Reforming Medicaid," 68. In percentage of poor children covered in 1980, states varied from Massachusetts with a high of 72% to Wyoming, that was low with 20%. Texas covered 25% and Florida 34%. The average for rural mountain states was 32% and for the deep South also 32%.

5

Maturity and Trouble

The 1980s were a time of profound change in the Medicaid program—in structure, purpose, and modes of adaptation. By the end of the decade, the program had "matured," *i.e.,* looked more like and suffered from ailments akin to those of Medicaid today. Yet it was incomplete change, with more begun or intended than accomplished; much that came about in response to an external stimulus; and unintended consequences were many times more important than sought objectives.

Three factors especially important in accounting for the unplanned nature of this transformation were the partial—and soon abandoned—Reagan "revolution" in domestic policy; the domestic economy and fiscal policy; and the polycentric[1] nature of the Medicaid program.

The Omnibus Budget Reconciliation Act of 1981 (OBRA '81) was a coup for the incoming administration. With one bold and well executed maneuver, it got the president's domestic program off to a swift start and left the Democratic opposition shocked and awed. It was a defining episode: setting the major issues and largely establishing the modes of dispute and resolution in a number of domestic policy areas, including Medicare and Medicaid. Yet, like many coups, this one left important underlying institutions and habits relatively undisturbed, failed to rally much of its own putative support and helped provide the stimulus and the resources for a counter-mobilization.

This theme of a partial revolution followed by counter-mobilization is important in the development of Medicaid policy from 1981 onward. The administration's broad strategy for tax and budget reductions included entitlements along with discretionary programs, with entitlements divided into the big, "middle-class" ones—Social Security and Medicare—and the "welfare" entitlements—AFDC, food stamps, and Medicaid.[2] Deferring the particulars for now, OBRA '81, though a major victory for the Reagan administration, still included a major defeat—a deflecting of the

145

proposal to convert Medicaid from an entitlement into a block grant.[3] This did not elevate Medicaid to the status of a "third rail," but did gain for it a kind of wary deference, and a strengthening of the tendency to go to Medicare for budget savings.

Medicaid did not come through unscathed. The administration's "hard cap" of five percent on federal matching funds for Medicaid was defeated, with three years of percentage reductions adopted instead. With continuing inflation, the percentage cuts would have been trivial. But with deflation and a sharp recession, they were onerous. Medicaid growth was also constrained indirectly by lowering AFDC eligibility. In addition, OBRA '81 sharply reduced authorizations for health service grants and direct support for community health centers and mental health treatment centers. As a consequence of these combined factors, the OBRA cuts were harsher than anticipated and Medicaid growth, corrected for inflation, was flat or "zero" for three years, in a time of recession and great need.

An unintended consequence of this added hardship was to create opportunities for Medicaid expansion. Tight eligibility for AFDC tended to hit children, mothers, and preventive medicine. Cutting back on health grants and services in a time of recession put additional strains on "safety-net" providers and state institutional budgets. And recession increased the demand for federal aid, not a reduced match, so that states could cover shortfalls in their own revenues and help laid-off workers and their families.

In the scheme of OBRA '81, the budget cuts for Medicaid would be off-set, in part by increased flexibility in the form of "program" waivers that would allow states limited authority to restructure their own programs. Sec. 1915(b),[4] the so-called "freedom of choice" waiver, allowed states to make use of service delivery modifications such as primary care case management, provider service panels, and other managed care arrangements. States were also given increased authority to modify payments for institutional providers and, under Sec. 1915(c)[5]—the "home and community-based services" waiver—to cover services in non-institutional settings. In addition to more flexibility for the states, other prime objectives were to reduce the institutional bias of Medicaid programs and foster cost-conscious decisions on the part of Medicaid recipients.

The new waivers encouraged a number of experiments and minor program modifications but did not become major vehicles for inducing competition or restructuring Medicaid programs for more than a decade, in part because of their limited nature and the administration's own policies. They did mark an increasing shift from the 1970s' emphasis upon claims paying and cost reimbursement to the use of payments as a way to shape service delivery systems and adapt them to meet specific needs and manage services.[6]

OBRA '81 fell short of its objectives in some ways, especially in reaching the level of budget reductions mandated by the first budget resolution. There were also unintended consequences from what it did accomplish. As noted, the Medicaid reductions, combined with other factors, were harsher in their impact than anticipated so that attention soon turned from further reductions in Medicaid to providing for unmet needs among workers, children, the unemployed and the disabled. Also, passage of OBRA '81 and the Reagan tax cut[7] removed most of the impetus for the alliance of Republicans and "Boll Weevil" Democrats and, with that, the *de facto* Republican control of budget and tax policy. The election of 1982, one year later, again consolidated Democratic control of the House of Representatives.

House Democrats, buoyed by electoral gains, sought in 1983 to advance their domestic agenda with a number of initiatives, including health insurance for unemployed workers and a revived and expanded version of an earlier Child Health Assurance Program (CHAP). These initiatives failed for different reasons, but they opened new prospects for Medicaid modification and expansion.

With a severe recession and over ten million jobless, health insurance for the unemployed was a popular proposal and received bipartisan support in both the House and the Senate, though not from the Republican administration.[8] An alternative to CHAP, introduced by Sen. Robert Dole, would have extended Medicaid to unemployed workers in states with high jobless rates.[9] These initiatives failed at the time, but were revived in the later COBRA legislation.[10] They also raised the larger question of what role Medicaid should have in extending health insurance to workers who had lost their coverage because of temporary unemployment.

In 1983, legislative bills were introduced in both houses to broaden Medicaid coverage for poor women in a first pregnancy. The House bill was the more comprehensive, and included infants and children along with expectant mothers. These bills were important precedents in other ways. Coverage for pregnant women and children was a high visibility issue, supported by the Children's Defense Fund and a broad national coalition. They chose Medicaid as a vehicle for this initiative rather than a health services grant. And they preferred the reconciliation bill for that year, in part because bills relating to maternal and child health were targets for amendments hostile to family planning or abortions.

Child health legislation failed to pass in 1983 because—among other difficulties—the Congress defaulted on its reconciliation instructions and there was no reconciliation in 1983. However, there was in 1984 and CHAP passed as part of the "Medicare and Medicaid Budget Reconciliation Amendments of 1984," which were folded into the Deficit Reduction Act of 1984 (DEFRA).[11]

These amendments succeeded at a time when both deficit reduction and administration efforts to shift spending from domestic to military programs were strong, providing an early example of Medicaid's ability to swim against prevailing fiscal currents.[12] The CHAP legislation was notable also because it *mandated* extension of Medicaid eligibility beyond mothers with dependent children to include poor pregnant women (not yet mothers), pregnant women in two-parent families even though not receiving welfare, and children up to age 5, living in one- or two-parent families.[13]

CHAP was a small, initial demonstration of what could be accomplished with this technique of combining budget reconciliation and incremental amendment of Medicaid—an approach that proved enormously adaptive and productive for a number of years, extending into the next decade. It was easy to expand a category gradually: for instance, by permitting then mandating coverage for infants, children up to age five, to 18, and then 21. In like fashion, eligibility for the elderly and those with disabilities could be raised up to the federal poverty level,[14] services paid for by Medicaid increased or upgraded, and various mandates imposed with respect to particular populations, standards of care, monitoring for fraud and abuse, and so forth.[15]

With the Reagan administration and deficit reduction providing impetus, the reconciliation process a vehicle, and congressional Democrats most of the detailed content, the effect over a decade was to transform Medicaid, at least in broad outline, into much the program that we know today. Originally a program exclusively for the categorically eligible public assistance recipient, Medicaid became, in fact, a program for those living in poverty and for the uninsurable and families of the working poor and unemployed. From an earlier (and necessary) focus on claims processing and payment, Medicaid moved increasingly into oversight, quality assurance, and modification of service delivery. In addition to an increased waiver authority, the Medicaid program was enriched with incremental modifications that enabled legislators, administrators, and program directors to adapt creatively to meet the health care needs of the poor, disabled, and underserved. During this period, Medicaid came of age as a political institution, with a recognized, if not always honored, place in state programs and governors' awareness, along with a growing professionalism and collective consciousness among Medicaid officials, advocacy groups, and federal-state institutions. In various ways, Medicaid was becoming a program of national health insurance for the poor.

There were problems with this rapid, opportunistic, and politically tendentious method of growth. Medicaid, like crabgrass, was good for coverage, but it was spotty and at times worked to the detriment of other options—such as safety net hospitals and clinics.[16] Also, the federal match tended to be addictive and, some thought, took too much from state budgets, even though for worthy and tempting opportunities. With their growing size, Medicaid budgets invited political struggles over cost containment, the directions and shaping of Medicaid programs, and the roles and prerogatives of the state and federal governments.

One important effect of these initiatives was increasingly to national-ize the Medicaid program, whether by enforcing national standards or regulations or by expanding eligibility and coverage and leveling them upward by some nationally applicable amount. Regulatory provisions such as EPSDT[17] or nursing home standards were irksome in their com-plexity and seeming obliviousness to local practices or perspectives. Waiver requirements were also a sore point and often seemed to take away with one hand what another had given. And the Medicaid expansions of eligibility, even when optional and bringing new federal dollars, had strings attached and different priorities from those the states themselves would have chosen.

Whether one regarded these developments as good or bad, there is no question that they seemed calculated to transform Medicaid and make it much more of a national program. For a time, the governors and state Medicaid directors supported or acquiesced in these developments. In 1984, the addition of coverage for pregnant women and children was welcomed, even though a mandate and not optional. OBRA '86, which greatly expanded coverage for pregnant women, children, and the dis-abled, was also well received. But the grumbling started with OBRA '87 and began to assume crisis proportions by 1989.

As usually the case with Medicaid, this crisis began and then deep-ened because of a conjuncture of events. An underlying cause was the rapid growth of Medicaid expenditures, which averaged 16.9 % a year between 1987-91,[18] and were generally the fastest growing element in state budgets and the largest in some. In 1987, the Democrats regained control of the Senate, and with the health subcommittees in House and Senate working effectively in tandem, a series of budget reconciliations followed that steadily expanded Medicaid eligibility and added mandate upon mandate, covering the disabled in addition to pregnant women and children, providing transitional coverage for welfare recipients, strength-ening EPSDT, imposing nursing home standards, and adding many new options which soon became requirements.

An egregious episode was the passage of the Medicare Catastrophic Coverage Act in 1988 and its subsequent repeal by OBRA '89. The MCCA protected Medicare beneficiaries in various ways, but especially with a requirement that states pay for the premiums, deductibles, and co-pays of elderly and disabled Medicare beneficiaries poor enough to qualify for Medicaid—a provision that turned a Medicaid buy-in option into a new mandate. Then came OBRA '89, which repealed the MCCA, but left standing the Medicaid obligations, *without* the additional Medi-care coverage in MCCA—such as prescription drugs—that would have lightened the burden for state Medicaid programs. In effect, the states got no help, only an additional burden.

By 1989, most of the states and their governors were at elevated levels of alarm and outrage, over what they perceived as a lengthening train of abuses with a lack of redress. Even as OBRA '89 was making its way through Congress, the National Governors' Association—meeting in Chicago—was voicing its discontents and endorsing a near-unanimous resolution that called for a two-year moratorium on federal Medicaid mandates.[19] A stock complaint was that Medicaid was eating into funds for education and other state services. Other arguments were that Med-icaid, with its institutional bias, was a poor way to provide preventive health care; and that its coverage for the uninsured competed with and tended to crowd out employer based health insurance.[20] The governors appealed to the president and the Congress to find ways to meet the ris-ing costs of Medicaid and to provide coverage for the 37 million then uninsured in the United States.

Meanwhile, some of the states, in the American tradition of self-help, were devising ways of meeting their financial distress: especially developing additional sources of funds matchable as state expenditures, through provider donations and taxes, "disproportionate share" distributions, intergovernmental transfers, and so forth. Beginning as early as 1985, these practices grew apace and eventually exploded during the period 1990-92, especially in response to the recession.

Repeated efforts by the Congress and the administration curbed these practices but did not entirely eliminate them. The abuses and the scandals raised were bad enough at the time. They also had lasting consequences, in the poisoning of federal-state relations and the loss of trust in and support for the Medicaid program. But these disreputable episodes were symptomatic of a much more fundamental issue: of how to sustain, and what to do about, an increasingly expensive entitlement that had grown by responding to morally imperative health care needs but exceeded limits that many state governments and federal authorities are willing to support.

The historic fact that Medicaid was a weakly institutionalized system made it highly adaptable, especially to incremental change. The entitlement status was important—rather like precedent in the common law—to consolidate gains and provide a base for additional growth. Because of this capacity for adaptation and growth, the Medicaid program could be transformed in the 1980s, both by extension in eligibility and coverage and through an increased federal involvement in service delivery modification. The NGA protests of 1989 and the various DSH stratagems were indications that this transformation might be moving too far and too fast. They marked the beginning of serious tension and partisan difference over federal-state relations, the role of Medicaid, and of its entitlement status. These events also illustrated the difficulties of curbing or redirecting incremental growth—when it extends too far or develops undesirable tendencies—with a lack of agreed upon institutions or procedures for system reform or "restructuring" of the Medicaid system.[21]

The Reagan Administration, the Congress and OBRA '81

The first year of the Reagan administration was enormously influential in setting the domestic policy agenda and in shaping, often perversely and unintentionally, the way in which later initiatives developed. That is not to say that the administration succeeded in all that it attempted, especially not with the Medicaid program. As for Medicaid, the administration's failures were more important than its successes. A brief description of the political environment and some of the events during this first year helps to understand this paradox and its importance.

Republicans and many Democrats believed that the newly elected President Reagan had a mandate for moving domestic policy in a conservative direction. He had campaigned avowedly and enthusiastically on a platform of lower taxes, a smaller and less intrusive federal government, and a stronger defense. The national election of 1980 was generally seen as a mandate for change in these directions. Ronald Reagan won all but 49 electoral votes, and with an absolute popular majority, even though John Anderson, an independent, took seven percent of the vote. Republicans gained twelve Senate seats, retaking the Senate for the first time since 1952. They also displaced a number of leadership and high seniority Democrats with conservatives and southerners. In the House, they gained 35 seats to bring the count to 243-192. This left them 26 seats short of a majority, but enough for House Republicans to join with southern Democrats and create a working majority on occasion and for some issues. In addition, the election showed that the new president had strong and broad coattails, further strengthening the sense of mandate.

The Reagan administration picked up where the Nixon and Ford administrations had left off, but with important differences. One was that President Reagan had a mandate, a Republican Senate, and a robust possibility of support in the House. Another was that the Reagan domestic agenda was more ambitious and more partisan. In domestic policy, Richard Nixon had sought mainly to limit Great Society programs, counter Democratic initiatives with moderate counterproposals of his own, and reorganize and manage the executive branch more sensibly and efficiently. In contrast to this modest domestic agenda, President Reagan and his chief aides aimed to change the role of the federal government in the lives of Americans and the way in which they thought about this relationship. They were revolutionaries in the sense that they intended to undo much of the past, to alter the direction and activities of the federal government, and to make these changes stick.[22]

This administration meant to "make a difference" and it *was* different from any preceding administration in its self-conscious espousal of and adherence to an "ideology"[23] or set of fixed principles and the extent to which transitional activities and the initial organization of the executive branch were centered upon the "strategic implementation" of Reagan's announced agenda.[24]

An important consideration in organizing the administration was the personality and style of the new president. Unlike Richard Nixon, who valued expertise and took a lively interest in policy, Reagan was deeply committed to a few principles that he championed and defended with tenacity and skill, but he preferred to delegate the details of substance and implementation to others. As a practical matter, that meant he needed subordinates he could trust to implement and steadfastly defend the conservative revolution and its principles once they had been ratified.[25]

President Reagan and his leadership team largely bought into the "window of opportunity" view of the presidency expressed by Lyndon Johnson. According to this notion, an incoming president had about one year when Congress would "treat you right," after which they would increasingly go their own way.[26] Closely related to this view was Richard Nixon's concern about the innate opposition between the president and his inner circle of White House advisers and the departmental secretaries and agency heads—who would over time to "go native," *i.e.*, be captured by their own bureaucracies and interest group constituencies.[27] Two slogans that expressed these points of view and were much used by the incoming administration were "hit the ground running," and "seize and hold." Leaving aside the military overtones[28] of such language, these pithy phrases meant that the new administration should be well organized in advance, be agreed about the objectives, and understand and be committed to their individual assignments in reaching them.

One way the Reagan administration "hit the ground running" in domestic policy was to assign key roles to the confidants with whom Ronald Reagan had worked for may years, especially the "troika" of Edward Meese, James Baker, and Michael Deaver. These were people Reagan trusted and who shared his vision, not campaign workers to whom he was indebted.[29] Over a year's advance work went into planning the structure and staffing of the sprawling Executive Office of the President, aiming especially to avoid past mistakes, increase the role of the president in policy making, accommodate to Reagan's personal style of decision making, and strengthen relationships with potential supporters in Congress.[30] Another important strategy, which largely begins with the Reagan administration, was to treat the election mandate as though it were a plebiscite on Reagan's policies, and especially some of the more radical ones. As history proved, this was a good way to get the president's agenda moving; but it could also lead—especially for a governmental system with separation of powers and checks and balances—to an unhealthy suspension of disbelief in which Congress and/or the president would support policies without sufficiently examining them. In keeping with that thought, the new administration did not, as was customary, postpone serious consideration of the budget until the next annual cycle. In December 1980, President Reagan with his advisers decided that they would lay out the grand strategy for domestic policy at the beginning of the new administration. This agenda required a frantic rush to meet the February deadline for the budget message—less than two months away—but would strike while the iron was hot.[31]

"Seize and hold" was an injunction not to lose ground once gained either to agency heads, the permanent bureaucracy, congressional sub-committees, or any combination of the above. Quite a bit of planning and organization fell under the rubric of ensuring that Reagan's legislative or administrative priorities were not preempted, diverted, or prejudiced by departmental or bureaucratic obstinacy or by new initiatives "bub-bling up" from below. Some of the measures included identification of key posts and staffing them with political loyalists; closely monitoring new program initiatives to ensure conformity with Reagan policies; and blocking attempts by administrative officials, high or low, to lobby Congress—for instance, during hearings on sensitive topics.[32] For the most part, these techniques built upon similar approaches during the Nixon administration, but with the difference that the Reagan administration was much more systematic in their application and enforcement.

Another aspect of administrative monitoring, especially important for Medicare and Medicaid was the central role given to the Executive Office of Management and Budget (EOMB) in the oversight and guiding of administrative activities. Again, there were precedents under Nixon and Carter but the role of EOMB was enlarged in the Reagan administration because of the central position of David Stockman as EOMB director, the increased importance of substantive policy in budgetary considerations, and the growth of rulemaking and research and development (R&D) in federal policy. Under Stockman, the four program associate directors (PADs)—carefully selected political appointees—were given line authority to enforce Reagan priorities in the development and implementation of the budget. The EOMB was charged by Executive Order 12291 with review of new regulations to ensure that they did not conflict with administrative policy, were not unduly burdensome, and could pass a benefit-cost test. Another executive order, EO 12498, gave the EOMB authority to review agency initiatives—such as demonstrations and waivers—likely to commit the administration to new and possibly undesirable expenditures.[33] These arrangements were often described as adjuncts to "top down" budgeting, but they were also implements in the war of the

Reagan White House against the departments—in other words, "holding ground" by assuring that policy moved downward rather than bubbling up from below.[34]

The Omnibus Budget Reconciliation Act of 1981

OBRA '81[35] was the first great victory of the Reagan administration, as well as the moving cause of a number of subsequent developments that continue to shape policy today. Yet it was a partial success and some of its most significant results were unintended, even perverse. In that respect, the episode illustrates the importance of "hitting the ground running," but also the wisdom of Murphy's Law ("If anything can go wrong, it will."), and of having a good "Plan B," since there may be bigger obstacles than expected and more casualties and unanticipated consequences along the way.

The fundamentals of President Reagan's fiscal policy were (1) a large tax cut; (2) a major defense buildup; and (3) an anti-inflationary monetary policy and a balanced budget. According to David Stockman, this agenda "had been given *a priori*," that is, not as a proposal to debate but as an assignment to be achieved in its entirety and as fully as possible. Accomplishing the first two agenda items of a tax cut and a military buildup without inflation or a deficit would be a reach; and Stockman acknowledged later that the plan was "riddled with contradictions."[36] However that may be, these contradictions were not so apparent at the time, especially while scrambling frantically to meet the February 18th deadline for the president's budget message. A final plan was developed on time, but it left unresolved differences between supply-side theorists and monetarists, took favorable growth estimates, assumed unrealistic budget savings, and failed to plan for what might go wrong.[37] Stockman said later that he would never have gone forward with their original plan had he known in advance how large a deficit the plan would create and how deep the budget cuts would have to be in order to offset a deficit of that size.[38] All that may have been so, but the imperative of moving fast made early closure essential and precluded pauses for reflection and reality checks.

Use of the reconciliation process as a vehicle for the Reagan domestic agenda may seem obvious, though it was less so at the time. Prior to OBRA '80, reconciliation had not been used for major program changes and even in 1980, such changes were relatively trivial. Moreover, the full-blown process was ponderous, protracted, and lent itself to incrementalism and bipartisan log-rolling more than the decisive, top-down action that the incoming administration desired.[39] But David Stockman, who was leading the administration's effort, liked the budget reconciliation process because it minimized the leverage of interest groups and congressional sub-committees and concentrated the voting into a few plebiscitary up-or-down decisions. It could also, with some tinkering, move quickly.

Early in March 1981, Stockman and Pete Domenici, chairman of the Senate Budget Committee, agreed upon a basic strategy with three elements. Budget reductions were to come first, to help sell the tax cut and to improve the odds for delivering a no-deficit budget. A second part of the strategy was to lead with the Republican Senate and achieve an early and convincing win for the Reagan agenda. To further this aim, the budget process was radically compressed by issuing reconciliation instructions along with the first budget resolution thereby getting a decisive vote and a mandate to the authorizing committees to start cutting *all* the programs the administration had recommended for surgery.[40] This step would, in a strong sense, be a ratification of President Reagan's mandate by the Senate. The third part of the strategy was to consolidate Republican support in the House and seek to win over conservative Democrats, mostly southern ones, taking advantage of the Senate victory and the favorable political momentum.

This plan succeeded perhaps too well in the light of subsequent developments. With minor changes, the Senate accepted the president's plan and passed the first budget resolution with reconciliation instructions on April 2, 1981.[41] In the House, the Budget Committee initially reported a budget resolution of its own that expressed the Democratic consensus. This resolution largely ignored the president's budget, and would have gotten less than half the budget savings in the Senate version. It was quickly superseded when an alliance of Republicans and 63 conservative Democrats—dubbed "Boll Weevils"—won a floor vote and substituted their own version, known as "Gramm-Latta,"[42] which adopted the administration's budget figures and its own version of reconciliation instructions. This was later replaced by Gramm-Latta II, which was essentially the Senate version. But that is to get ahead of the story. Along the way the administration suffered two important defeats, both of which were significant for the future of Medicaid: one that would have established a cap on the annual increase in federal expenditures for Medicaid, and the other of which would have turned a large number of federal categorical health grants into block grants. Behind each of these, there was a history which helps explain their significance as well as why they were important victories.

A five percent cap on annual increases in federal funding for Medicaid was not a new idea. It surfaced repeatedly when savings in health care were discussed and had been seriously proposed in the Nixon administration. As for OBRA '81, it became an important issue in a curious, indirect way having to do with the general problem of entitlements. Especially with the Johnson administration and the Great Society, entitlement programs grew in number and program expenditure, so that by 1981 they amounted to roughly half of the federal budget. Since "entitlements" by then included not just Social Security, but also Medicare, Medicaid, veterans' benefits, food stamps, and AFDC, a great many people depended vitally upon them and they also cost a lot of money. The Reagan administration was proposing a big tax cut as well as an increased military budget which meant, almost inevitably, that Stockman and his Budget Working Group would have to reduce entitlements, since the sum of entitlements, the military budget, and interest on the national debt left only 15% of discretionary funding ($8 billion in 1980) from which to get $28 billion in 1981 savings. Either that, or increase the deficit.

Within the Reagan administration and among Republicans in Congress there were differences about whether to go after entitlements and, if so, which ones. Some, like David Stockman and Phil Gramm, were alert to the entitlement issue. In fact, the two of them had, as House colleagues, collaborated on a budget proposal that would have trimmed entitlements in various ways, including a percentage cap on Medicaid and reducing cost of living adjustments (COLAs) for federal retirees.[43] At the time, President Reagan was only dimly aware of entitlements as such and—much in point—was reluctant to take on Social Security or Medicare, especially early in his administration. Moreover, he was committed to protecting the "social safety-net," a rubric that was interpreted to include Social Security (but not SSI or SSDI), Unemployment Insurance, veterans' benefits, and Medicare. Sometimes referred to as "main street" or "middle-class" entitlements, these were distinguished from the "welfare" entitlements, which included Medicaid, food stamps,[44] and AFDC. The groupings were interesting and not just for their budgetary applications, since they sharpened once again the division between the poor and the middle-class and left the fair-minded to wonder how those who used such terminology conceived of a "safety-net," whom it was intended to serve, and how much commitment there was to it.[45]

According to David Stockman, he and his Budget Working Group first asked Richard Schweiker, the new secretary of the Department of Health and Human Services (DHHS), to come up with $2 billion in cuts from programs under his jurisdiction. When Schweiker demurred and sent along "185 pages of bureaucratize on why it couldn't be done," they turned especially toward the "welfare" entitlements. Medicaid was included in this group and received the same treatment meted out to the rest: across-the-board percentage cuts.[46]

This casual or even contemptuous treatment of Medicaid upset two important congressional members, Sen. Robert Dole (R., Kans.) and Rep. Henry Waxman (D., Cal.)—the first over dollars, and the latter mostly over entitlement status. Sen. Dole, although making a name for himself as a fiscal conservative, still cared about Medicaid and the poor. And with Medicaid expenditures growing at a rate of 15% a year[47] a 5% cap seemed too drastic. He pushed for and got an amendment to the Senate budget resolution raising the Medicaid cap to 9%, which was stretched farther by ratcheting the minimum Medicaid match down from 50% to 40%.[48] Henry Waxman was bothered most by the prospect of losing the entitlement status, since cuts in funding could be won back once the Republican tide receded, but losing the entitlement could be permanent, with incalculable losses for the program and its recipients.[49] Accordingly, he and his staff—especially Karen Nelson and Andreas Schneider—set out to get rid of the cap.

In this and subsequent legislative engagements, Rep. Henry Waxman had (and has) a number of assets. Before coming to the Congress in 1976, he served as chairman of the Health Committee in the California Assembly and acquired there a knowledge of health policy and skills in log-rolling and coalition building especially useful for health-related legislation. Among other accomplishments, he had co-authored the Waxman-Duffy Act, which brought much needed oversight and regulation to managed care and HMOs in California. He was rock-solid with his Los Angeles constituency and had run for and been elected—despite his lack of seniority—to the chairmanship of the Health and Environment Subcommittee of the Commerce Committee, [50] which had broad jurisdiction over health programs generally, as well as over Medicaid and Part B of Medicare. The subcommittee attracted members interested in health legislation, which helped to report out bills Waxman favored. He was also well known—especially among health policy advocates—for retaining one of the best staffs in the Congress. With a parent committee chairman (John Dingell) who shared his interests in health,[51] and the strategic jurisdiction of the Commerce Committee, he could often leverage his resources and find a vehicle and allies for some unlikely piece of health or Medicaid legislation. In addition, he was almost always part of a conference on health legislation, and his persistence and skills as a conference negotiator were legendary.[52]

Another important reason for the success of Henry Waxman and his staff was their ability to work with the given: the immediate context, the legislative process, the key actors, and the interests at stake.[53] For this particular issue of a Medicaid cap, the immediate context was, of course, the stunning coup executed by David Stockman, the House Republican minority, and the Democratic "Boll Weevils." Accordingly, a first step for the Committee was to carry out their reconciliation instructions. These were "mandatory" under the budget resolution, but achieving compliance depended on the good faith of the separate authorizing committees—controlled in the House by Democrats. Broadly, the Democratic strategy was to go along with the budget resolutions, but to do it in a way that protected their own priorities. Alert to this strategy, David Stockman got the top House Republicans and the administration to work toward a "Gramm-Latta II" tax bill that would defer, in some measure, to the House committees, but had in it, among other savings, nine entitlement "reforms," including a percentage cap on Medicaid, and turning a large number of categorical grant programs into a few block grants.

For Henry Waxman and his staff, the most disturbing part of the reconciliation instructions was the "hard" cap on Medicaid, which, in their view, wiped out the program's entitlement status.[54] Their response was to meet the mandated $1 billion savings, but to do it in a way that kept the entitlement status and, they hoped, did no permanent damage to the program. The formula they developed would reduce the federal payments by 3% in fiscal year (FY) 1982, 2% the next year, and 1% in the third year. These cuts could, in turn, be reduced by 1% each for (a) an unemployment rate 50% above the national average; (b) having in force a qualified hospital cost review program; and (c) fraud/abuse or third-party collections equal to 1% of the state's federal payments.[55] This formulation, when added to savings from the health care "block grant" proposal, would meet the reconciliation target of $1 billion, kept the Medicaid entitlement intact, and would go away after three years.

The proposal appeared to be headed for an easy passage with bipartisan support, especially because of Henry Waxman's assiduous efforts to enlist Edward Madigan, the ranking Republican, and other sympathetic Republicans on the subcommittee. As the vote neared, David Stockman intervened with a series of telephone calls to Madigan who reluctantly withdrew his support. Eventually, the Waxman version passed both the subcommittee and the full Commerce Committee; but it was clear that the entitlement issue was far from settled. Central to the Gramm-Latta II strategy was to pass a substitute to the Democratic reconciliation bill, incorporating the key entitlement amendments.

Democrats on the Commerce Committee had done some advance planning of their own and decided, early on, to write a reconciliation that included the health care provisions in a bill for the whole commit-tee. This step would not only assure broad support, but would create an aggregated bill with a "take it or leave it" protection for the components of the bill—in other words, a bundle of reconciliation agreements hard to do without if the whole reconciliation were to succeed.[56] Central for this venture was a natural gas bill under the jurisdiction of the Commerce Committee. With a deal brokered by Phil Gramm, then a Democrat, the southerners agreed to support the Commerce Committee proposal as a whole—illustrating the importance of the committee's broad jurisdiction as well as the strangeness of the bedfellows that politics makes.

This strategy of aggregation was important for the legislative outcome, since a good many people wanted the Commerce bill to succeed. Also, by this time a number of governors and "Gypsy Moth"[57] Republicans in the House were beginning to realize that a 5% cap—even a 7% or 7.5% cap then being offered by Stockman—could be a bad deal for them,[58] especially with the recent Medicaid rate of growth. As support for Gramm-Latta II weakened, the pressure grew to save it by separating it from the administration's Medicaid proposals. When this was done, the Commerce bill passed easily, with the irony that Rep. Phil Gramm was, unintentionally, a major factor in thwarting an important objective of his own bill.[59]

The Senate went to conference with their initial proposal of a 9% cap and a reduction of the minimum federal match from 50% to 40%. In conference, this formula was changed—largely through Sen. Dole's influence—in favor of 3% in the first year, 4% in the second, and 4.5% in the third. The reduction of the federal match was dropped; and the 9% was kept only as a first year ceiling above which a cost-sharing bonus would not apply.[60] The entitlement survived.

Block Grants

The block grant proposal was part of OBRA '81 because collectively, health grants, along with a number of other categorical grants-in-aid were targeted for steep cuts; but the block grant proposal was of greatest significance, not as a money-saver, but as an expression of views held by President Reagan and shared by many Republicans about federalism and the role of the federal government.[61] The same, of course, could be said of some Democrats, especially with respect to health policy. In other words, the amount of money at stake was not large, but the symbolic and practical consequences for health were important.

Some of the background for the block grant initiative was that federal grants to the states, localities, and private service agencies had grown enormously in number, variety, and programmatic impact, beginning with the Roosevelt New Deal and taking a great leap forward with Lyndon Johnson's Great Society. Initially, many of these grants were "block grants," that is, broad and supportive of state efforts without much in the way of mandated objectives, except to spend the money for "public health" or "maternal and child health." But the purpose of such grants was, usually, to get a state, locality, or service group to support program activities favored by the federal government, so that, over time, requirements were added and grants made narrowly categorical, earmarked with "set-asides," and directed to cities rather than the states or targeted for specific projects or populations. Also, the number of grants grew from 132 in 1960, costing about $7 billion, to over 500 in 1980, and costing, in the aggregate, more than $91 billion.[62] Meanwhile, the dependence of the states upon federal grant support had grown tremendously, since 1960 when one-tenth of state programs were supported or underwritten by federal grants to 1980, when one-fourth were.[63] States complained about excessive categorization that stymied their efforts and distorted priorities, about complexity and inefficiencies, and about being undermined by grants to the localities and private organizations. And they protested loudly and at length about intrusions by the federal government at the behest of "new social, moralistic, and single purpose" groups arriving in Washington and adding their claims to the existing hordes of interest and advocacy groups.[64]

A persistent theme in these complaints was that functions needed to be sorted out anew as between the federal and the state governments. This project had been addressed in the Eisenhower, Johnson, and Nixon administrations, but without much effect. In 1981, President Reagan had a mandate for change and assigned high priority to this issue.[65]

The administration's block grant proposal would have compacted 88 categorical grants into seven block grants: two each for health and education, and one each for social services, nutritional assistance, and energy and hardship. Other grants in community development and Indian Affairs would be partially consolidated and put on a list for future block-granting. Five year savings were expected to be $24 billion.[66] It was a comprehensive and drastic initiative and well-designed to meet the administration's objectives of governmental reduction and decentralization. At the same time, little advance thought had been given to how the reconciliation instructions would play in each of the separate authorizing committees.

As with other elements of the reconciliation bill, the plan was for the Senate to lead and, by its example, encourage the House to walk in paths of righteousness. In the Senate, the main burden fell upon the Labor and Human Resources Committee, traditionally liberal, but since the Republican turnover in 1981 now Republican, with Sen. Orrin Hatch as chairman. Sen. Hatch did not do well in that role, in part because he was inexperienced, but also because he confronted on his committee Sen. Edward Kennedy—whose favorite issue was health—and eight liberal Republicans, including Sen. Lowell Weicker (Ct.) and Robert Stafford (Vt.), each of whom had strong categorical interests that they were determined to protect.[67] Eventually, chairman Hatch got support for a much compromised pair of block grants regarded as only marginally better than nothing by the administration. Seeking to strengthen his conference delegation, he then bungled a scheme to block Stafford as a conferee, and found himself, after considerable delay, leading the conference delegation with a sorely disgruntled member from his own party and confronting Henry Waxman on the other side. Hatch then compounded his past errors by opening the meeting with a number of "non-negotiable" demands that moved no one. With that kind of approach and a weak and insecure chairman, Waxman simply let Hatch flounder about for awhile, with the humiliating result—for Hatch—that Howard Baker, the Senate majority leader, intervened and asked Stafford to draft a compromise bill while he and Pete Domenici began negotiating a deal with Henry Waxman.[68] All of which explains in part why Waxman had such a central role with respect to the block grants as well as the percentage Medicaid cap.

The administration's proposal collapsed 25 categorical health grant programs into two block grants: one for health services and the other for preventive health. Health services included mental health, maternal and child health, and alcohol and drug abuse along with community and migrant health clinics. The second block grant was traditional preventive health services such as hypertension screening, water fluoridation, rat control and prevention of lead-based paint poisoning. Also in this group were some highly controversial programs, such as childhood immunization, family planning, adolescent pregnancy prevention, and VD prevention and control. The target was to cut funding by 25%. In exchange, states would have much greater freedom to spend the money as they pleased.[69]

Henry Waxman was unhappy with the administration's block grant proposal on several accounts. He was especially concerned that—without federal categories of aid—larger and more popular programs would crowd out smaller but equally vital ones, such as mental health and family planning, that were notoriously weak politically, especially at state levels. Popular programs were lumped together with unpopular and contentious ones, which would tend to invite controversy over health service grants generally and provide a handy excuse for spending less money on health and more on highways, education, and prisons. Another important consideration for him, especially relevant to Medicaid, was the adverse effect that block granting and an overall 25% cut in funding would have on the health safety-net and on the development of service delivery options for Medicaid recipients at the local level.[70]

Faced with this unpleasant offering, Waxman made common cause with Edward Madigan, the ranking Republican on the subcommittee, and developed an alternative proposal with three block grants devised to make sense programmatically and win support politically. The prevention block grant was similar to the administration's proposal, but with some protections for hypertension and local emergency medical services, support for which was unpopular with organized medicine. A second block grant included the existing maternal and child health programs along with hemophilia and genetic research, lead-paint poisoning, sudden infant death syndrome (SIDS), and adolescent pregnancy prevention. The third block grant combined mental health and alcohol and drug abuse clinics and services. Added to the redesign was some earmarking, a three-year maintenance–of–effort requirement, and the barring of clinic closures for two years.[71]

The Waxman-Madigan proposal provided separately for continued federal support of community health centers, with an illustration of the kind of ploys sometimes used in such legislative games. This was also a block grant, with funding going directly to the states and matching funds required, but with a proviso that the CHCs would continue to be funded by the federal government if the states failed to put up matching funds. Only West Virginia chose this option, but did not qualify because it used other federal funds for a match.[72]

A number of grants, originally part of the administration's proposal, were simply left out and continued as categorical programs. These included migrant health centers, childhood immunization, adolescent VD prevention, and family planning. Family planning is worth special mention because of the continuing controversy over abortion and reproductive counseling and the impact of this issue upon Medicaid policy. Although not included in the health services block grant, the family planning grant was endangered. President Reagan wanted it terminated and congressional Republicans sought, at the least, to have it included in the health services block grant then leave the matter up to the states, where its future would have been uncertain. In that same year, Sen. Jeremiah Denton, a freshman Republican senator from Alabama, introduced the "Adolescent Family Life Act," intended to "promote chastity" as a way of preventing pregnancies among teen-agers. Since this bill originated in the Senate Labor and Human Resources Committee, Democrats looked to Sen. Edward Kennedy to deal with it, but his sister, Eunice Shriver, was a strong supporter of the chastity approach, so Kennedy negotiated with Denton rather than seeking to kill the measure. Ultimately it survived, largely because Henry Waxman agreed not to oppose the bill if Denton would, in return, support him on family planning.[73] Both bills passed; but it proved to be an expensive victory.

The defeat of the Medicaid cap and the administration's block grant proposal were important victories for the congressional Democrats in a year when they had few. After the Reagan administration lost on the Medicaid entitlement—and on Social Security as well—Medicaid was treated with a wary respect. The entitlement issue did not arise again until the last years of the Bush administration and, then, only as an incident to national health insurance proposals. The health care block grant compromise endured, without dismantling the existing framework or block-granting additional categories.

There was a bitter aftermath to these victories, brought about especially by the recession of 1981-82 and by other administration policies. As part of the original deal, the budget cuts were high: 3%, 4% and 4.5% for Medicaid and 25% for the block grants. Democrats in the House and Senate agreed to these figures at a time when the basic rate of inflation was about 10% a year. But Paul Volcker, chairman of the Federal Reserve Board, had little faith in the "supply side" economics of the White House and administered a strong dose of classic "monetary" policy—raising interest rates and restricting the money supply. The sharp recession that followed had the expected deflationary impact as well as lower federal and state taxes and an increasing deficit. State Medicaid programs were caught in a triple squeeze: declining state revenues, increasing numbers of unemployed and uninsured, and federal Medicaid program cuts now reckoned in deflated dollars. Because of welfare "reform," an additional 441,000 lost their health insurance; yet Medicaid enrollments remained basically the same.[74] And cuts in health service grants weakened and rent the safety net that Medicaid recipients and the uninsured often relied upon.[75]

Some of these results were not intended, but they had important effects on the future of Medicaid policy by creating sympathy for the recipients and a sense that the Reagan administration had gone too far; increasing the backlog of unmet need; and reducing the role of health grants which made Medicaid increasingly the program of first and last resort for poor people in need of health care.

Waivers: Managed Care and Home and Community-Based Services

Chapter 2 of Title XXI of OBRA '81, entitled "Increased Flexibility for the States," deals primarily with waivers, especially managed care (Sec. 1915(b)) and home and community-based services (Sec. 1915(c)). But it opens with Sec. 2171(a), which included a list of services that must continue to be covered and expands other services, especially for children and pregnant women. After several minor flexibility amendments, Sec. 2175 (Sec. 1915(b) in the Medicaid statute) takes up the "freedom of choice" waiver, so called because the Medicaid statute's freedom to choose any qualified and willing provider could, under appropriate circumstances, be "waived." That freedom, of course, might have little meaning in situations where providers were refusing to take Medicaid recipients. One purpose of managed care, in that respect, was to increase and assure access to care. Another idea was that these recipients would become more active in helping to contain costs. The terminology also suggests that the Medicaid recipient, in surrendering a valuable freedom, is owed benefits and protection in return, and not just a "voucher" to hunt for a willing provider.

The major provisions of Sec. 2175 allowed waivers under which states could:

1)   Set up a case management or specialty referral system that restricts the providers from whom a recipient can receive care [important for partial systems].

2)   Allow a locality to act as a central broker in assisting individuals to select among competing health plans [negotiate with plans; organize, regulate elections, enrollment].

3)   Share with recipients, through provision of additional services, cost savings from more effective medical care.

4)   Restrict providers to those who comply with payment, quality, and utilization standards set forth in an appropriate state plan.

This text seems disjointed, obscure in its references, and needlessly elaborate if what is intended is a waiver to encourage Medicaid MCOs. But it needs to be understood in relation to the underlying policy issues and the legislation as a whole. Initially, both the administration and the Senate, in keeping with the "flexibility" approach dispensed almost entirely with mandatory services or such requirements as statewideness and comparability. Medicaid was to become a block grant, so that waivers would seldom, if ever, be needed. Seen in this context, the 1915(b) and 1915(c) waivers were not so much devolution to the states as they were a way of retaining some control over programmatic changes. In fact, the mandated services[76] and the textually difficult Sec. 2171(a) was part of a successful effort by the House Commerce Subcommittee to add exceptions to existing mandates and protective legislation so that these waiver provisions could be limited and monitored.

Sec. 2175 is cautious about managed care with hints of the continuing struggle for the soul of Medicaid managed care and HMOs. At the time, health care liberals tended to see managed care as a way of increasing access and moving toward more coordinated and comprehensive health care, while conservatives, including a number within the Reagan administration, saw managed care, and especially HMOs, as ways to promote competition, privatize activities, and save money. The Commerce Committee report took note of these aims in saying that states would be expected to "document the cost-effectiveness" of their projects but also that waivers should be approved only if "access to care is maintained or improved ..." and invoked "coordinated and comprehensive care" as the justification for restricting "freedom of choice."[77] As for cost containment, there may have been a presumption that managed care would save money, but there was no budget neutral requirement initially specified[78] as there was for home and community based services waivers. Managed care waivers were supposed to be "cost-effective and efficient and not inconsistent with the purposes of this title" and the secretary was instructed in some cases to make a finding and directed to monitor plans and terminate them (after a formal hearing) if they were out of compliance. As another indication of wariness, managed care waivers had to be renewed after two years, which assured timely review.[79]

Home and Community-Based Services Waivers

The HCBS waiver (Sec. 2176; 1915(c)) was intended primarily to provide a community or home based alternative to nursing home care, which was expensive and often unsuitable. This legislation tracked closely an earlier initiative from Rep. Claude Pepper (D., Fla.) and the House Special Committee on Aging—first begun in 1977 to extend and liberalize the home health care benefit for Medicare and other community based services for the elderly. The Carter administration also supported community-based services: for instance, in the Comprehensive Older Americans' Act Amendments of 1978 and the Mental Health Systems Act of 1980. To some extent, Sec. 1915(c) followed a trend, though coming later in the course of this development.[80] It is of interest, in passing, that 1915(c) was primarily aimed at nursing homes although it proved to be of much more importance for the mentally retarded and developmentally disabled than for nursing homes.[81]

Neither the administration proposal nor the Senate report contained a similar provision since their approach was to increase flexibility without waivers—prohibiting abuse rather than a review *ex ante*. OBRA '81 had protections along with the waiver: requiring a "plan of care" and determination of need for the services included and assurances with respect to providers, health and welfare of the recipients, and fiscal accountability. Not included in the final legislation was a Commerce Committee proposal for a "comprehensive assessment" of anyone applying for Medicaid coverage in a SNF, ICF, or ICF/MR, a right to a fair hearing for any person aggrieved by their assessment, and some hortatory language about putting the recipient's health and welfare ahead of cost containment considerations.[82]

The framers of this waiver authority were aware that home and community based care might well cost more than institutional placement, especially if unpaid caregivers (such as spouses or children) were not available, so they added several cost containment features.[83] One was a "budget neutrality" provision—permissive as such requirements go—to the effect that "the average expenditure per capita" for such waivers should not exceed the expenditure the state "reasonably estimates" would be spent without the waiver.[84] Another restriction was a "determination" that "but for the provision of such services," the individual would require "the level of care" provided in a SNF, ICF, or ICF/MR, the cost of which could be reimbursed under the State Plan."[85] Readers are invited to parse this language for themselves, though let it be said that it occasioned considerable difficulty in application.

In recognition of the difficulty and complexity of organizing home and community based services, the Commerce Committee recommended, and Congress adopted, a three-year term for such waivers (in contrast to the two years for the 1915(b) managed care waivers). Some of the ambivalence about waivers is conveyed, though, by the special data requirements imposed upon the states for the HCBS waivers and the provision that "the Secretary" report to Congress not later than September 30, 1984 on the implementation and experience with the managed care waivers.[86]

Disproportionate Share (DSH) Allowances

Special allowances for hospitals, ICFs and SNFs were included under the "flexibility" amendments (Chapter II). As noted earlier (*supra,* 130), the background for the DSH allowances was the Boren Amendment of 1980, which established the "reasonably cost related" test for state rate-setting for SNFs and ICFs, with some murky language added to indicate the limits of state discretion. In 1981, at the insistence of Rep. Henry Waxman, the Boren Amendment was itself amended to add hospitals to its protection and to require that the reimbursement "take into account" those hospitals that serve a "disproportionate number of low-income people with special needs."

As written, this provision was remarkably broad and indeterminate, and was largely ignored by the states for a number of years.[87] The original formulation deserves brief comment. The provision was put in because of a concern that the combination of federal Medicaid cuts and state payment modifications might bear too heavily on hospitals serving Medicaid patients, the poor, the uninsured, and those with special needs.[88]

At the time, the term "health care safety-net" was not yet in vogue. But a major consideration in adding this particular provision was to protect large, often inner-city and public hospitals in urban centers such as Los Angeles, New York City, Chicago, Philadelphia, and the District of Columbia. Considerable thought was given to both the "disproportionate share" concept and to the language, which, it should be noted, included the poor and those with special needs and not just a disproportionate share of Medicaid patients.[89] In effect, then, Medicaid policy was moving to support the health care safety-net, though with practice leading theory.

Other Provisions

Title XXI of OBRA '81 ("Medicare/Medicaid and Maternal and Child Health") contained many more amendments, but only a few that were especially important for tracking future Medicaid policy developments.

A welcome change for the states was Sec. 2181 (a)(1) which repealed the EPSDT penalty of 1% of federal AFDC payments for failure to inform AFDC families about the program or provide the mandated screening, diagnosis, and treatment. The penalty had much aggrieved the states, was not systematically assessed or collected, and—as noted by the Commerce Committee Report—did not work. With the repeal came new hortatory language about informing Medicaid eligibles under age 21 of the screening and treatment services, and assuring that these would be available either directly or by referral.

OBRA '81 included a number of relatively minor provisions aimed at curbing inappropriate utilization, overcharging, and fraud and abuse.[90] Notable in this respect was the authorization of "civil monetary penalties" (CMPs) as a sanction—important because the existing criminal penalties were so cumbersome and punitive that they were not used. The thought was, of course, that CMPs might be both more acceptable and more useful. Accordingly, Sec. 2105(a) added to Title XXI of the Social Security Act a provision for a CMP of $2000 for each item or service improperly claimed as well as assessments of two times the value claimed. The secretary was directed to inform the state agencies involved with Title XXI of any final determinations and they were authorized to bar any person involved from future participation in the Medicaid program.

The repeal of the Mental Health Systems Act of 1980 could probably be described as an over-determined event. The original concept, developed under the Carter administration was therapeutically advanced and structurally ambitious.[91] It especially took account of the growing numbers of deinstitutionalized and homeless psychotics and the awareness that many of those with mental illnesses are chronic sufferers who will never get well, so that non-institutional care for them would require a battery of community-based services, active outreach, and effective coordination. Had the MHSA been implemented, it might have provided a template of general application, not only for those with a mental illness, but also for others with disabilities. As it was, community mental health centers survived, though drastically reduced in funding, and mental health was made part of Alcohol, Drug Abuse, and Mental Health, a public health type of grant, which distanced mental health as a therapeutic category from national leadership in the field and inevitably led to an increased reliance upon the Medicaid program both for funding and for structuring service delivery.

Pregnant Women and Children

Initiated in part as a response to OBRA '81, a campaign to expand Medicaid coverage for pregnant women and children not only recovered ground lost because of the 1981 legislation, but radically transformed the coverage of maternal and child health for Medicaid recipients. This change was equally as remarkable for the way in which it was achieved: by a strategy of sustained incrementalism that made use of deficit reduction politics and the budget reconciliation process and an alliance of east and west coast health care liberals and southern governors and advocacy groups. It was an outstanding example of turning lemons into lemonade—unfavorable circumstances to good account.

Under the Reagan administration and with the Senate controlled by Republicans, one favoring circumstance was that national health insurance was not even remotely being considered. This worked to the advantage of Medicaid policy, since attention could turn to Medicaid as such, rather than postponing Medicaid enhancements or reforms on the theory that Medicaid would be born again with national health insurance. With NHI "off the table," Medicaid became, to some extent, a surrogate—a way to broaden eligibility or improve benefits as well as, for some, to continue the struggle for NHI.[92]

OBRA '81 and policies of the Reagan administration helped the advocates for pregnant women and children in several ways. Both the Medicaid cap and the block grant proposal tended to disenchant and to mobilize a number of governors and state delegations within the Congress. A second such effort, in 1982, associated with New Federalism and devolution made the governors and the states even more aware of their stake in Medicaid. Also in 1982,[93] the recession and the percentage reductions in Medicaid matching funds and the block grants began to bite deeply, generating sympathy for the poor, the unemployed, and the uninsured as well as a sense that the administration had gone far enough, and perhaps a bit too far.[94] In a curious way, these episodes seemed to confirm the entitlement status of Medicaid, by making that status an issue, fighting over it, then passing legislative compromises that seemed, at least implicitly, to ratify the notion of entitlement.[95]

The state of the economy and unemployment became critical issues in 1982 and 1983. By 1983, 10.9% of the workforce was unemployed, a higher percentage than at any time since the Great Depression. One effect of the recession—which lasted from late in 1981 until the middle of 1983, was loss of health insurance by laid-off workers. As of December 1982, eleven million workers had lost their health insurance, a number that rose to 19 million when dependents were included.[96] Voters expressed some of their discontent about this and other matters in the November 1982 elections, with one consequence that both Democrats and Republicans sought ways to replace the temporary loss of health insurance. Ultimately, no legislation was passed, in part because congressional debates continued so long that the economy improved and the issue became moot.[97]

The episode was of special interest because it raised the question of what role Medicaid should have in such a situation and because of a House bill[98] and what its fate revealed about the political dynamics of such situations. One approach, proposed by Sen. Robert Dole, would have been to extend Medicaid to cover some of the unemployed. This option raised complex issues of federalism and existing eligibility requirements. It was also strongly opposed by organized labor because it reeked of poverty and welfare and might require unemployed workers to meet stringent income and assets tests. As an alternate approach, Henry Waxman advocated a new temporary entitlement—but this was generally opposed because it would be open-ended and likely to be self-perpetuating. Instead, the House bill provided for a temporary block grant, to be repealed after October 1, 1985. It would require states to maintain their existing level of effort for Medicaid and give preference to pregnant women and children under five years of age. As a way to help the neediest states, only a 20% state contribution was required. There were many specifics, but two other major provisions were of broad interest. One was a requirement that employers of 25 or more provide 90 days of open enrollment for laid-off spouses and family members of covered workers. The other was to authorize grants to the states for FY '84 through FY '86 to support providers of last resort.[99] These features give a sense for the politics of such arrangements. They also anticipated some elements of the later COBRA provisions for health insurance for laid-off workers and possible approaches to an often-discussed Medicaid counter-cyclical benefit or fiscal subsidy.

The recession of 1981-83 contributed to the future of Medicaid in an indirect and somewhat perverse way. For an item, economic hardship registered at the polls in the national election of 1982. The Republicans lost 26 seats in the House, ending any future prospect of forging another working majority with the support of Boll Weevil Democrats. They lost only one seat in the Senate, but came close to losing others. An important result of this electoral shift was that a number of Republicans in both the House and the Senate were more open to bipartisan collaboration on health and social issues than in the previous Congress.

Meanwhile, there were secular trends within Medicaid that needed attention and that were, to some extent, both strengthened and made more visible by the recession and by OBRA '81. From the beginning, Medicaid had suffered from an "institutional bias"—too many in institutions and too much spent on costly institutional care as compared with amounts spent for preventive and acute care. Over time, as the population aged and as more persons with disabilities were added, this imbalance grew sharply. Data from ASPE, for instance, indicated that between 1972 and 1982 the total expenditures for the aged, blind, and disabled grew from 62% to 70%, with the result that 30% of Medicaid recipients accounted for 70% of the total expenditures, while the AFDC-related population (acute care, women and children) which was 66% of the Medicaid population got only 26% of the program expenditures.[100] Nursing home residents alone (including ICF/MR), only 7% of the numerical total, were almost half of all Medicaid costs.[101] Moreover, the gap between the number living in poverty and those covered by Medicaid continued to grow along with differences among the states in eligibility criteria, coverage of the medically needy, and Medicaid expenditures.[102]

By 1982, many states had begun tightening eligibility criteria and cutting back on services. OBRA '81 made matters worse. Some states that historically had spent generously on health opened their Medicaid rolls and took advantage of the waiver provisions to add new services;

but overall, eligibility contracted sharply in 1982, in part because welfare reform had reduced AFDC eligibility by 441,000 families.[103] Medicaid spending (in constant dollars) was essentially flat for three years; many states added co-pays and reduced coverage and services; and disparities continued to grow. Hardest hit were the poorest states and the AFDC families.

By 1983, the political situation had changed considerably. With the election of 1982, Democrats were firmly in control of the House and Republicans in the Senate had become more moderate in their stance. Some states were rescinding earlier Medicaid cuts and once more expanding eligibility and coverage. Following OBRA '81, interest in the plight of poor mothers and children grew, with some southern governors even appealing for federal mandates, which they could use to bargain with their own legislatures.[104] With this opening window of opportunity, the Children's Defense Fund began a campaign for an updated version of the child health assurance program, concentrating on pregnant women and infant care and drawing attention particularly to the high level of infant mortality in the United States.[105]

The Washington-based Children's Defense Fund was one of the relatively new advocacy groups that did not stop with lobbying and coalition building within the Washington beltway but mounted broad-based and high visibility appeals to help build a national movement. The issue of infant mortality was chosen for its shock value as well as its broad appeal. It was shocking enough: The United States, which liked to describe itself as the richest nation on earth, at 11.2 deaths per 1000 births, was higher than Sweden, Japan, Denmark, Spain, and tied with England for eighth place.[106] After declining for years, infant mortality in the United States had leveled off and was, at the time, climbing again. No surprise: it was especially high in the South, in large cities, and among non-white, young, single mothers, the unemployed and uninsured.

Health care for pregnant women and infants had wide appeal. Professionals liked it. It appealed to pro-life groups as anti-abortion and to the economy-minded as a way to avoid complicated pregnancies and premature births. And it connected with a broadly based movement among southern governors and public spirited citizens wishing to do something about the regional scandal of high infant mortality and lack of pre-natal care among African-Americans in the South.[107]

Early in 1983, a second, more modest version of the Child Health Assurance Program was introduced by Henry Waxman and passed by the Commerce Committee.[108] In was strongly backed by the Children's Defense Fund and supported by advocacy groups such as the American Association of Pediatrics, the American Public Health Association, and the U.S. Catholic Conference. It took an incremental approach, seeking primarily to induce states that had not already done so to take advantage of some liberalizing interpretations of categorical eligibility for pregnant women and children that many, even a majority, of states were already following.[109] States that did so would get a 100% match (full reimbursement) for instituting a program of comprehensive maternal services.[110]

The bill itself was comparatively minor, but important as the beginning of a campaign. By way of advance preparations, Henry Waxman had already gotten an allotment of $200 million in the FY '84 budget resolution. Lloyd Bentsen, an ally on health issues in the Senate and the ranking Democrat on the Senate Finance Committee, had a similar bill to require state Medicaid programs to cover first-time pregnant women who could qualify for Medicaid after the birth of the child. To provide some cover for his bill, Waxman sought to attach it to the Medicare budget reconciliation proposal. But the amendment was blocked, and his bill died along with the reconciliation bill itself.[111] In 1983, Congress failed to complete the reconciliation process for the first time since the passage of the Budget and Impoundment Act of 1974.

CHAP was important in the development of a winning strategy. Waxman and his legislative aides believed strongly that everyone should have health insurance. As a practical matter, doing something about that during the Reagan administration meant that Medicaid, not originally intended for that purpose, would have to be adapted to provide health care for the poor—that is, go beyond narrow categorical eligibility. So they set about to expand and equalize Medicaid eligibility, beginning with pregnant women and children and building incrementally on established categories of eligibility, especially those where states were already pressing against existing limits. The budget resolution and reconciliation process was the chosen vehicle especially because—as a legislative vehicle—it was reliable, low profile, and allowed its users to influence the design of the programs being funded.[112] The reconciliation conference, which was vitally important for Medicaid, also played to Waxman's strengths as a coalition builder and negotiator.[113]

Basic to this incremental strategy was the idea of starting small with an eye to future expansions.[114] The first installment, in the Deficit Reduction Act of 1984 (DEFRA), fit this prescription well. Essentially, the House version replicated the CHAP provisions, including the 100% federal support. The Senate version, more incremental, required states to cover first-time pregnant women meeting AFDC income and resource requirements. The conference took some of both: adopting the four categories included in CHAP and the House bill and making these mandatory, but at the existing matching percentage. An important change, that is likely to escape notice, was making eligibility dependent upon income and resource standards as opposed to actually receiving assistance, which was a much smaller number of eligible persons.

The outcome seems minimal enough, though in 1984 the champions of Medicaid won a good bit more, especially in the category of bad things that did *not* happen. 1984 was a big deficit reduction year and one in which President Reagan hoped to shift resources away from domestic spending toward a military build-up. In the president's budget, both Medicare and Medicaid were targeted for hits, with mandatory co-pays for hospitals and physicians' services slated for Medicaid along with a permanent 3% reduction in the federal match as a follow-on to the OBRA '81 scheduled reductions, then in their last year. Title X, the family planning program, was also under renewed attack—as part of the continuing opposition to abortion, family counseling, and contraception—and could be used to hold hostage any legislation dealing with pregnant women and children. In short, CHAP could easily get waylaid.

The situation displayed to advantage the potential of the incremental approach when used with skill. On legislation like this, Henry Waxman would consult with the Democratic Budget Committee chairman, Leon Panetta, who tended to be generous toward health care for the poor. In this instance, he also sought David Stockman's assent, discussing with him his own initiative along with Stockman's desire to impose a temporary "freeze" on Medicare Part B physicians' fees, which fell under Commerce jurisdiction.[115] Even so, the bill was no "slam dunk" since it dealt with pregnancy and would be considered along with family planning, then under attack. Waxman arranged a trade: he supported Sen. Jeremiah Denton's (R., Ala.) pro-chastity approach to family planning in the House in return for the senator's agreement to oppose defunding of the family planning program in the Senate,[116] and was able to present his own bill as a compromise proposal since it was pro-life and would save money.

As for other matters, neither the House nor the Senate liked the administration's co-pay provision and it died quietly in the conference.[117]

The 3% permanent reduction was a more serious matter and the Senate accepted the reduction, but for three years rather than permanently. This was also dropped in the conference— according to Henry Waxman, after "intense" discussion and negotiation.

In 1984, President Reagan had asked the Congress to join with him in reducing the federal deficit by $100 billion through FY '87. In seeking that goal, DEFRA raised taxes but achieved three year spending cuts of only $13 billion, most of it from entitlements, with $7 billion from Medicare. Medicaid contributed savings of a mere $22 million (while adding $455 million to outlays).[118] This difference came in part from the Medicare Part B physician fee freeze and additional savings that could be realized as the Medicare PPS was implemented but also from the fiscal and political reality that Medicaid savings were hard to come by. In this respect, DEFRA was important for setting a precedent about apportionment of savings as between Medicare and Medicaid. In succeeding years, both Congress and the administration tended to look upon Medicare as a "piggy bank" and to come there because that was where the money was.[119]

In 1986, there were two omnibus reconciliations, the Consolidated Omnibus Budget Reconciliation of 1985 (COBRA) which started early in 1985 and passed in March, 1986 and the Sixth Omnibus Budget Reconciliation of 1986 (SOBRA), enacted in October, 1986. Both of these made important changes in the Medicaid program. Several related developments and non-events were also significant.

Aside from its sheer complexity, another reason that COBRA'85 did not pass in 1985 was the adoption of the Gramm-Rudman-Hollings Amendment.[120] This act, aimed at eliminating the deficit, provided for mandatory annual deficit reduction targets with a special "sequester" procedure of a percentage reduction when appropriations exceeded budget resolution targets by more than $110 billion. Several categories of expenditure were exempted, such as the national debt and Social Security. In 1985, Democrats were making an issue of the plight of the poor and unemployed and pressed successfully for additional exemptions, especially AFDC, food stamps, and Medicaid, though not Medicare.[121] Medicaid was exempted, though Gramm-Rudman tightened the budget process and made funds generally scarcer and negotiation for off-sets more difficult.

On the positive side were the relatively amicable relations with the Republican Senate on Medicaid issues, and especially with the Senate

Finance Committee. Aside from the fact that the Senate was not strongly partisan—even less so in the wake of the 1984 election—the Senate Finance Committee was largely bipartisan by tradition, and had eleven Republicans to nine Democrats, a non-partisan staff, and several Republicans who were prone to side with Democrats on health issues.[122] The chairman, Robert Dole, and the ranking Democrat, Lloyd Bentsen, were, respectively, the Senate majority and minority leaders. In addition, Pete Domenici (NM) and Bob Packwood (Ore.) on the Budget Committee were disposed to be helpful on health issues and, even prior to the 1986 Democratic takeover of the Senate, they and Sen. Bentsen could often discover a way to fund Medicaid programs when the House Ways and Means Committee was not disposed to do so.[123]

One provision that was tangential to Medicaid but important indirectly was the COBRA requirement that employers of 20 or more extend coverage to laid-off workers for up to 18 months and up to three years for workers' spouses and dependents who would otherwise lose their insurance because of the death, divorce, or the worker's becoming eligible for Medicare. Beneficiaries could be charged up to 102% of the group rate for insurance. Employers who failed to comply would face penalties that could include loss of the tax deduction for their contribution.[124] This COBRA provision was similar to earlier House and Senate proposals for dealing with loss of health insurance, but noteworthy especially because it built upon insurance provided by employers of 20 or more and ignored poverty as such.

Both COBRA '85 and OBRA '86 (SOBRA) extended eligibility for pregnant women and children. In 1984, DEFRA gave states an option of covering pregnant women in two-parent families who otherwise met welfare standards. COBRA now *required* states to cover them. SOBRA then broadened this by *allowing* states to offer Medicaid to pregnant women, infants up to age 1, and by incremental stages, children to age 5 in families below the federal poverty level (FPL) but not qualified for welfare. Eligibility was also extended beyond pregnant women and children to increase coverage for the elderly and disabled: COBRA *allowed* states to cover hospice care for terminally ill Medicaid recipients; and SOBRA *allowed* states that already covered pregnant women and children to extend Medicaid to elderly and disabled persons who were below the poverty level but above SSI limits.[125] Then, following Democratic victories in the election of 1986, much of the optional coverage for women and children and for the elderly and disabled was changed into federal mandates.

A highly visible, and sometimes resented, feature of this process was this characteristic "Waxman two-step": first offering the states an attractive option and then mandating it permanently and for all the states, rich or poor, willing or unwilling.[126] On the other hand, a major purpose of this legislation, aside from expanding eligibility, was to fill in the unseemly gaps and equalize eligibility across the states; and the two-step process would broaden the acceptance of improved practices—already adopted by many states—before mandating them.

In addition to expanding and equalizing eligibility, the strategy was also to ratchet it upward and to move the criterion for eligibility beyond "receiving assistance" to "otherwise qualified" for welfare or SSI, and then to the federal poverty level. The latter is particularly interesting because, unlike categorical eligibility or SSI, it acquired a statutory foundation primarily because it was national, considerably higher than SSI eligibility, and was a convenient benchmark.[127]

Not to be missed in this development is that it amounts to a partial though historic severing of the link between public assistance and Medicaid, as far as pregnant women and children are concerned. This separation received statutory sanction in SOBRA ('86) which allowed states to extend coverage to all pregnant women, infants up to age one and then by annual increments, up to age five with incomes below the federal poverty level but above AFDC income eligibility. It also contained the puzzling provision that states would not be allowed to reduce their AFDC payment levels as a means of extending Medicaid coverage (Sec. 9401).[128] Preceding these low-profile but important changes was some history involving southern ladies and southern governors who got together on regional health and welfare issues.

Although the southern push for child health developed in a number of different states and through the efforts of various groups and community leaders, an early impetus came from Gov. Richard Riley of South Carolina who was then chairman of he National Governors' Association and also a leader among Southern governors on health issues. He worked in his home state though an Advisory Committee on Human Resources and its staff director, Sarah Shuptrine. Seeking to extend Medicaid to the uninsured, especially children, they were stymied by an imposed budget cap and the formidable technicalities associated with Medicaid eligibility determination and enrollment. One way out this quandary, they perceived in 1982, was an unexplored pathway in the Medicaid statute itself, which linked welfare and Medicaid eligibility but did not in terms set any lower minimum for the state's contribution—which would allow them to cover pregnant women and children with very low public assistance payments, much below the going rates. Exploiting this loophole, they were able to double the AFDC eligibility level for Medicaid without increasing the state's cash payments. After this initial success, South Carolina went on to pass (in 1985) a Medical Indigents' Assistance Act which received a modicum of national recognition for the state as a Medicaid leader.[129]

The years following OBRA '81 were hard times for Medicaid recipients in the South with recession and percentage cuts in the FMAP adding their bite to traditionally penurious levels for welfare eligibility. One result of this adversity was to generate widespread regional interest among advocacy groups, community leaders, and elected officials in providing some help for the uninsured.

In this effort several other governors associated with Riley included Lamar Alexander (Tenn.), Bill Clinton (Ark.) and Mike Castle (Dela.), some especially active in the Southern Governors Association. They were particularly aggrieved by the 1981-84 caps on Medicaid and sought ways to work around them. Their primary interest was coverage for the uninsured, but they realized that raising public assistance eligibility levels would be a hard sell at best and might be impossible because of racial politics and anti-welfare sentiments. Their decided to go with children and use the issue of infant mortality as both widely attractive and less divisive.[130]

With consensus on this approach, the Southern Governors' Association and the Southern Legislative Conference formed a Southern Regional Task Force on Infant Mortality which had on its board a number of notable southern ladies, including Honey Alexander, Hillary Clinton, and Lynda Bird Johnson Robb. This body deliberated with governors' staffs over reports and options, and developed a report, "For the Children of Tomorrow." A final meeting over the adoption of the report was tense, with AFDC advocates fearful about a loss of political leverage and assistance money and governors concerned about race and the welfare issues.[131] Breaking the welfare link—a step negotiated behind the scenes—was the way to get around this impasse. The provision in SOBRA, allowing coverage based upon the FPL, came directly from that meeting.[132]

Also important in 1986 was the extension of this approach to include the elderly and disabled: first in COBRA with the addition of hospice care for terminally ill Medicaid patients and then, in SOBRA, permitting states that covered pregnant women and children to include the disabled and elderly with incomes above SSI but below the FPL.[133] Financially, this was not as large a step as it might seem, since all but a few who were qualified for SSI were automatically eligible for Medicaid;[134] but the disabled and their advocates were by this time becoming increasingly visible and politically influential and this measure helped to support the next steps in legislating for these categories.[135]

Along with this legislative strategy, as it matured, came increased involvement in the structure of service delivery, including micro-management of state Medicaid policies: as noted, by encouraging hospice and HCBS waivers for chronically ill institutionalized patients. Other forms of intervention in 1986 included directing states to formulate policies for organ transplants and requiring them to cover home care for some ventilator-dependent individuals. Going along with these efforts to modify service delivery were liberalizing provisions, such as extending renewals for HCBS waivers to five years instead of three and allowing states to provide eligible pregnant women with a broader range of services than those available to other Medicaid recipients. This mode of policy making lent itself to deep federal involvement with health care service delivery, and even impelled it.

The next year, 1987, brought additional changes in Medicaid as well as related developments that profoundly affected Medicaid policy. In this respect, 1987 can be seen as a maturing of policy and beginning a transition to a new phase. Most of the former category will be discussed more fully in the next section; but in the most general sense, they combined help for the elderly and disabled along with a quickening pace in the extension of benefits to pregnant women and children.

In a large sense, the elderly were in for attention because of the ill-fated Medicare Catastrophic Coverage Act (MCCA), that occupied much of the health policy agenda in 1987. In addition, OBRA '87 included a major overhaul of the Medicare/Medicaid nursing home regulations, upgrading facility, staffing, and training requirements. Non-institutional care for the elderly and disabled was also addressed. A new waiver specifically authorized home and community-based services for the elderly if institutional care would otherwise be required.[136] Other waivers—and especially the HCBS for the developmentally disabled—were simplified and liberalized in a number of ways.[137]

OBRA '87 further increased coverage for pregnant women and children, building in stepwise fashion upon existing law, but with new approaches. For pregnant women with infants up to one year of age, states were given the option of extending coverage up to 185% of the FPL. For children up to five years of age (born after Sept. 30, 1983) states were allowed to extend coverage immediately up to 100% of the FPL rather than phasing it, one year at a time. Coverage was mandated for all children under age six whose families met AFDC means and income tests, with coverage optional through age eight. Additional measures sought to improve access to medical services of pregnant women already covered.[138]

This gradual and relentless extension of Medicaid coverage continued in 1988 and 1989. In 1988, coverage of pregnant women and infants up to age one in families below 75% of the FPL was mandated by July 1, 1989, rising to 100% of the FPL for the following year. In 1989, mandatory coverage of children up to age six was raised to 133% of the FPL. These were also the years in which the Medicare Catastrophic Coverage Act was passed and repealed, with major consequences for Medicaid, of which more later. Two other important pieces of legislation of importance for Medicaid were welfare reform in 1988 and the legislative clarification and strengthening of EPSDT.

The welfare reform legislation, a huge statute with the disarming title of "Family Support Act of 1988" (PL 100-485) included provisions requiring states to extend child care and provide a year of transitional coverage for families who had received welfare for three of the preceding six months but had become ineligible because of increased earnings or expiration of earned income disregards.[139] The statute also required every state to operate AFDC-UP programs, which extended welfare benefits to two-parent families if the principal wage earner were unemployed. These changes, though relatively modest, were significant as additional attenuations of the public welfare-Medicaid linkage.

More important was the reformulation of EPSDT. First legislated as part of the Social Security Amendments of 1967 (*supra,* 77), EPSDT had a troubled history: plagued by uncertainty about its scope and intentions, lacking effective means of enforcement, and much resented by the states, especially when federal officials tried to enforce its requirements or collect penalties for non-compliance.[140] Especially troublesome was the "T"—getting treatment to follow diagnosis.

The EPSDT amendments, Sec. 6403 of OBRA '89, attacked these issues comprehensively and expansively,[141] defining terms, spelling out obligations, and coming down hard on anticipatory diagnosis and treatment of at risk children, including obstacles to their growth and development, not just existing pathologies or diseases. "Treatment" received itself a treatment that has become famous, or notorious, depending on the point of view. Sec. 6403(a) in particular mandated any medically necessary treatment for conditions identified through screening and/or diagnosis, even though such services were not covered in the Medicaid state plan.[142] In addition, states were required to report annually to the secretary on the populations served and the services provided; and the secretary was directed to establish participation goals for each state to help assure that by FY '95 initial and screening services would be in place for 80% of the eligible Medicaid population. A final and important point was that states not meeting this and other obligations would be out of compliance with the Medicaid program.

In the summer of 1989, even before the passage of OBRA '89 with its additional mandates, the National Governors' Association was calling for a two-year moratorium on new mandates, and urging that the Congress "work with them" on a bipartisan basis to resolve their differences. Protests by the NGA are not always to be regarded seriously, but the grounds for the complaints were portents of important change. The governors said, first, that even with the matching funds, Medicaid was taking too large a share of state budgets and impinging too heavily on other programs in a time of relative hardship and fiscal stringency. They also argued that Medicaid was not the best vehicle for expanding health care for pregnant women and children or the uninsured[143] and that Congress ought to step up and see what it could do about universal coverage or national health insurance.[144] Viewed in this light, the action of the governors was an indication that Medicaid expansion might be reaching a limit. Also, their stand helped to redirect attention to NHI as well as shift it from Medicaid.

Despite these signs of discontent, OBRA '90 continued to press onward with Medicaid expansion, adding the biggest increment yet: coverage for all children through age 18 in families below 100% of poverty. This process was to begin July 1, 1991 and continue over 12 years, ending in 2003. This and other mandates in OBRA '91 were expensive—they would cost the states more than $17 billion over the next five years— leading Governor Bill Clinton, for one, to complain that Congress was making mandates "the vehicle for achieving universal coverage using the states' credit cards as the financing mechanism."[145]

An important innovation was the Medicaid drug rebate, which required manufacturers to enter into drug rebate agreements with the secretary for drugs reimbursed by Medicaid. Federal matching funds would be denied for any drug expenditures not covered by such an agreement.[146] This new program was expected to save about $2 billion over the next five years. The drug rebate provision was accompanied by a requirement that the states establish drug review boards to review drugs prospectively for appropriateness and contraindications as well as retrospectively for inappropriate use or prescription practices.

A development of administrative significance was the establishment in HCFA of a Medicaid Bureau in 1990 headed by a Director. This move was prompted in part by the growth of Medicaid program responsibilities, largely as a result of the Waxman amendments. Especially important, though, was the view of Gail Wilensky, the new HCFA administrator, who was appointed in 1990. She believed strongly that Medicaid was primarily a state program, radically different from Medicare, and needed representation and structuring as a separate administrative entity.[147]

In 1990, Congress also passed the Budget Enforcement Act,[148] a comprehensive revision of the budget process aimed especially at more effective deficit reduction. One of its many provisions established a "pay-as-you-go" (PAYGO) procedure whereby entitlements such as Medicare and Medicaid would be required to provide offsetting reductions or revenues within the same category of "direct spending." This requirement, which could have affected Medicaid spending drastically, was said to have been passed as a restraint on Henry Waxman. Former aides denied this, though they said that the scramble for funds got worse after 1990—primarily because of the unhappiness of state people with federal mandates and general resistance to the increasing costs of the Medicaid program.[149]

Elderly and the Disabled

The elderly and the disabled as Medicaid recipients share some common characteristics that help to explain both their importance for Medicaid policy and the special challenges they present. Most significantly, they typically involve chronic illness and often institutional care. Therefore, they are expensive as compared with pregnant women and children.[150] Also, in many instances, they are "institutionalized," for example, in nursing homes or mental hospitals, and many or most would be better off and less costly if treated in some kind of community or ambulatory setting.[151] For the elderly and disabled, then, there is a special issue of service delivery or of design, along with eligibility and coverage. With

Medicaid, furthermore, service delivery can be an especially difficult because of such factors as the pre-existing "institutional bias" of Medicaid and because of federalism, including the politics and economics of state-federal relations as well as the time lags and deflection of purpose involved in implementation.

The Elderly and Nursing Home Reform

Nursing homes as an infant industry were nurtured by federal government programs such as public assistance with its vendor payments, the Hill-Burton Hospital Survey and Construction Act, and the Kerr-Mills medical assistance program. Early on, with the combination of pecuniary temptation and lack of regulation, nursing home reform emerged as a prominent national concern, publicized especially by a series of hearings begun in 1965 by Sen. Frank Moss (D., Utah), chairman of the newly created Subcommittee on Long Term Care,[152] and continuing over the next decade. Despite his efforts and those of distinguished public servants and dedicated advocacy groups, nursing home reform was a fitful process—often quickened by scandals or tragedies, but then slowed or halted by the entropy of interest group politics, the electoral cycle, or extraneous events that shifted attention elsewhere.

It took more than 20 years to develop and pass comprehensive nursing home reforms, in part because of this fitful and sometimes retrograde process. The Moss Amendments of 1966 (*supra,* 79-80) were incorporated into the Social Security Amendments of 1967, but then progressively weakened in the course of implementation.[153] In 1971, President Nixon responded to a growing clamor over nursing homes with an eight-point program that incorporated some of the best thinking of the time; but the president lost interest following the election of 1972 and its aftermath.[154] In the Carter administration, nursing homes were a principal reason for and focus of the fraud and abuse legislation of 1976. HCFA also published proposed regulations in July 1980 that were suspended as one of the first acts of the incoming Reagan administration, but later became the basis for the comprehensive legislation of 1987—and therein hangs quite a tale, as the saying goes.[155]

A major priority of the Reagan administration was regulatory relief, including getting rid of "midnight regulations" promulgated in the last weeks of the Carter administration. One day after President Reagan took office, the acting secretary of HHS, Donald Frederickson, suspended a patients' rights regulation issued two days earlier by Patricia Harris, the outgoing secretary.[156] As part of a larger plan, the Reagan administration immediately established a task force on regulatory relief with Vice President George H. W. Bush in charge, to develop policies and specific targets for deregulation. Among regulatory systems identified as overweening and largely or entirely dispensable were PSROs, health planning, and nursing home regulations. One of the first actions of the task force on nursing homes was to dispense with the patients' rights bill. The members decided, furthermore, that their review would be based not upon the existing Carter administration regulations but the previous ones, developed under the Nixon administration and in effect since 1974. They also raised the prospect of a selective privatization of the survey and certification process. After soliciting public comment, the task force largely closed the doors to any further participation by interested parties, although serial leaks of memos kept outsiders informed and strengthened their views that unconscionable steps were being planned.[157]

With the benefit of hindsight, it is astonishing that the Reagan administration, in its deregulation initiative, would have chosen—along with PSROs and health planning—to take on nursing home regulation, with all the passion and pathos that could arouse. But it did. Waxman staffers have said that they could scarcely believe this fat, slow pitch coming across the plate, but they intended to make the most of it. The issue quickly got national attention from advocacy groups all the way from the National Citizens' Coalition for Nursing Home Reform and the National Association of Social Workers to the American Federation of State, County and Municipal Employees and the United Auto Workers. Despite these warning signs,[158] the administration refused to back off, even as opposition built over the summer of 1982. In October, HHS published its own set of rules, which Congress promptly suspended for a year. As a compromise, Congress and the administration agreed upon a study by the Institute of Medicine.

The study,[159] which took almost three years to complete, helped the cause of nursing home reform immensely. It was thorough and authoritative. The twenty-person Committee on Nursing Home Regulation, which oversaw the study and signed off on the report was made up largely of people connected with academic medicine, health policy research, or not-for-profit health care and likely to favor a pro-regulation approach. Ultimately, it endorsed pretty much the views of nursing home reform advocates and helped create a groundswell of support for reform. In fact, it served as a platform from which the NCCNHR launched its national campaign in June 1985, with movie actor Kirk Douglas as the keynote speaker.[160]

The legislation, which passed as part of OBRA '87 three days before Christmas, followed closely the IOM recommendations and remains today largely intact as the most comprehensive nursing home reform ever passed. Among its leading provisions were:

- Elimination of the distinction between SNFs and ICFs as of October 1, 1990. Thereafter, all Medicare or Medicaid nursing homes must meet the same requirements for provision of services, rights of patients, staff, training, and administration.
- Quality assurance—with plans of care and periodic comprehensive assessments of residents' ability to perform activities of daily living; and required services including physician, nursing, special rehabilitation, pharmaceutical, dietetic, and dental services; and a program of activities to meet residents psychological and social needs.
- Residents' rights—to choose a personal physician; to be informed in advance about transfers; to be free from coercion or physical restraints; to privacy, communication, and to "reasonable accommodation" of individual needs and preferences; to complain without fear of reprisal; to a prompt resolution of grievances; and to a hearing on appeal of an involuntary transfer.
- Staffing and training:—minimum requirements for staff (1 RN 8 hours/day; 1 LPN 24 hours/day) and nurses aides must complete an approved training and competency evaluation program.
- Survey and certification—states are responsible for certifying compliance with service mandates, residents' rights, and administrative standards; unannounced surveys on an average of 1/year but not less often than every 15 months, by a multi-disciplinary team and based upon DHHS protocols. States to maintain adequate staffs and procedures for the survey and certification, but with a federal match of 90% in FY 1990, reduced to 75% after 1992.
- Enforcement and sanctions—provided for emergency takeover of facilities and for intermediate sanctions including denial of payments for new residents, civil monetary penalties for each day of non-compliance, and temporary takeover of management.

Ultimately, the new regulatory authority was even more prescriptive than the HCFA proposed regulations that had been superseded by the Reagan administration. One of the small paradoxes of this whole affair was that it was a regulatory review under the Carter administration that alerted anti-regulatory interests[161] and a regulatory review by Vice President Bush's Task Force on Regulatory Relief that initiated a huge and successful campaign for comprehensive reform. With this victory, there were reasons for ambivalence. The nursing home regulations were enormously prescriptive and have given rise to continuing controversy, evasions, and enforcement by means of costly and protracted lawsuits. At the time, industry representatives—including the more public-spirited NFP sector—urged that lack of adequate reimbursement, Medicaid cuts, and labor market shortages of nurses and other nursing home personnel were a large part of the problem—all of this raising an issue that surfaced later, of how much effort should be devoted to regulating an institution that, arguably, shouldn't continue to exist.

Mental Illness and Mental Retardation

One aspect of the Reagan-Bush era that is remarkable, especially in the light of Medicaid related activities in the 1970s and 1980s, is how little attention mental illness and mental retardation received in the 1980s. In part, this was because these concerns were largely dealt with by Medicaid under the categories of "disability" or "developmental disability." But it also owes much to an historic asymmetry: that for mental retardation there was the ICF/MR and no similar facility for mental illnesses. The way this difference played out provides a good example of how relatively insignificant initial decisions that seemed prudent at the time can compound into sizeable disasters when left unchanged.

The ICF/MR was established in a little noticed final paragraph of a 1971 bill authorizing a burial benefit for deceased Social Security beneficiaries. Though relatively minor, the ICF/MR was an instance in which a mustard seed flourished. At the time, state welfare directors, as well as national advocacy groups were struggling with problems created by the Social Security Act's exclusion of funding for "inmates of public institutions," and seeking money for institutional placements of the mentally ill and mentally retarded.[162] Lloyd Rader, the Oklahoma welfare director, had been a pioneer in services for the mentally retarded and had, over time, seen to the development of three large, public institutions for the mentally retarded that were in chronic need of funds. He believed, as a matter of policy, that Medicaid would be an appropriate source of funding.[163] Other states joined in and Rader—who was influential with congressional powerbrokers from Oklahoma, Arkansas, and Louisiana—had little trouble in getting his amendment passed.[164] At the time, he was insistent upon a program of active treatment and upon downsizing of the physical facilities. Later, funding was opened for private institutions as well.

The establishment of an institutional concept along with Medicaid eligibility coincided roughly with increased visibility for mental retardation and the developmentally disabled and national and local advocacy for deinstitutionalization, community based facilities, strong family involvement, and normalization and education to the extent feasible.[165] The ICF/MRs soon became the fastest growing form of institutional care, even threatening to become a form of re-institutionalization; but they could be structured as small residences in campus-like settings and helped supply a source of funding for the HCBS waivers,[166] so that a relatively satisfactory balance of institutional and non-institutional care could be achieved and even facilitated.

To a considerable extent, the elements of an adequate service delivery model were present at an early stage, and there for later legislation to build upon incrementally. The 1915(c) HCBS waiver authority was so heavily used for the mentally retarded and developmentally disabled that by 1989, two-thirds of all HCBS funds were targeted to this population. In 1984, Congress initiated a three-year program of grants to the states to coordinate services for the mentally retarded and severely handicapped.[167] Revised regulations for ICF/MR facilities in 1988 addressed not only physical facilities, staffing and required services and quality improvement, but put an increased emphasis upon active treatment and increased self-determination.[168] The Medicare Catastrophic Coverage Act of 1988 mandated coverage for "dual eligibles" and strengthened EPSDT, both of which were of enormous benefit to the mentally retarded and developmentally disabled. In 1990, a Medicaid option of community living arrangements for the mentally retarded was authorized. Also in 1990, the Americans with Disabilities Act passed (*infra,* 199), which was broadly important for persons with disabilities seeking to work and live in the community, outside institutional walls.

Mental Illness

Mental illness and Medicaid were quite a different story, largely because of two historic accidents. One of these was the "institutions for mental diseases exclusion," an odd relic that had its roots in the Social Security Amendments of 1950 (*supra,* 221n169). These amendments authorized reimbursement for vendor payments made by a state for medical services for welfare recipients. At the time, Congress excluded patients in mental institutions from receiving payments for old age assistance, not because of a prejudice against the mentally ill, but because mental hospitals, along with tuberculosis hospitals, had traditionally been the responsibility of the states and Congress thought they should remain so.[169] As a consequence, the states continued to pay full freight, with their own dollars, for patents in mental hospitals while they received Medicaid matching for nursing home patients—which led to wholesale transfers of elderly mental patients to nursing homes. Subsequent legislation corrected for this by allowing Medicaid coverage for the mentally ill over 65 years of age. Mental health services could also be covered in general hospitals, but room and board were not included. Then, in 1972, coverage in IMDs was extended to Medicaid eligibles under the age of 21. These steps, of course, left the large question of what happened to the mentally ill between the ages of 21 and 65 or to those under 21 who were mentally ill but not institutionalized. To compound this mess, IMDs were not defined, and it was not until the MCCA of 1988 that this was more or less clarified when Congress specified that the lower limit on an IMD was 16 beds. This opened the way for smaller, residential type institutions. But not until OBRA '90 did Congress extend coverage for mental health *services* to those under 21. In practice, all of this meant, for the decade of the 1980s, that chronic mental illness in a mental hospital was covered for those under 18 and over 65, while those between 21 and 65, if chronically and/or severely ill could receive long-term care from a nursing home or other institution not classified as an IMD; be admitted to a general hospital for diagnosis or an acute episode, but not for long-term care; and be covered for physicians' clinical services in small facilities or group homes, but not[170] for room and board; and not for services if the facility had more than 16 beds.

The IMD exclusion hampered Medicaid related developments in mental health directly by creating a wall of separation between state public institutions and Medicaid funding and indirectly by diverting policy efforts toward getting rid of the IMD exclusion rather than concentrating more on other possibilities for funding, including but not limited to Medicaid.[171] Another historic development was the Reagan administration's block grant initiative that put mental health together with alcohol and drug abuse and cut back drastically on health grants to the states. This was also a time when the initial community mental health movement was aging and declining in public support and the mental health constituency was divided over underlying concepts of therapy.

These developments affected mental health policy for the entire decade. One flaw in the original community mental health centers conception was that it oversold "deinstitutionalization," largely because of a failure to take adequate account of the chronic nature of severe mental illness and, therefore, of the need for community-based maintenance and supportive services, even including "reinstitutionalization" as needed. The IMD exclusion, by denying Medicaid funding, added a powerful incentive to deinstitutionalize, whether or not there were adequate community facilities, services, or case-management available. The block grant legislation drastically cut federal funds and repealed the one piece of legislation—the Mental Health Systems Act—specifically designed to address this general problem. Mental health advocacy groups spent much of their time and effort in trying to get rid of the IMD exclusion and improve supporting changes in housing, employment and education—all of which was good in itself, but did not exploit the potential of Medicaid or implement the next generation of service delivery capabilities.[172] The Reagan administration also cut back on federal money for community mental health centers and began purging disability rolls, concentrating especially on mentally ill persons alleged to be inappropriately certified as "disabled," which added yet another cohort to the "deinstitutionalized" mentally ill, many of them living with distraught relatives or spouses, wandering the streets, or being housed in temporary shelters, jails, or prisons.[173]

As for mental health policy during the 1980s, Medicaid was notable mostly for its absence. Expansion of Medicaid eligibility and the gradual adoption of the FPL rather than welfare eligibility or receipt of payments as a criterion helped the mentally ill, along with others. A few states secured waivers for programs aimed at preventive care, case management, and community support for deinstitutionalized patients.[174] Congress mandated additional money for DSH hospitals, some of which were IMDs.[175] The MCCA left behind a significant mandate of coverage for the dual eligibles; and revision of EPSDT gave mental health agencies a stimulus and some leverage to demand treatment; but aside from these instances, Medicaid was of little importance for mental health policy, even though of great help for the developmentally disabled and other categories of disability. Most of the action with respect to mental illness and the poor took place under different auspices: under the AD-AMHA block grant, laws to protect mentally ill patients in institutions from neglect and abuse, in "Baby Doe" legislation, re-authorization of the Older Americans' Act, and in small inserts or addenda to provisions dealing with employment, housing, or rights of the disabled under the Americans with Disabilities Act.

One small but significant development was the State Comprehensive Community Health Services Act of 1986,[176] which authorized $10 million in grants to the states to implement comprehensive plans for community-based care for individuals with chronic mental illness. This scheme tracked closely the theory and many provisions of the Mental Health Systems Act of 1980, though with a $10 million authorization—little more than "budget dust"—it seemed designed mostly to keep an idea alive than to implement it.[177]

Other Disabilities

Medicaid "disability" includes all ages from the very young through the elderly, a range of physical conditions and diseases, and both the working and non-working. As for numbers, the mentally retarded and the mentally ill were by far the largest categories, but "other disabilities" included such physical conditions and diseases as blindness, paraplegia, cystic fibrosis, cerebral palsy, muscular dystrophy, autism, spina bifida ,emphysema, and AIDS. Those afflicted with a recognized condition or disease that met the definition of "disability"[178] and survived the income and assets tests were, with some exceptions, eligible for Medicaid.[179] Broadly, people within these categories were helped in the 1980s, along with others, by eligibility extensions, by new optional services, and by waivered initiatives in the states. Also, Medicaid recipients benefited from the large amount of attention the whole issue of disability received during the decade, including a four-year campaign that culminated in the comprehensive Americans with Disabilities Act. For the most part, Medicaid policy with respect to these other categories—other than mental retardation and mental illness—moved along in the familiar categorically incremental fashion; but several of the most important developments came about in unexpected ways.

The Karie Beckett Waiver and Beyond

The development of the Katie Beckett waiver makes a good story, remarkable both as an example of a caring and persistent mother and as an illustration of how a "majority of one" can sometimes prevail with a program like Medicaid that—along with its eccentricities and irrational constraints—provides opportunities for creative manipulation.[180]

The heroine of this story is Julie Beckett, an Iowa housewife and school teacher, whose infant child Katie—born in March 1978—contracted viral encephalitis that left her paralyzed, often on life support, and subject to *grand mal* seizures. While visiting her daughter in a long-term care hospital, Julie Beckett was disturbed to note that she and her husband were the only parents there, and that one child next to Katie had been there for five years and another for thirteen years. In this and other sections she noted how children that got attention and stimulus would be up and about, even after major surgery, while Katie seemed depressed, would relapse, and go back on her ventilator. She and her husband resolved to get Katie out of the hospital and find a way to treat her at home.[181]

Paying for home treatment was another matter. There was no question that Katie was disabled. She had no income. Under Medicaid regulations in 1979, she could be treated at home, but all the countable resources of her parents would be "deemed" (attributed) to the child to pay the medical expenses. If she were in an institution for more than 30 days, though, none of the parent's income would be deemed to her. Simply put, she would be covered by Medicaid in the hospital, but not at home.

The Becketts nevertheless took Katie out of the hospital and started caring for her at home, working through the state Medicaid director, Donald Herman, and writing to their local congressman, Tom Tauke—and, for good measure, to Sen. Edward Kennedy as well. They soon discovered that they had become locally famous, mostly because of money raised on their behalf by the parish church. Rep. Tauke took the issue back to Washington where he got a sympathetic reception, but was told that it would take two to three years to do anything about Katie. HCFA said that nothing could be done without legislation. Tauke persisted. On an airplane with Vice President Bush, he pointed out how a solution might be part of the administration's anti-regulation campaign. Shortly thereafter, Carolyne Davis, the HCFA administrator, took up the matter more formally with the vice president who then walked her into the Oval Office. According to report, when told that this was a situation that needed fixing, the president said, "Well, Carolyne, that's your job." She put together a committee. Shortly thereafter, she used the Katie Beckett story in a news conference as an example of hidebound regulations. Seizing an opportunity, veteran reporter Daniel Shorr asked whether this meant that the government would be paying for home care. That was not in the script. But the next day, a swarm of reporters gathered at the hospital and the secretary called to release Katie from the hospital and to ask the Becketts whether their home could handle the amount of electric current that would be needed.[182]

The "Katie Beckett" waiver became Sec. 134 of Subtitle B of the Tax Equity and Fiscal Responsibility Act of 1982 (TEFRA),[183] and is sometimes referred to as the "TEFRA waiver."[184] Under this option, a child under 19 years of age meeting the Medicaid test of disability and eligible for Medicaid if institutionalized would be eligible for home care benefits so long as the estimated cost to Medicaid is no higher than it would be if the child were institutionalized.[185] The option went into effect on October 1, 1982, less than one month after TEFRA became law. Initially, these were "model waivers" with a limit of 50 on the number that could be granted. Iowa applied for several of them, but the response was slow, in part because neither the families nor the county intake workers knew anything about them.[186] On this, Julie Beckett and her advocacy and support group, Family Voices, worked with volunteers and with the state university at Ames to get out the word and help with the processing.[187] Despite their efforts, a 1985 study by the Congressional Research Service indicated that successful applications of this type had not been numerous, either for the Katie Beckett "model waiver" or the more generic 1915(c) HCBS waiver. Seventeen Katie Beckett and 95 HCBS waivers had been approved, but the latter mostly for case-management of the elderly disabled and the mentally retarded and developmentally disabled.[188]

Alcohol and Drug Abuse; HIV/AIDS

Alcohol and drug abuse and HIV/AIDS are dealt with together because they are both important health problems that for different reasons were not seen initially as core responsibilities for Medicaid but, with some important exceptions, illustrate the adaptability of the Medicaid program. More generally, both underline the importance of a broad residual coverage that can be deployed with low political visibility to meet some emerging and important needs.

Alcohol and Drug Abuse

Medicaid made no provision, as such, for the treatment of alcoholism, drug addiction, or substance abuse. None of these topics was even mentioned in the original statute or in Supplement D. The Social Security Amendments of 1972 did address the issue, but only to say that neither alcoholism nor drug addiction would qualify as *disabilities* without a medical diagnosis of that condition and active treatment in an appropriate unit.[189] This exclusion left undetermined what "medical conditions" could be covered. Alcoholism and drug addiction were classified as illnesses by the DSM, but coverage via that route was skimpy and often inappropriate.[190]

States explored whatever options might be open. Substance abuse qualified as a mental illness according to the DSM so that acute episodes or institutional care in facilities with less than 17 beds would seem to qualify. Mental health clinics generally were not covered, though in-patient residential care for drug abuse and alcoholism was sometimes available, but with a requirement of JCAHO accreditation that excluded most facilities. General hospitals with psychiatric units could be used for acute episodes and some drugs were available. An EPSDT "wrap-around" could be tapped, especially by psychologists, social workers, and other non-medical staff. A rehabilitation option was selectively available. But any of these depended very much on what a particular state offered by way of optional services[191]—which often did not include substance abuse.

As providers sought to take advantage of these various options, states would appeal for guidance to HCFA, where some case-law was gradually developed for substance abuse. In 1990, Sen. Daniel P. Moynihan (D., NY) sought clarification from Gail Wilensky, the new HCFA administra-tor, about what services were available to treat crack cocaine addiction.[192] She responded, minimally, that Medicaid eligibles were covered for inpatient hospital care and other mandatory Medicaid benefits, and that regulations expressly prohibited any "arbitrary" limiting or denials of services because of the "type" of illness or condition.[193] Three months later, guidelines were sent to the state Medicaid directors setting forth a number of Medicaid benefits that were available:

- Primary care, including physicians' services, clinics, and pharmaceu-ticals (*e.g.*, methadone).
- Inpatient hospital services for acute symptoms, detoxification, and drug-related medical complications.
- Rehabilitation services in hospitals, clinics, and inpatient facilities in psychiatric hospitals and nursing homes.
- Home and community based services under waivers.
- As part of EPSDT.
- Managed care "freedom of choice" waivers 1915(b).
- Case management including specialized day treatment.

The Senate Finance Committee codified the substance of these guide-lines in OBRA '90, adding the following new language to Sec. 1905(a) of the Medicaid statute: "No service (including counseling) shall be excluded from the definition of 'medical assistance' solely because it is provided as a treatment service for alcohol or drug dependency."

This evolution shows how pathways to coverage could be gradually opened but it tends to obscure the fact that there still remained huge treatment gaps, that availability of sources of treatment varied greatly from state to state and community to community, and that many such services simply were not available, because of a lack of facilities or health care professionals who would treat addicts or alcoholics. There were, of course, substance abuse block grant funds (which usually did not keep up with inflation) but no equivalent of the walk-in community mental health centers, little residential treatment, or supportive rehabilitation and social services.[194]

HIV/AIDS

The HIV/AIDS saga begins according to most accounts in June 1981, with a report in the *Morbidity and Mortality Weekly Report* of five cases of *pneumocystis carinii* pneumonia among homosexual men. Prior to this, there had been isolated reports of *Kaposi's sarcoma* in young, homosexual men in New York City, San Francisco, and Los Angeles. But the MMWR was read in public health circles and the article awakened wide interest. During 1981, there were additional reports of *Kaposi's sarcoma* in the medical literature. A CDC task force on AIDS was formed. And the NCI convened a meeting specifically on KS.[195] Almost a decade later, with the passage of the Ryan White Act, Congress responded with legislation that is generally acknowledged to be comprehensive and well designed, though past due and underfunded. Along the way, Medicaid—that comfort of the poor and the afflicted—had little to do with this tragic epidemic, at least until late in its development. Those who were close to the events differ in their views: some say that demagogic politics and hatred of homosexuals and drug addicts delayed action; others that, considering the difficulties, events moved about as quickly as could realistically have been expected. It is not our purpose to resolve that dispute, but rather to put some of these developments in perspective, along with the role played—or not played—by the Medicaid program and how this relates to the larger picture.

One important part of the context is to realize how little was known about this epidemic in its early stages. What to make of these odd variants of pneumonia and skin cancer? Were they related and, if so, were they indicators of an epidemic? How was it spread; and what was the pathogen? Whom did it affect and what was its course? From a historical perspective, it is well to recall that HIV/AIDS as a disease affecting human beings had never been identified as such and that it proved to be one of the most mysterious pathogens in medical history. Also, recent experience with the swine flu episode under the Carter and Reagan administrations showed the folly of proceeding without a sound biological foundation.[196]

Another impediment was the National Institutes of Health, which despite its disease-related titles, looked with disfavor upon disease-targeted research as opposed to more general, basic research. In this respect, Robert Gallo's decision to concentrate the work of his tumor cell laboratory on AIDS and then upon a retrovirus was bold and risky but an essential element of ultimate success. In May 1983, less than a year after AIDS was identified as a syndrome, two articles published in the *Journal of the American Medical Association* stated that a retrovirus was the likely AIDS pathogen. Shortly thereafter, the assistant secretary of health, Dr. Edward Brandt, made AIDS the top priority for the Public Health Service.[197] About the same time, Henry Waxman and Ted Weiss (D., NY) opened hearings in Congress on AIDS with the strong implication that a new phase had begun.[198] The point being that this phase of the AIDS response was probably pushed along as quickly as the nature of the problem and the constraints of orderly scientific progress would permit.[199]

Even though the virus had been identified with reasonable certainty, it was not obvious how best to proceed, especially with the enormous perplexities still remaining. In April 1984, for example, the HHS secretary, Margaret Heckler, predicted enthusiastically—some would say fatuously—that a blood test for HIV would be available within six months and a vaccine in two years. A test was available within a year; but we are still seeking a vaccine. Identifying the virus was only a beginning. What should be the next steps? And what should be the priorities as between aiming for an effective therapy and/or vaccine, caring for those already ill, public education and prevention, or aiding state, local, and volunteer efforts.[200]

No doubt, had we known more, we could have done better. But nothing approaching an effective therapy for HIV/AIDS was available during the first decade of the epidemic. As it was, lacking a grounded consensus about the nature and size of the task, developing a comprehensive strategy was especially difficult and the downside consequences of betting heavily on the wrong prospect could have been disastrous. Moreover, HIV/AIDS was not, like the polio epidemic, a disease that randomly stuck innocent children across the country. It was a loathsome affliction spread by marginal groups—primarily homosexuals or drug users—concentrated in a few large, urban areas, pursuing an unpopular lifestyle and, in the view of some, getting what they deserved. Even the development of preventive strategies aroused primal passions not unlike those common to the abortion controversy.[201] Under these circumstance, the kind of sub-optimizing strategy that developed seems, at least arguably, to have been prudent and perhaps right.

Since funds for PHS activities were highly categorized, one of the first needs in confronting the AIDS crisis was a source of discretionary funds that could be used to pursue targeted priorities. Even as the May 1983 JAMA articles were published, Henry Waxman began hearings on a Public Health Emergency Act,[202] which established a $40 million contingency fund for research into the cause, treatment, and prevention of public health emergencies. Edward Brandt, as assistant secretary for health, was in charge of the departmental efforts on AIDS research. Since he understood well the difference between an authorization and an appropriation, he developed his own strategy to free up some funds. A first step was to appoint an Executive Task Force on AIDS, one function of which was to decide which AIDS-related programs could be phased out and what new ones should be formed. These recommendations were sent in a memo to Secretary Heckler along with his request for supplemental funds. As a result of this ploy—and despite administration cuts in PHS funding—AIDS research for the first 3 1/2 years was funded solely through existing PHS authorizations.[203]

Getting from this stage of significant interest among a few key leaders to making HIV/AIDS a national priority was still a big reach. The epidemic—if that's what it was—was still localized, with significant visibility in a few metropolitan centers. Aside from a probable identification of the pathogen, even scientists knew little about HIV/AIDS. Popular knowledge and understanding bordered upon superstition.[204] And mass opinion was not broadly sympathetic, remaining until as late as 1987 in the phase of "denial, blame, and punishment," rather than one of understanding and help.[205]

Several developments changed this situation, among them an increased awareness of the horror of the disease and the plight of the affected and of its innocent victims. A second was the determination and skill of the gay advocacy and action groups and of a few key figures in the Congress and the administration.[206] The disclosure in 1984 that Rock Hudson, the film star, was being treated for AIDS was an important catalytic event. His death and the subsequent campaign, led by celebrities such as Elizabeth Taylor, gave national visibility to this issue and associated President Reagan with the cause—if not enthusiastically, at least with muted antipathy.[207]

Whatever the relative contribution of these factors either severally or together, 1985 marked a legislative thaw with an appropriation of $230 million for research and special projects related to AIDS, a significant amount in a year that spending freezes were imposed upon a number of DHHS programs. This increase was followed by an additional $200 million for AIDS research in 1986 and with almost a billion more for HHS and CDC in 1987 for activities related to AIDS.

Meanwhile, as funding continued to increase, some fissures opened within Congress and the administration as well as among the HIV/AIDS advocacy groups. Within the government, differences came to a head in 1987, largely over the issue of AIDS/HIV testing and anti-discrimination protections. On the one side were administration health officials, especially Brandt, Koop, and Mason, who framed the issue in terms of a public health threat and people in need of medical treatment, and members of Congress, such as Waxman and Weiss in the House and Kennedy and Weicker in the Senate who seconded the health argument and saw confidentiality and protection against job discrimination as both humane and good practice from a public health perspective. Within the administration, this view was strongly opposed by Secretary of Education William Bennett and by representatives of the religious right, most notably Gary Bauer, who opposed initiatives such as distributing prophylactics and needle exchanges as endorsements of immoral lifestyles. They also argued that HIV/AIDS testing should be mandatory for selected populations and that positive results should be disclosed to public health officials. President Reagan generally supported money for research but waffled on the testing issue and eventually opposed the majority bill in 1987. Within the Congress, the opposition was led by Rep. William Dannemeyer (R., Cal.) an influential and high-ranking member of the Health Subcommittee and by Sen. Jesse Helms (R., NC) one of the wiliest and most effective tacticians in the Senate.

In 1987, Congress increased appropriations but failed to pass legislation on AIDS testing or anti-discrimination measures, largely because of the successful maneuvering of Helms and Dannemeyer. Instead, the House and Senate voted, almost unanimously for a national AIDS Task Force.[208] In 1988, the Democratic majority divided the work and let the

House do the heavy lifting on the testing issue and the Senate deal with funding. Following this strategy, the House passed a bill strongly endorsing voluntary testing with guaranteed confidentiality which the Senate watered down to the extent of striking the confidentiality guarantee and requiring mandatory testing for federal prisoners. A factor in this divided outcome was President Reagan's failure to endorse the recommendation of his own commission[209] that had come out for voluntary testing and protection against discrimination. In any event, the outcome of the testing issue gives point to the concern of health officials that AIDS not become a battle over "values" and ideology and suggested further that additional efforts in this direction might prove costly and futile.

As is so often the case with Congress, the next step forward took a new turn, especially with the passage of the Americans with Disabilities Act of 1990.[210] Disabilities were a topic of broad concern that Congress had worked on for years and that had strong support from President Bush. Much of the initiative within Congress came from the Labor and Human Resources Committee, which had sole jurisdiction,[211] and where a bill had already passed in 1989. The ultimate legislation, which was an omnibus bill covering employment, public services, accommodations, transportation, and health services, was passed and signed into law in August 1990.

Primarily through the efforts of the Health Subcommittee the protections of the act were extended to persons "regarded as having a disability" which included individuals with disfigurements and—as understood by both Henry Waxman and William Dannemeyer—individuals with HIV/AIDS. Aggrieved parties were given the same remedies that had been made available under the Civil Rights Act of 1966.[212] By itself, the provision did not specifically deal with the issue of testing, but it did help remove the most significant objection to testing, which was the fear of job discrimination, including discharge.

Another source of distress, other than job discrimination, was the lack of insurance or access to health care and social services. Medicare was of no help to non-poor people under 65 years of age unless they could qualify under SSDI, which took two years and five months: a five-month waiting period to qualify for SSDI benefits and then two years of receiving the benefits.[213] Moreover, Medicare benefits were primarily oriented toward acute care, lacking the nursing, housekeeping, and care coordination needed by AIDS victims—although that might not matter since they would probably be dead before they qualified. As for Medicaid, single males or females would have to qualify as "disabled," which would typically be only with full-blown AIDS. In addition, many AIDS victims were not poor and not yet attuned to the idea of "spending down" and then seeking whatever Medicaid providers or services that might be available to them. Beyond that, there were huge problems of access: getting experimental drugs or finding a doctor, a dentist, or a hospice or health care facility that would accept AIDS sufferers in various stages of dying. Under these circumstances, many in the gay community devised ways to take care of themselves with collection depots, "buddy" systems, and makeshift hospices. They also lobbied and demonstrated, sometimes quite imaginatively, for instance organizing huge, peaceful demonstrations commemorating dead friends and teaching themselves the necessary science and health policy to lobby effectively before state legislatures and congressional committees.[214]

With respect to treatment or care, a comprehensive response to HIV/ AIDS evolved slowly and, initially, in a fragmented and incremental way, involving Medicaid, health care grants, and state, local, and private initiatives. The Ryan White Act of 1990 is generally regarded as the important breakthrough, though there were important steps along the way that illustrate the dimensions and complexities of mounting an attack on this perverse and terrible disease. In February 1985, the Social Security Administration issued an interim regulation that allowed a professionally qualified diagnosis of AIDS or ARC to establish "presumptive disability" for SSDI/SSI. This was a step in the right direction, but less helpful that it might seem because the Social Security Administration followed the restrictive CDC definition which recognized only full-blown AIDS and severe related conditions.[215] The next year, OBRA '86 authorized the DHHS secretary to grant HCBS waivers for Medicaid recipients who were AIDS/ARC[216] or chronically mentally ill and who would otherwise have to be hospitalized—although, as yet, relatively few AIDS victims could qualify for Medicaid.[217] In 1987, a supplemental appropriation act authorized $30 million in grants to the states to help pay for the experimental drug AZT—although this particular drug was eventually to prove ineffective as a therapeutic agent.[218] Then, in 1988, Congress authorized a major program of research, grants for home and community based services, for demonstration projects, for training professionals, and for a national hotline and information and education network. This legislation helped build the infrastructure for the comprehensive approach then developing, but—important to note—before successful drugs had been developed.

The Ryan White Act of 1990 is important and interesting in a number or ways. The full title is "The Ryan White Comprehensive AIDS Resource Act of 1990", usually shortened to the "Ryan White CARE Act.[219] Ryan White was a high school student who was barred from attending school and died of AIDS contracted from a blood transfusion. The "Ryan White" was added to the title late in the legislative process at the instance of Sen. Orrin Hatch who wished to call attention to victims of HIV/AIDS who were neither homosexuals nor drug users.[220]

The Ryan White Act resembled the earlier Mental Health Systems Act in several ways. It was comprehensive; it sought to deal primarily with a single, particularly troublesome disease (and related co-morbidities); and it attempted to provide a template for, or relate and coordinate, the efforts of public and private entities and state, local, and community organizations. It built upon antecedent experience: that of local communities in administering AZT grants; demonstrations funded by HRSA and the Robert Wood Johnson Foundation; and studies of big city social organizations, the "buddy" systems, clinics, and private clubs. Hearings on comprehensive legislation began in 1988 and a bill containing many of the features of the eventual Ryan White Act cleared the House but was blocked that year by Jesse Helms in the Senate. Some of the delay was useful: Sen. Kennedy, with members of his staff, visited community programs, local physicians, hospitals, and medical schools to learn about local experience.[221] Also, more was learned between 1988 and 1990 about the progression of the disease from HIV to full-blown AIDS and about new drugs and their effectiveness.[222]

The statute is complex, but its philosophy and main objectives can be briefly summarized. It stressed support for, and making use of, the local infrastructure of care-giving agencies; project grants with a strong emphasis upon consortia; comprehensiveness and continuity of care; and community based organization along with targeting, set-asides, and planning. Other distinctive features were emergency funds with early deadlines for distribution, the use of "in kind" matching, and a special fund for hospitals with high (20%) case-loads of HIV/AIDS patients. This approach, reminiscent of the "War on Poverty," was balanced with a strong state involvement. Half of the emergency funds went to metropolitan areas to be distributed by public health authorities and HIV health services planning councils; the other half, via the HHS secretary, to the states with many of the usual procedures and safeguards associated with formula grants, such as set-asides, required services, and assurances of compliance.

Title III, the special contribution of the House, put great emphasis upon early intervention and treatment with an array of formula grants earmarked 35% for testing, consultation, and referral and another 35% for diagnosis and treatment. It stressed outreach, assistance in establishing eligibility, and case management to coordinate services. As for reporting, the House sought to limit requirements to statistical information, but the final compromise left additional disclosure requirements up to the states.

Compared to the Ryan White Act, the Medicaid response to HIV/AIDS was modest: authorizing waivers and supporting grants for HCBS. One of the most important reasons was, simply, eligibility: Medicaid wasn't set up to take care of young, childless, middle-class males, and adjustments such as "presumptive eligibility" were limited in their effect by such obstacles as restrictive definitions of AIDS and "medical necessity," waiting periods and spend down requirements, and the hassle of multiple applications and periodic renewals. For these reasons many AIDS victims viewed Medicaid as irrelevant, and relied on safety-net institutions and their own resources.[223]

As the AIDS epidemic matured, with more impoverished and disabled, and with AIDS and related diseases spreading to the poor, addicted, and women and children, many more qualified, so that eventually, 40% to 50%, according to various estimates, were eligible for Medicaid at some stage.[224] States also made good use of the Medicaid waiver authority to target coverage, move patients from expensive hospital care to community-based services, and to manage care. Seen as an exercise in federalism, the AIDS effort is an interesting case study in melding approaches; but it also illustrates the terrible price sometimes paid because of Medicaid categorical eligibility.

The Medicare Catastrophic Coverage Act

The Medicare Catastrophic Coverage Act of 1988 was another of those instances in which legislation about national health insurance or Medicare had large, unintended, and detrimental consequences for Medicaid. In brief outline, the original MCCA protected Medicare beneficiaries against catastrophic medical expenses in part by providing that Medicaid would pay for Medicare premiums, deductibles, and co-pays for Medicare beneficiaries below the FPL.[225] This additional burden on Medicaid would be partly offset by a Medicare pharmaceutical benefit paid for by a Medicare Part B premium increase. Largely because of the premium increase—which was progressive and upset middle- and upper-class Medicare beneficiaries—most of the MCCA was repealed in 1989, before it could go into effect, leaving in force the mandated supplement for poor Medicare beneficiaries, without the pharmaceutical benefit as an offset. Unlike the Cheshire cat in *Alice in Wonderland*, this disappearing act did not leave a smile, but a continuing burden that has grown over time.

In an obvious sense, the MCCA—as the title indicates, was an effort to remedy the lack of such coverage under the original Medicare Act: coverage for lengthy hospital stays or home health care, for the absence of a pharmaceutical benefit, and for the cumulative burden of co-pays and deductibles which could be catastrophic for beneficiaries of limited means and with lengthy and severe diseases. By itself, this lack of catastrophic coverage was a problem that grew more severe as health care expenses steadily outstripped other costs of living, but it was made worse by the health care cost containment measures of the Reagan administration. With national health insurance off the table, impulses toward health care reform turned toward amending Medicare and Medicaid by incremental extensions of health insurance or improvements in benefits. With Democrats in control of the House after the 1982 elections, health initiatives began to sprout, along with a Senate proposal for Medicare catastrophic coverage.[226] Few of these initiatives went forward, largely because of the Reagan administration's firm commitment to health care cost containment, the Republican Senate, and David Stockman's strategic role as OMB director. One exception was Rep. Henry Waxman's extensions of coverage to pregnant women and children. Another was a catastrophic initiative for Medicare that began within the administration, largely because of Otis Bowen and circumstances surrounding his appointment as secretary of DHHS in 1985.

The circumstances were that Margaret Heckler had become an embarrassment as secretary of health and human services and the Reagan administration saw in Otis Bowen—a family physician, state legislator, and popular two-time governor of Indiana—a distinct plus and a way of recouping some political losses. For his part, Dr. Bowen was not eager to leave his comfortable retirement, but could be persuaded if promised political support for a catastrophic coverage bill that would be, for him, a memorial to his first wife who had died after a long, painful, and expensive struggle with cancer.[227] He consented to come, but only after President Reagan agreed to include a plug for catastrophic care in his State of the Union address in February 1986.

Secretary Bowen's proposal was comparatively modest, aiming only to eliminate existing Medicare limits on acute hospital stays and put a cap of $300 on annual out-of-pocket expenditures for physician services. This would have been financed by an additional Medicare premium of $12 per month. It had no additional benefits: no long-term care, home health, or prescription drugs. To help Medicare beneficiaries meet some of the additional costs, Bowen proposed "individual medical accounts" (IMAs), which could be used to accumulate a fund to pay for nursing home care.[228] Modest though it was, this plan was strongly opposed by insurance companies because of its potential impact upon the lucrative "Medigap" insurance market. As a result, President Reagan only mentioned catastrophic insurance in his State of the Union address, asking for a report by year's end rather than moving toward early introduction of a bill.

President Reagan's maneuver gratified the insurance companies and some conservatives, but turned out to have been a tactical blunder. In November 1986, the Democrats again won control of the Senate and that brought Lloyd Bentsen (Tex.) to the chairmanship of the Finance Committee and Edward Kennedy to head Labor and Human Resources. Within the House, Fortney (Pete) Stark took over as chair of the Ways and Means Health Subcommittee, which began a lengthy collaboration within the House between Waxman and Stark. At the same time, major changes within the administration weakened some of the opposition to expansive health care proposals: Otis Bowen replaced Margaret Heckler as HHS secretary; David Stockman departed and was succeeded by James Miller; and William Roper, who was not replaced as White House health adviser, left to become the HCFA administrator. In net effect the support for health services and insurance was strengthened relative to advocacy for budget restraint and presidential priorities such as de-regulation and privatization.

The administration quickly lost control of the catastrophic coverage issue as health subcommittees of Commerce, Ways and Means, and Senate Finance ignored Secretary Bowen's version and wrote their own bills, adding big ticket items such as prescription drugs and home health care and increasing inpatient hospital and skilled nursing coverage. Sen. David Durenberger (R., Minn.) sought to add an outpatient mental health benefit and Rep. Claude Pepper proposed a long-term care benefit. Although neither of these was adopted, this kind of extravagance led Secretary Bowen, at one point, to send a letter warning that Congress had distorted "the concept the President endorsed," of an "acute, catastrophic benefit under Medicare." Instead, he said, the bill had become a "vehicle for modifications and add-ons to the basic Medicare program."[229] Some of these provisions were added to win support and others because they helped the beneficiaries. In any event, Congress had also lost control of its own bill which ultimately proved fatal because of the constraint laid on by the president that the legislation had to be budget neutral and paid for by the beneficiaries.[230] The whole story is lengthy and complex, but can be summarized briefly.

In 1987, neither the Democrats nor most of the Medicaid constituency cared much for Secretary Bowen's minimalist version. They were more interested in add-ons, especially prescription drugs and long-term care. The latter was too much of a reach and Claude Pepper was persuaded to postpone it; but prescription drug coverage had wide backing, including the AARP, Henry Waxman, and especially James Wright, the newly elected speaker of the House, who prevailed upon the Ways and Means Committee to include prescription drugs. This inclusion along with other add-ons—such as increased hospital, skilled nursing, and home health care benefits added greatly to the total cost and—because of the administration's budget neutrality requirement—to the amount the beneficiaries would have to pay through increased premiums, deductibles, and/or co-pays. This burden upon the beneficiaries would, of course, be hard on the poor among Medicare recipients, especially the elderly and disabled. An alternative, which was something of a fad at the time, would be to make the Medicare Part B premium progressive: that is, have a "means test" for the better off and make them pay more, perhaps a figure approximating the value of the their Part A benefit. This would help, but it would still leave the poor heavily burdened.[231] In this context, Henry Waxman proposed that an existing option, the Medicare buy in, be turned into a mandate for a "Qualified Medicare Beneficiary," (QMB) which would obligate the state Medicaid programs to pay for premium, deductibles and co-pays for Medicare beneficiaries with incomes below the official poverty level.[232] Ultimately, Congress did both, with some significant consequences.

To pay for the benefits, Congress created a progressive supplementary premium or surtax, which applied to all Medicare beneficiaries paying more than $150 in federal income tax, and which would rise with income until it reached $1050/person in 1993.[233] Affluent elders were angry, and a number of advocacy groups were even more outraged on their behalf—because they would be paying a surtax for benefits most of them already had through their own employer-sponsored insurance or Medigap policies. Mass demonstrations and a national campaign attacking the MCCA ensued. A particularly unsavory memory was a "grass roots" National Committee to Preserve Social Security and Medicare, headed by James Roosevelt, that swelled the ranks of protesters by telling them, falsely, that all Medicare beneficiaries would have to pay the surtax. At one point, Dan Rostenkowski, the Ways and Means chairman, was trapped in his own car by angry demonstrators shouting and beating on the roof and sides of the car. Within one year, the MCCA was repealed—the first and only time that Congress has rescinded a major social benefit.[234]

A second part of the story is that the MCCA was not entirely re-pealed. Congressman Waxman and his allies lobbied hard to keep the Medicaid provisions and they were retained, as they had been written, by repealing the rest of the statute but leaving Title III intact.[235] This was a mixed outcome, seen largely as making the best of a bad situation. Several points are worth noting. The QMB coverage was a mandate, not an option—although states had the option to take coverage beyond the FPL. In addition, the Medicaid program was taking on an expensive additional population—especially the elderly and disabled—without benefit of a Medicare supported drug benefit, which was repealed, in 1989, along with the Medicare sections of the MCCA. Nor did it stop there: as with pregnant women and children, dual eligibility could be extended and was, with the creation of "Special Low Income Medicare Beneficiaries" (SLMBs)—for whom Medicaid paid Part B premiums for Medicare beneficiaries up to 120% of FPL—and with similar installments over the next decade.

A contribution of Title III that survived the repeal was Sec. 1864 that dealt with long-term care. This was a logical extension since long-term care was the major component of catastrophic expense and both Medicare and Medicaid beneficiaries suffered from lack of access or the rigors of "spend down" regulations.[236] This legislation, which originated with the Waxman subcommittee, involved small and technical issues such as counting and attribution of income and resources, but it made important and lasting changes.

One part of the legislation related to "spousal impoverishment": *i.e.*, the extent of a spouse's responsibility for the nursing home costs of a wife or husband who has been institutionalized. Here, the committee sought to eliminate anomalies, such as one spouse having all or no responsibility, establish some national standards, and assure that the "community spouse ... has income and resources sufficient to live with independence and dignity."[237]

Of more importance and interest was an amendment (generally known as 1902(r)(2)) that permitted states in their Medicaid eligibility determinations to use methods for income and resource determinations that were less restrictive "and not more restrictive" than those used for SSI determinations or AFDC cash assistance. This particular provision had a long and clouded history,[238] but it was important in the present context because it enabled states to make more generous allowances for medically related expenses or assets needed, for instance, to support community living without having to follow the more restrictive SSI rules or HCFA's interpretation of their applicability. Also, aged, disabled, and many families and children could become eligible by counting less of their income or assets *without* having to raise Medicaid eligibility across the board. This provision did not immediately "open the floodgates," but over time most or all of the states took advantage of it and it was a significant factor in enrolling large numbers of elderly, disabled, and children and families in optional categories.[239]

Dual eligibility grew over the next decade until it covered seven million beneficiaries by 1999, and accounted for $63 billion, or 35% of total Medicaid spending. By way of contrast, dual eligibles cost Medicare $50 million, or 24% of that program's total expense.[240] Looked at from one perspective, this evolution served dire medical need and represented another tribute to the adaptability of the Medicaid program. But it also amounted to an enormous shifting of responsibility from the federal government to the states and, in that respect, lit a long fuse.[241]

DSH and Related Adventures

Disproportionate share (DSH) funds were established for Medicaid hospitals in 1981 as part of the Boren Amendment, as a way to compensate and help sustain hospitals serving large numbers of Medicaid and/or no-pay patients. For a number of years, hospitals paid little attention to the program and both HCFA and the Congress sought in various ways to encourage wider use, for instance, by establishing the category of "DSH hospitals" and allowing states flexibility in designating these hospitals and setting payment levels and tolerating or encouraging such devices as hospital taxes or donations to raise funds for DSH payments and Medicaid matching.[242] Following a HCFA ruling of 1985, West Virginia was the first to take advantage of the donation option. The state had been so hard hit by recession and loss of tax revenues that it was unable to meet even its low Medicaid matching rate. West Virginia's resort to provider donations was strongly defended in Congress by the Health Subcommittee of House Commerce that sought to write in some limitations but also argued that the state was stripped for cash and was using the money raised in this fashion to cover pregnant women and children, support increased Medicaid hospital lengths of stay, and augment payments to DSH hospitals within the state.[243] The Subcommittee noted with approval a decision by the DHHS Appeals Board upholding the state of Tennessee in a similar proceeding.

By 1990, a good many other states had gotten into this DSH game and were tempted to make the best of it because of rapidly growing Medicaid budgets, federal mandates, and a sharp economic recession that lasted from August 1990 until the middle of 1992. By then, Medicaid DSH had become an industry, growing from $1.4 billion in 1990 to $17.5 billion in 1992, and accounting for 15% of total Medicaid spending in that year and, in some states, two and three times that percentage.[244] The speed and pandemic nature of this development attracted attention, especially in Washington; and both Congress and the administration set about to curb this growth, though not to kill off DSH entirely. They were, as history records, partly successful. States showed remarkable capacity to adapt and come back for more. So the federal authorities would try again, and again. DSH or related methods have continued, though much reduced in number and overall significance. And the DSH experience provides a good example of how the flexibility and loopholes in our American system of fiscal federalism enable venturesome and public-spirited officials to work a power of good. They also reward the shrewd and greedy, punish those who live by the rules and make do with their share, and breed lies, hypocrisy, distrust, and cynicism.

A bit of historical perspective is useful. Some of the earlier tax and donation schemes seemed both innocent and unobjectionable. For instance, Pennsylvania used a tax on hospitals to establish a fund for needy safety-net hospitals; and West Virginia asked for donations to get enough money to keep its Medicaid program running. But in their more developed form, DSH schemes were less benign, as a simplified example illustrates.

> State A requests a donation or imposes a tax on a hospital of $10 million. The state then makes a DSH payment of $12 million to the hospital, either as a lump sum or by means of increased Medicaid rates. This nets the hospital $2 million and "costs"

the state $2 million. The state then claims the $12 million as a "legitimate" Medicaid expense and, assuming a 50% match, receives $6 million from the federal government. Final result: the provider netted $2 million from the transaction; the state is ahead by $4 million; the federal government is out $6 million; and Medicaid recipients may or may not benefit from this transaction.[245]

Whatever the ultimate rights and wrongs of the matter, the potential of these schemes for abuse, for explosive growth and raids upon the federal fisc and for eroding mutual trust and upsetting federal-state relations led to watchful monitoring and then to forceful intervention by both the administration and the Congress.

In September 1991, HCFA published regulations that would have banned voluntary contributions and sharply limited provider taxes.[246] Congress had its own legislation under consideration and had already authorized provider taxes. Moving quickly and ignoring a veto threat, the House passed House Resolution 3595 by a vote of 348-71, blocking the administration's rules until September 30, 1991. Meanwhile, the National Governors' Association—restive and complaining over mandates and recession hardships—intervened and negotiated yet another version with the administration. After much fine-tuning to accommodate specific states, this became the basis for The Voluntary Contributions and Provider-Specific Tax Amendments of 1991.[247]

The Act was notable, in part, for introducing a kind of policy-making by crisis negotiation that characterized many high–level decisions about Medicaid in the 1990s. As to substance, the statute established a limit of 12% of a state's Medicaid expenditures on the amount of DSH payments that would be matched; disqualified provider donations for federal matching and made provider taxes difficult; regularized intergovernmental transfers; and required states to submit annual reports on amounts received from provider donations or taxes or from local governments.[248] Of course, the Act did not settle much: its lasting importance was to set a percentage limit on DSH contributions and to redirect the search for DSH funds into other channels.

The first permutation was to rely more on intergovernmental transfers (IGTs), which worked much the same way as taxes or donations except that the initial contributions would come from public institutions such as county and municipal public hospitals, state mental institutions, or state university (medical school) hospitals. This scheme was popular for several years, until Congress became concerned with how much DSH money was being retained by the states or bestowed upon hospitals not truly DSH-eligible. These concerns were addressed in OBRA '93, which restricted DSH payments to hospitals with a Medicaid census of 10% or more. It also limited the amount of DSH payments for a single hospital to the total of its losses from no-pay patients and unreimbursed Medicaid costs.[249]

The states soon found ways around these limitations. One was to fold DSH payments into 1915(c) managed care waivers so as to avoid hospital specific limits and establish legitimate DSH eligible expenditures that would otherwise be lost in a managed care reimbursement system.[250] But the major development following OBRA '93 was to exploit the Medicaid upper payment limit. This particular scam was based upon a perversion of the existing law, which established as an "upper payment limit" for Medicaid what "would have been paid under Medicare principles."[251] There was no standard method for calculating this figure and these limits applied to large, aggregate categories such as inpatient hospital services, nursing home services, and ICF/MRs. This allowed states to pay up to an aggregate total in a particular category but select providers within the group (such as safety-net hospitals) collect provider taxes or IGTs, pay specific providers an inflated rate, still retain a generous amount for themselves, and avoid the DSH laws and regulations.

Legislation continued throughout the 1990s and into the next millennium, with some ground gained but the war by no means over. In April 2005, for instance, the GAO and the newly appointed DHHS secretary, Michael O. Leavitt, complained of "creative accounting" and gimmicks designed to conceal the "recycling" of federal dollars and inflating Medicaid payments so as to claim more federal funds. Local officials asserted that their activities were "entirely legal," that they had documented expenditures for everything they claimed, and that if anyone was aggrieved it was the states and local communities and providers staggering under burdens of poverty and uncompensated care.[252]

No doubt there is an unresolved difference. Some state Medicaid officials, especially in low DSH states, liken the fiscal relationship to the federal income tax and the distinction between tax avoidance and tax evasion. In their view, they stay within the law, "pay their taxes" so to speak, and what is left is for them to spend, according to their best judgment, for the benefit of their own Medicaid recipients. It seems a reasonable point of view, and if all were like these states there would be less of a problem. But there are abuses: states that spread DSH money around like political spoils and use it for non-health purposes, even for highways and football stadiums.

From another perspective, the Medicaid entitlement is like a double covenant: one between the state and the federal government, to implement the Medicaid program faithfully; and the other with the Medicaid recipient, to fulfill an obligation to him or her.[253] And to many of this school, DSH schemes and the like are excusable if used sparingly and scrupulously but otherwise are violations of a trust and akin to theft.

In time, Congress and the Administration reduced the significance of DSH by about half. Yet it is a perennial problem and likely to erupt in times of economic recession or unusual cost pressures, when it can lead to distrust, intergovernmental conflict, and political explosions.

A Note on Process

Over the twelve years between 1980 and 1992, the Medicaid program was transformed from its original welfare-linked, claims paying model into a dynamic program that reached beyond welfare eligibility, encouraged service delivery modification, and became much more immediately involved and aggressive with respect to access, quality, and cost of care. It was a period of expansion, waivers, and mandates:[254] extending eligibility and coverage for pregnant women and children and various categories of persons with disabilities; waivers to deinstitutionalize, manage care, and contain costs; and mandates to include new groups, add services, and implement regulations. This second stage of evolution could also be described as a maturing of the program—becoming more like the entity we know today and growing into an administrative competence and a stable set of activities and objectives. Putting it another way, it became the Medicaid program that we argue about and take as a baseline for policy recommendations. That said, some observations may be worth making about the way in which we got to this point.

Legislation affecting Medicaid during this period was, almost without exception, developed and passed under conditions of divided government and by use of the budget reconciliation process. The Carter administration was an exception to these statements, but President Carter was primarily interested in hospital cost containment and national health insurance, not Medicare or Medicaid as such. With national health insurance off the table in the Reagan and Bush administrations, Democrats turned to Medicare and Medicaid. The budget reconciliation process worked well for them, enabling a Democratic House to move forward on Medicaid issues even with a strong, conservative president and a Republican Senate. When Democrats regained control of the Senate in 1987 they could go farther and faster, to enact an expansive Medicaid agenda that, by 1990, was beginning to raise serious questions about overreaching and getting ahead of the states and some of their own Medicaid constituency.

The budget reconciliation process, like the perennial social security amendments of an earlier era, was a powerful legislative engine. It was good for passing the budget and tax bills since it facilitated incremental changes, set legislative timetables and deadlines, and ended with an up-or-down plebiscite. These were properties that also made it useful for dealing with Medicare or Medicaid; but like most tools, it was good for some operations, not others, and could be overworked.

A great strength of the budget reconciliation process was that it facilitated opportunistic coalitions in support of politically weak causes—such as health care for indigent pregnant women, children, and those with disabilities. But the process was less good at assuring that newly added parts work as intended or work together or for the whole system. It tends to produce partial solutions which give rise to wasted effort, discontent, and the need for additional intervention. For instance, the home and community based services waiver, intended mainly to provide an alternative for nursing homes, served mainly to benefit the ICF/MRs, even as much of the policy effort was taken up with nursing home regulations. As eligibility was expanded and benefits increased for various Medicaid populations, little related effort was made to address rising costs. The managed care option, featured in OBRA '81, was eventually used to good effect, but not until the 1990s, when Medicaid costs and access problems had reached crisis proportions. One of the most dramatic instances of a partial solution was the addition of the "dual eligible" mandate, an important step forward, but seen as hard and unfair by the states without additional federal support such as a pharmaceutical benefit. In fact, much of DSH money was used to plug holes or compensate for Medicaid omissions or lack of adequate support—such as IMDs or safety-net services for the uninsured—which gives point to the observation that amendment by increments may be the best option under the circumstances, but its limitations need to be understood and taken into account.

The reconciliation process was better for centralizing power and moving efficiently than for diffusing understanding and consent. It was more effective for implementing the majority's will than for building consensus within sub-committees and across party lines. As the committee system tended to give too much voice to the particularistic and the parochial, the reconciliation process tended to give too little. Also, it was annual—or nearly so—and toward the end of this twelve-year period, mandates and major new changes piled one upon another, so that many states felt that Washington was bent upon centralizing the system and not listening to their grievances. It was a system headed for trouble.

Notes

1. It is "polycentric" in the sense that, unlike Medicare, it is a federal program, involving 50 states, the District of Columbia, and 4 territories.
2. President Reagan and others within the administration were wary about any assault on the "big entitlements" of Social Security and Medicaid. They were taken on—with scant success—largely because of Reagan's inflexible commitment to a major tax cut, the failure of Congress to deliver on its reconciliation targets, a sharp recession, increasing pessimism about the "rosy scenario" of "supply side" economists, and a huge projected out-year deficit which was, back then, regarded as unacceptable.
3. The only major defeat with respect, specifically, to OBRA '81. The administration also suffered a defeat over Social Security, but that was not part of OBRA '81.
4. Sec 1915(b) refers to the Medicaid statute. In OBRA '81, it was Sec. 2175.
5. Sec. 2176 in OBRA '81.
6. John D. Klemm, "Medicaid Spending: A Brief History," *Health Care Financing Review*, 22 (1) 2000, 105-112, at 108.
7. Economic Recovery Tax Act of 1981, P.L. 97-34.
8. Richard Sorian, *The Bitter Pill—Tough Choices in America's Health Policy.* New York: McGraw-Hill, 1988, 80.
9. *Ibid.,* 82.
10. Provisions in the Consolidated Omnibus Budget Reconciliation Act of 1985 (COBRA), P.L. 99-272, that allowed workers to extend their insurance for 18 months after non-voluntary loss of employment.
11. P.L. 98-369.
12. In 1984, and in most subsequent years, Medicare would absorb much larger budget cuts than Medicaid.
13. The legislation was notable for several reasons: 1) covering pregnant women, not yet mothers; 2) covering them if they were poor enough for welfare—though not actually enrolled and even though the state might not offer welfare to them; and (3) coverage even though living in a two-parent family.
14. The Federal Poverty Level (FPL) was higher than the Supplemental Security Income (SSI) eligibility level and, in most states, than the state income eligibility.
15. For illustrations, see *Congressional Quarterly Almanac,* 1991, 1282-83. Between 1981 and 1990, the Medicaid program grew in numbers from 21.6 million to 25.2 million and in annual total state and federal expenditures from $25.8 billion to $72.5 billion.
16. Medicaid payments and DSH funds helped these institutions, but Medicaid programs and especially Medicaid managed care could often displace grant-supported safety-net institutions—for instance, hospitals and clinics with a religious affiliation.
17. Early and Periodic Screening, Diagnostic, and Treatment.
18. John Holahan, Teresa Coughlin, Leighton Ku, David Heslam, and Colin Winterbottom, "Understanding the Recent Growth in Medicaid Spending," in Diane Rowland *et al. ,* eds., *Medicaid Financing Crisis: Balancing Responsibilities, Priorities, and Dollars*. Washington, D.C.: AAAS Press, 1993, 23-42 at 24.

19.   "Medicaid: Moving Too Fast?," *Medicine and Health, Perspectives,* September 6, 1989, 1.

20.   *Ibid.,* 3, 4.

21.   Note in this connection, difficulties with precedent in the common law, as well as the many techniques and institutions that deal with needed modifications and reforms in this polycentric and incremental system.

22.   The initiative was often described as the "Reagan Revolution," and later conservative Republicans spoke of "completing the Reagan Revolution." Note also David Stockman's exalting of "ideology" (principles or political philosophy) over pragmatism or politics. Cf. Stockman, *Triumph of Politics.*

23.   "Ideology" was the term commonly in use, though the ideas involved were less articulated or comprehensive than in most ideological systems.

24.   Chester A. Newland, "Executive Office Policy Apparatus: Enforcing the Reagan Agenda,' in Lester M. Salamon and Michael S. Lund, *The Reagan Presidency and the Governing of America.* Washington, D.C.: Urban Institute, 1985.

25.   Bert A. Rockman, "The Style and Organization of the Reagan Presidency" in Charles O. Jones, *The Reagan Legacy: Promise and Performance.* Chatham, NJ: Chatham House Publishers, 1988, 3-29 at 11.

26.   Charles O. Jones, "Ronald Reagan and the U.S. Congress: Visible Hand Politics," *Ibid.,* 30-59 at 34.

27.   Nathan, *The Administrative Presidency;* also *The Plot that Failed: Nixon and the Administrative Presidency* New York: Wiley, 1975.

28.   Such language might apply, for instance, to a paratrooper assault in hostile territory.

29.   Edward Meese was assigned responsibility for long-term vision, James Baker for immediate legislation and administrative implementation, and Michael Deaver for politics and public relations.

30.   Some specific activities included reviewing the Nixon and Carter administrations, consulting with the National Academy of Public Administration and with public administration experts, and use of volunteer task forces and "think tanks" to interview executive branch officials and decide what changes to recommend. Cf. Newland, "Executive Office Policy Apparatus"; also, Charles L. Heatherly (ed.) *Mandate for Leadership—Policy Management in a Conservative Administration.* Washington, DCL: Heritage Foundation, 1981.

31.   Stockman, *Triumph of Politics,* 76 ff.

32.   Peter M. Benda and Charles H. Levine, "Reagan and the Bureaucracy: The Bequest, the Promise, and the Legacy, in Jones, *The Reagan Legacy,* 102-142; also Heatherly, *Mandate for Leadership,* esp., David Winston, "The Department of Health and Human Services," Pt. I, 245-306.

33.   David Kleinberg, a former PAD, said that with this authority they could see everything that went on in HCFA. Interview by Smith, April 1, 1988; also Donald Moran, January 5, 1988.

34.   Benda and Levine, "Reagan and the Bureaucracy," 106 ff; also, interview with Donald Moran, January 5, 1988.

35.   P.L. 97-35, August 13, 1981

36.   Stockman, *The Triumph of Politics,* 82.

37.   *Ibid.,* 94. An early version came to be known as "Rosy Scenario," descriptive language now in common usage.

38.   *Ibid.,* 94.

39.   An omnibus bill of this sort (involving a number of authorizing committees) required each house to pass two separate budget resolutions (with conferences)

to be followed by "reconciliation instructions" directing the authorizing committees to come up with the necessary changes in the law to meet the agreed upon budget limits. Moving on another track, separate committees worked on the tax legislation to raise the revenue needed to meet expenditure projections and other fiscal objectives.

40. Stockman, *The Triumph of Politics*, 159-160.
41. As Stockman pointed out, the Senate Budget Committee was not quite the "rubber stamp" that a 20-0 approval of the Reagan budget proposals would make it seem. Senate committees have a tradition of individualism and moderate and conservative Republicans along with Democrats objected to various provisions of the initial budget resolution. Winning over the Budget Committee took hard and persistent work by the chairman, Pete Domenici (NM), and by the majority leader, Howard Baker (Tenn.). At one critical point, the Committee voted 12-8 against the initial budget resolution on the ground that it was squishy on the deficit. It took some masterful brokering and maneuvering to produce a consensus vote. *Ibid.,* 166-167.
42. After Rep. Philip Gramm (D., Tex.) and Delbert F. Latta (R., Ohio).
43. Stockman, *Triumph of Politics*, 56.
44. Food stamps were not strictly an entitlement, but were often treated as such.
45. As an illustration, 70% of the $35.2 billion initial savings from OBRA '81 came from programs earmarked for the poor. *Congressional Quarterly Almanac, 1981* 461.
46. Stockman, *Triumph of Politics,* 158-59.
47. with inflation estimated at 9-10% a year. Cf. *Congressional Quarterly Almanac, 1981,* 478.
48. Sorian, *The Bitter Pill,* 29.
49. Interview by Moore and Smith, Jan 25, 2005.
50. Then the Committee on Interstate and Foreign Commerce. The committee's name changed a number of times, but to avoid confusion, it will be referred to as the "Commerce Committee."
51. Though they often clashed over environmental issues.
52. It was said that he could outlast anyone in conference negotiations; also that he "never had to go to the bathroom." In this vein, it is interesting that a number of conferences in which he was involved concluded well past midnight, even in the early morning. He was credited with a "phonographic" memory, meaning that he had almost total recall of briefings for committee hearings or for negotiations.
53. Edmund Burke would have appreciated their methods, if not the results.
54. In a narrow sense, the entitlement was capped, but was still an "entitlement" because the federal government was obligated to provide for eligible recipients—up to the cap. This may seem a distinction without a difference, but the notion of a "capped entitlement" has a long history.
55. *Congressional Quarterly Almanac 1981,* 477. Sorian, *The Bitter Pill,* 25-26.
56. Henry Waxman interview by Moore and Smith, January 25, 2005.
57. "Gypsy Moth" Republicans, like the "Boll Weevil" Democrats disagreed with the majority of their own party on a number of issues.
58. Richard Sorian, *The Bitter Pill, op. cit.,* 31.
59. There was a Broyhill Amendment that would have restored the administration version of Medicaid cuts to the reconciliation bill, but he failed to offer it when it appeared that the votes weren't there to support it. *Congressional Quarterly Almanac 1981,* 480.

60. The formula was that savings between actual expenditure and a 9% cap (for the first year) could be shared, but only to offset the annual percentage cuts of 3%, 4% and 4.5%. According to Henry Waxman's account, Sen. Dole was both sympathetic and helpful in keeping the entitlement, but felt a strong obligation to reach the reconciliation target. Interview by Moore and Smith, Jan. 25, 2005.

61. Cf. Richard P. Nathan *et al., Reagan and the States.* Princeton, NJ: Princeton University Press, 1981, 5 ff.

62. *Current Conditions of American Federalism*, U.S. Congress, Hearings before the Committee on Government Operations, House of Representatives, 97th Congress, 1st Session, 1981, 1.

63. *Ibid.,* 2.

64. *Ibid.,* 5.

65. Cf. James W. Ceaser, "The Theory of Governance of the Reagan Administration," in Salamon and Lund, *The Reagan Presidency.* 57-87 at 79-82.

66. *Congressional Quarterly Almanac 1981,* 464.

67. For Weicker, it was mental retardation, and for Stafford, education programs and community health centers. Sorian, *The Bitter Pill.* 46.

68. *Ibid.,* p. 50; *Congressional Quarterly Almanac 1981*, 464.

69. though with state plans, set-asides, and reporting requirements.

70. Interviews by Moore and Smith of Henry Waxman, Jan. 25, 2005; Karen Nelson, Jan. 15, 2003; and Howard Cohen Apr, 2, 2003. The point being that Medicaid provides funds, but people also need health care facilities, a place to go for services.

71. Sorian, *The Bitter Pill,* 81.

72. In 1986, the CHCs reverted to federal funding as before. *Ibid.,* 51.

73. *Ibid.,* 53.

74. Charles N. Oberg and Cynthia Polich, "Medicaid: Entering the Third Decade," *Health Affairs,* 9(3), 83-96, at 87.

75. The Reagan administration shut down dozens of community health centers; a number of alcohol and drug abuse clinics were closed or never started; the Mental Health Systems Act was repealed and budget cuts forced many mental health clinics to close; maternal and child health clinics suffered and the infant mortality rate remained where it was, one of the highest among advanced nations.

76. Most importantly, Sec. 2171 broadened coverage for pregnant women, children under 18, and SSI recipients. It also continued the requirement of basic services.

77. Omnibus Budget Reconciliation Act of 1981, U. S. Congress, *Report of the Committee on the Budget to Accompany H.R. 3982,* 97th Congress, 1st Session, H.R. 97-158. 308.

78. This was later added at the insistence of OMB.

79. Henry Waxman was well acquainted with managed care and had co-sponsored a bill regulating HMOs and other MCOs in California. He saw advantages to managed care but believed that it needed supervision.

80. In 1980, the Commerce Health Subcommittee held hearings on this particular topic and introduced the Medicaid Community Care Act of 1980, which failed to pass, although much of this bill was incorporated in the Commerce Committee's response to the OBRA '81 reconciliation instructions. *HRpt 97-158,* 317; also *Medicaid Community Care Act of 1980*, Hearings before the Subcommittee on Health and Environment of the Committee on Interstate and Foreign Commerce, House of Representatives, 96th Congress, 2d session or HR 6194, June 10, 23, 1980. GPO: 1980.

81. Andy Schneider, interview by Smith, Feb. 14, 2005.

82.	Omnibus Budget Reconciliation Act of 1981, 319.

83.	Because estimated expenditures beyond the reconciliation limits would be scored by CBO against the Committee. Andy Schneider, interview by Smith, Feb. 14, 2005.

84.	Sec. 2176(c)(2)(D).

85.	Sec. 2176(c)(1).

86.	Sec. 2175(d)(2).

87.	By 1985, only 17 states had sought DSH funds. In 1983, Congress added Medicare DSH along with the prospective payment system. OBRA '87 defined DSH hospitals and set Medicaid and low-income utilization rates to qualify for DSH payments but also allowed states to designate additional hospitals as DSH eligible and set the reimbursement rates, without putting any limits on federal participation. Despite this encouragement, DSH payments were still relatively insignificant as late as 1989, although by then the stream was beginning to swell.

88.	Andy Schneider, interview by Smith, Feb. 14, 2005.

89.	Also added was a provision that "individuals eligible for medical assistance" should have "reasonable" geographic access to inpatient hospital services of "adequate quality," and a "step-down" provision for Medicaid similar to that for Medicare.

90.	Some related provisions were (1) allowing Medicaid programs to contract with PSROs, with a 75% match for expenses; (2) authorizing the secretary to withdraw approval of drugs for Medicare/Medicaid with a determination that the drug was "less than effective" (Sec. 2103(a)(1)(3)), authorization for the secretary to withhold *Medicare* payments from providers unresponsive to state efforts to collect overpayments or seek information about the overpayments (Sec. 1855(a)(4)); eliminating Medicaid payments for inpatient hospitalization not ordered by a physician (except from an ER) (Sec. 2164(a); 5)), allowing Medicaid matching for transition grants for closure of underutilized services (Sec 1884(c)(2)).

91.	Thomas E. Bryant, interview by Smith, Nov. 10, 2002. The MHSA was premised, in part, upon NHI expectations.

92.	For example, Henry Waxman and his staff made no secret of the fact that they believed universal health insurance to be a good thing and were working toward that end. Others, such as Sen. Edward Kennedy and Sen. Lloyd Bentsen shared this view. So did a number of advocacy groups, and especially the Children's Defense Fund.

93.	"New Federalism" was the major domestic initiative of the administration's second year. Much of the emphasis of this initiative was "devolution," which included—as one element—attempting to separate federal and state responsibility and funding. An expression of this was a proposed "swap" in which the states would take over responsibility for AFDC and the federal government would take the Medicaid adult categories. In a second version, the administration proposed that it take Medicaid acute services with the states responsible for long-term care. This approach revealed especially the divisions between states with high vs. low utilization rates as well as the complexities of developing a formula to resolve these differences. Note in all of this the role of federalism as a conservative defense, much as James Madison conceived it. Cf. David R. Beam, "New Federalism, Old Realities: The Reagan Administration and Intergovernmental Reform," in Salamon and Lund (eds.). *The Reagan Presidency,* 415-442.

94.	Henry Waxman, interview by Moore and Smith, Jan. 25, 2005; Marina Weiss, interview by Moore and Smith, May 2, 2003.

95. One observer— in the EOMB at the time—notes that, paradoxically, OBRA '81 tended to legitimate much of the Great Society. Lynn Etheredge, telephone interview by Smith, March 21, 2004.
96. Sorian, *The Bitter Pill,* 75.
97. Sorian alleged that David Stockman's insistence that either Congress or the insured workers pay for the relief package was calculated largely as a means to stall decision until the economy improved. *Ibid.,* 8; also, *Medicine and Health,* April 25, 1983, 1.
98. "Health Care for the Uninsured Act of 1983," HR 3021; HRpt 98-236.
99. The committee report did not employ the "safety-net" concept, though it clearly contemplated these hospitals as providers of last resort. Among their qualifications was that they be in areas with high unemployment or a medically underserved area, that they serve a disproportionate share of no-pay patients, and that they provide services without regard to the patient's ability to pay. The committee report provides an illustration of a concept developing from practical experience. HRpt 98-236, 43-45.
100. Marilyn Rymer and Gerald Adler, *Short-Term Evaluation of Medicaid: Selected Issues,* Office of Research and Development, Health Care Financing Administration, Department of Health and Human Services, July 1982, 2.
101. *Ibid.,* 7.
102. *Ibid.,* 20; also, John F. Holahan and Joel W. Cohen, *Medicaid: the Trade-Off between Cost Containment and Access to Care* (Washington, D.C.: Urban Institute, 1986), 98-99.
103. The CBO projection was 687,000. *Congressional Quarterly Almanac 81,* 473.
104. Henry Waxman, interview by Moore and Smith, January 25, 2005.
105. *Congressional Quarterly Almanac 83,* 419.
106. "Infant Mortality," *Report Prepared by the Congressional Research Service for the use of the Subcommittee on Health and Environment of the Committee on Energy and Commerce,* Committee Print 98-J, 98th Congress, 1st Session, June 1983, 22.
107. Sarah Shuptrine, interview by Moore and Smith, July 16, 2003.
108. *Congressional Quarterly Almanac 83,* 419-421.
109. These options were liberalizations of strict categorical eligibility: 1) allowing a state to "deem" a first-time pregnant woman (not yet a mother) eligible if the child, when born, would be considered dependent; 2) a two-parent family could be considered eligible if the principal earner were unemployed (AFDC-UP); 3) extending eligibility to children under 18 (or under 21 at state option) who qualified as "Ribicoff" children or a member of a qualified two-parent family; and 4) extending eligibility to pregnant women in two-parent working families whose children, if born, would be eligible as "Ribicoff" children. Another provision prohibited deeming the parent's income to a pregnant adolescent so that the pregnant teen-ager could qualify for Medicaid and thereby for maternal services. Cf. *"Infant Mortality," op. cit.,* 43-44.
110. States that already had such options in effect would be forgiven 1/2% of the OBRA '81 reduction.
111. The Waxman strategy was to offer CHAP as a floor amendment to the Ways and Mean reconciliation bill that would be included as part of the larger reconciliation tax bill. But this maneuver required a favorable rule allowing the amendment to come to the floor on the next to last day of the session. With the usual end-of-session log-jam, this would have given Waxman's bill precedence over others waiting in line, so the rule was not allowed. With this denial, CHAP and the reconciliation

bill both failed to pass. There were many other reasons for this failure to pass a reconciliation bill in 1983, but CHAP was an important one.

112. Karen Nelson, interview by Moore and Smith, January 15, 2003 The reconciliation process was vitally important because any Medicaid legislation standing alone, especially if it cost money, would have almost no chance for passage. Reconciliation was annual, moved quickly, and was not subject to a Senate filibuster. It could be used for major legislation, but was also well adapted for small, almost invisible incremental changes.

113. The reconciliation conference involved huge and complicated budget and tax provisions that took enormous amounts of time and energy to negotiate so that Medicaid would get only a few minutes at the end of lengthy and exhausting negotiations, at which point few members would be involved or aware of the policy and technical issues.

114. Karen Nelson, interview by Moore and Smith, January 15, 2003. At a somewhat later date, the concept of "strategic incrementalism" came into vogue.

115. Henry Waxman, interview by Moore and Smith, January 25, 2005.

116. *Ibid.,* also, *Congressional Quarterly Almanac 1984,* 465.

117. A third try without success. The House provision would have prohibited co-pays outright; the Senate omitted any provision.

118. *Congressional Quarterly Almanac 1984,* 150-152.

119. Henry Waxman, interview by Moore and Smith, January 25, 2005; Marina Weiss, interview by Moore and Smith, May 1, 2003. At the time, the "Willie Sutton" principle was often invoked. Sutton was a notorious bank robber who, when asked why he robbed banks responded, "Because that's where the money is." Ways and Means staff would marvel as Medicare took whopping reductions and Medicaid came through unscathed, usually with substantial increases.

120. The Balanced Budget and Emergency Deficit Control Act of 1985 (PL 99-177, 1985), popularly known as "Gramm-Rudman-Hollings" or "Gramm-Rudman."

121. Henry Waxman said they "fought like tigers" for the exemptions. Interview by Moore and Smith, January 25, 2005.

122. Especially John Chafee (R.I.), David Durenberger (Minn.), John Heintz (Pa.) and Bob Packwood (Ore.) and, on some issues, Robert Dole (Kans.).

123. Quite apart from a desire to support particular programmatic ends—such as health care for pregnant women and children—budget reconciliation also involved building support for the tax bill, which took a great deal of negotiation and tit-for-tat.

124. *Congressional Quarterly Almanac 1964,* 256.

125. A good summary of this process can be found in the *Congressional Quarterly Almanac 1991,* 1282-83.

126. States found the dollars hard to resist, but that they distorted their priorities. Cumulatively, these mandates had a large impact and could be unsettling. One state official complained about getting their programs all decided for the coming year and then "Here would come Andy and Waxman again."

127. Cf. OBRA '81, sec. 672(2); and OBRA '86, sec. 9401. The FPL is sometimes rendered as "federal poverty line" as well as "federal poverty level."

128. *Congressional Quarterly Almanac,* 1986, 564.

129. Sarah Shuptrine, telephone interview by Moore and Smith, July 16, 2003.

130. *Ibid.,* also Linda Bilheimer, interview by Moore and Smith, October 1, 2003.

131. Bilheimer, *ibid.*

132. *Ibid.* Another important step was approval by the National Governors' Association. There, Strom Thurmond's staff was blocking the proposal. At one point, when the discussions between principals were heading for an impasse, Thurmond said

(referring to Shuptrine) that he would like "to hear what this pretty lady had to say." She based her pitch entirely on the money that would be saved by preventive health care which she knew was a priority for Thurmond and that approach (according to her) won him over. Sarah Shuptrine, interview by Moore and Smith, July 16, 2003.

133. Tying this option to coverage for pregnant women and children was a precautionary measure, added by the Senate, to prevent states from spending all their Medicaid money on nursing homes.

134. The major group being the states under Sec. 209(b) of the Social Security Amendments of 1972 that chose to continue with their own historic standards of eligibility. In 2000, eleven states. Cf. Schneider, *The Medicaid Resource Book,* 28.

135. Also significant was a provision authorizing the secretary to grant HCBS waivers for Medicaid beneficiaries afflicted with AIDS or who were chronically mentally ill. Hospice care for AIDS victims was made more accessible as were clinic services for the homeless. *Congressional Quarterly Almanac 1986,* 258.

136. This authorization was especially broad including, in addition to health services, homemakers and home health aides, adult day care, and respite help for family members. *Congressional Quarterly Almanac 1987,* 559.

137. "Freedom of Choice," Sec. 191915 (b), waivers were included, but attention was centered on the HCBS waivers for the elderly and disabled.

138. *Omnibus Budget Reconciliation Act of 1987,* House of Representative, Rpt. 100-495, 100th Congress, 2d Session, 1987, 730-37. These provisions included authorizing of demonstration projects to reduce infant mortality and morbidity, extending the length of post-partum services, and a maintenance-of-effort requirement prohibiting states that elected for optional coverage of pregnant women from lowering the AFDC eligibility level or requiring an AFDC application.

139. *Congressional Quarterly Almanac 1988,* 356.

140. Rosenbaum, "EPSDT History;" Larry Bartlett, interview by Moore and Smith, March 14, 2003.

141. Sec. 6403 was systematic and prescriptive in detail—much more so than the original legislation or many of the provisions in the reconciliation statute.

142. The operative language was "such other necessary health care, diagnostic services, treatment, or other measures described in Sec. 1905(a) to correct or ameliorate defects and physical and mental illnesses and conditions described by the screening services, whether or not such services are covered by the State Plans." Senator Bentsen (D., Tex.) was primarily responsible for this particular provision and for making available the necessary funds. Marina Weiss, interview by Moore and Smith, May 1, 2003; also Sara Rosenbaum, telephone interview by David Smith, March 10, 2005.

143. Alicia Pelrine then of the NGA staff, observed that Medicaid was not good for preventive care, that it had an institutional bias, and that it didn't stress case-management.

144. As an aside, George H. W. Bush had promised, during his campaign for the presidency, to expand eligibility for pregnant women and children to 185% of poverty. *Medicine and Health, Perspective,* September 4, 1989, 2; Democrats and Michael Dukakis, who ran against Bush for the presidency, also defended Medicaid stoutly.

145. *State Health Notes,* February 1991, 3.

146. *Ibid.,* November/December 1990, 5.

147. Gail Wilensky, interview by Moore and Smith, July 9, 2003.

148. Title XIII of OBRA '90, PL 101-508.

149. Andy Schneider, telephone interview by Smith, February 14, 2005.

150. Pregnant women and children are roughly 70% of the Medicaid population and account for about 30% of the payments. The elderly and disabled about 30% of the Medicaid population, are responsible for 70% of the payments. *Medicaid Source Book* 1993, 155, Fig. II-15; and 161, Fig II-17.

151. The "probably" is there because of the "woodwork effect" (previously undiagnosed or untended conditions that add to expense) and the alleged "savings" that make no allowance for the unpaid caretakers such as spouses and/or children.

152. A subcommittee of the Senate Special Committee on Aging (see note,   ). The plight of the aged, somewhat like that of the highways, has been a topic that brings legislators together. Agitation over this issue was important in leading to Medicare and Medicaid. Also, many legislators—Frank Moss, Claude Pepper, John Heinz, Edward Kennedy, and Charles Grassley, etc., gained recognition from their support of the aging and of nursing home reform.

153. Vladeck, *Unloving Care,* 59 ff.

154. *Ibid.,* 68.

155. Cf. Linda E. Demkovich, "Government's Nursing Home Rules—Better Care or More Bureaucracy?," *National Journal*, November 1, 1980, 1846.

156. Linda E. Demkovich, "Nobody's Happy over Administration's Attempt to Change Nursing Home Rules," *National Journal*, March 20, 1982, 502.

157. *Ibid.,* 505.

158. One obvious warning sign was the speed and extent of mobilization by advocacy groups, within the Congress and nationally, in opposition to the nursing home deregulation. There was also dissension within the administration: Richard Schweiker, then the DHHS secretary, had concluded that the earlier HCFA regulation had merit; and, later, HCFA drafts revived the patients' rights, though not as a condition of participation. Sorian, *The Bitter Pill,* 148.; Linda Demkovich, "Nobody's Happy over Administration's Attempt," 508.

159. *Improving the Quality of Care in Nursing Homes,* (Washington, D.C.: National Academy Press, 1986).

160. Elma Holder, telephone interview by Smith, January 30, 2003.

161. Linda Demkovich, "Government's Nursing Home Rules"—Better Care or More Bureaucracy," 1846.

162. Robert Gettings, interview by Smith, December 4, 2002.

163. Michael Fogarty and Charles Brodt, interview by Moore and Smith, August 11, 2003. In fact, some states were already claiming nursing home support for MR recipients under Medicaid, but the GAO had ruled this unlawful in the case of California. Robert Gettings interview, December 4, 2002.

164. Especially Sen. Henry Bellmon (R., Okla.), Russell Long (D., La.), Carl Albert (D., Okla.), and Hale Boggs (D. La.).

165. Wayne Smith, interview by Moore and Smith, Feb. 3, 2003; James W. Trent, Jr., *Inventing the Feeble Mind—A History of Mental Retardation in the United States.* Berkeley, Calif.: University of California Press, 1994; also, Burton Blatt and Fred Kaplan, *Christmas in Purgatory: A Photographic Essay on Mental Retardation.* Boston, Mass: Allyn and Bacon, 1966.

166. Wayne Smith, interview, by Moore and Smith, Feb. 3, 2003.

167. *Congressional Quarterly Almanac 1984,* 481.

168. *Medicaid Source Book, op. cit.,* 882.

169. Jeffrey L. Geller, "Excluding Institutions for Mental Disorders from Federal Reimbursement for Services—Strategy or Tragedy?" *Psychiatric Services*, Vol. 50 (2000), 1397-1403, at 1398.

170. *Medicaid Source Book,* 926.
171. Chris Koyanagi, telephone interview by Smith, March 22, 2005.
172. In some instances, when mental health agencies were more enterprising and secured Medicaid funding, states decreased or took away their block grant funds. *Ibid.*
173. "Abandoned," *Newsweek,* January 6, 1986, 14-19; Gerald N. Grob, *The Mad Among Us* (New York: Free Press, 1994), 302 ff; Edward D. Berkowitz, *Disabled Policy—America's Programs for the Handicapped.* New York: Cambridge University Press, 1987, ch. 4.
174. A small number of waivers were used to support patients in IMDs. Geller, "Excluding Institutions for Mental Disorders…",1399.
175. Among the justifications given for DSH schemes was that they provided a way to finance IMDs.
176. PL 99-660.
177. Chris Koyanagi and Howard H. Goldman, "The Quiet Success of the National Plan for the Chronically Mentally Ill," *Hospital and Community Psychiatry,* 42 (9),1991, 899-905 at 901. Earlier, in 1984, Congress directed the secretary to prepare a comprehensive plan for alcohol and drug abuse and, in other legislation, provided for planning and service grants for half-way houses, day care, and supervised work for deinstitutionalized mental patients. *Congressional Quarterly Almanac 1984,* 480-81.
178. "[A] medically determinable physical or mental impairment which results in marked and severe functional limitations, and which can be expected to result in death, or which ha lasted or can be expected to last for a continuous period of not less than 12 months." Schneider, *The Medicaid Resource Book,* 22.
179. The blind receive special treatment. Neither alcoholism or drug addiction qualify as disabilities.
180. Again, much like the common law.
181. Julie Beckett, interview by Moore and Smith, May 23, 2003.
182. *Ibid.*
183. PL 97-248.
184. This is more technically known as a "model waiver," a title which seems to mean little except that it isn't a large new class by itself.
185. Schneider, *The Medicaid Resource Book,* 23.
186. Donald Herman, interview by Moore and Smith, July 17, 2003. As a condition for these model waivers the state had to undertake to cover any other like cases arising in the state. In addition, they had to form councils to aid in allocating and processing the applications. A 1915(c) waiver would also have been an option, but the budget neutrality test, at that time, was more difficult to meet.
187. *Ibid.* As we were conducting this interview with Julie Beckett at the Omni Shoreham in Washington, Katie Beckett—who was there to attend a TTW meeting—appeared briefly with a friend and then went off, like any other active young adult, to explore the local setting.
188. Carol O'Shaughnessy and Richard Price, "*Medicaid "2176" Waivers for Home and Community-Based Care."* Congressional Research Service, Library of Congress, June 21, 1985 (mimeo), 6.
189. PL 92-603, Sec. 1611(e)(3)(A). Apart from the potential abuse of such a category of eligibility, this was a time when alcoholism and drug abuse were seen by many as defects of character rather than as illnesses.
190. *Diagnostic and Statistical Manual: Mental Diseases.*
191. Rita Vandevoort, telephone interview by Smith, July 16, 2003.
192. *Medicaid Source Book, op. cit.,* 979.

193. *Ibid.*

194. *Ibid.*, also, Shelley Gehsham, interview by Smith, July 24, 2003.

195. Sandra Panem, *The AIDS Bureaucracy*. Cambridge, Mass.: Harvard University Press, 1988, 9.

196. Richard E. Neustadt and Harvey Fineberg, *The Epidemic that Never Was—Policy Making and the Swine Flu Scare.* (New York: Random House, 1982.

197. Panem, *The AIDS Bureaucracy,* 31.

198. Apart from his interest in health, Waxman's Los Angeles constituency was an area with a high incidence of HIV/AIDS. The same was true of Weiss's Greenwich Village district. Jeff Levi, interview by Smith, January 28, 2003.

199. Panem, and Dr. Edward Brandt, (interview by Smith, August 12, 2003) who were close observers of the governmental response to AIDS, largely concur with this view. Others who have been more critical make the point that, along the way, the government could have done more about AIDS related diseases (ARC) and prevention (for instance, Jeff Levi; also, cf. Steven Epstein, *Impure Science—AIDS, Activism, and the Politics of Knowledge* (Berkeley, Calif.: University of California Press, 1996)). A further point: Robert Gallo might have been wrong. He was concentrating on a feline retrovirus, while the French scientist, Luc Montagnier, may have made the first identification of the human retrovirus. This issue of priority was protracted and rancorous, but two points seem clear: that Gallo *may not* have had the right virus and that it was good that foreign scientists were also working on the same problem. Without the earlier work on retroviruses by David Baltimore and Howard Temin, we might still be looking for the answer.

200. One distinctive and noble aspect of the AIDS epidemic was the role of local gay associations in caring for those already stricken and dying of AIDS.

201. Between 1984 and 1986, some of the fiercest debates were over prevention involving, for example, closing the bath houses in San Francisco, compulsory testing with disclosure for specific populations, and the use of needle exchanges or sterilization with bleach to prevent intravenous contamination.

202. The Public Health Emergency Act, PL 98-49, 1983.

203. Panem, *The AIDS Bureaucracy,* 87, 89.

204. For instance, many people believed that *giving* blood could lead to AIDS.

205. Lawrence O. Gostin distinguishes three phases: 1) denial, blame, and punishment, 1981-87; 2) mobilization and engagement, 1987-97; and (3) complacency, injustice, and unfulfilled expectations, 1997—present. This division is insightful and useful, although partial mobilization began almost immediately, reaching a high level of national organization and visibility by 1987.

206. Key figures were Reps. Henry Waxman (D., Calif.) and Ted Weiss (R, NY) and Sens. Edward Kennedy (D., Mass.) and Lowell Weicker (R., Conn.). Within the administration, Edward Brandt, ASH; C. Everett Koop, the surgeon-general; and James Mason, head of the CDC.

207. The role of President Reagan is unclear. Without question, he was slow to speak out sympathetically. When he did so, his statement was grudging and while he urged the establishment of a national commission on AIDS, and more research appropriations, he also came out for compulsory testing for immigrants, federal prisoners, and (by the states) for those seeking marriage licenses. Dr. Edward Brandt, a highly credible source, said that Reagan had proposed that he speak out earlier but had been urged not to do so for fear of inciting the religious right. Brandt and others also remembered the swine flu episode, made worse by politically inspired intervention by the White House. Interview by Smith, August 12, 2003.

208. *Congressional Quarterly Almanac 1987* 516.
209. Adm. James D. Watkins, chairman of the commission had said that discrimination against those testing positive was the foremost obstacle to progress in combating the spread of the epidemic. *Congressional Quarterly Almanac 1988,* 301.
210. PL 101-336.
211. In the House, four committees shared jurisdiction, which would have complicated the legislative process and multiplied the opportunities for attack by opponents.
212. This included the right of private parties to sue for enforcement, job restoration and back pay, but not for damages. A separate bill that included private damages was vetoed by President Bush.
213. Thomas P. McCormack, *The AIDS Benefits Handbook.* New Haven, Conn.: Yale University Press, 1990, 52.
214. Epstein, *Impure Science.*
215. Later modified in 1992, but even so, few qualified via this pathway. *Medicaid Source Book op. cit.,* 1098-1100.
216. AIDS Related Complex.
217. *Congressional Quarterly Almanac 1986,* 286.
218. PL 100-71.
219. PL 101-381
220. *Congressional Quarterly Almanac 1990,* 583, 586.
221. John Palen, interview by Smith, March 4, 2003; Michael Iskowitz, interview by Smith, March 12, 2003.
222. *Congressional Quarterly Almanac 1990,* 583.
223. Dennis Murphy, interview by Smith, February 18, 2003; Palen, interview by David Smith, March 9, 2003.
224. A recent estimate has 55% of persons living with AIDS and 90% of afflicted children covered by Medicaid. Andy Schneider, *The Medicaid Resource Book, op. cit.* 86.
225. More precisely, coverage would start at incomes 85% of FPL and be phased in up to 100% of FPL and assets up to the SSI level.
226. *New York Times,* March 25, 2005, A-12; April 8, 2005, A-28.
227. He had also chaired an earlier presidential commission on Medicare that recommended, as one item, consideration of a catastrophic insurance plan. Sorian, *The Bitter Pill, op. cit.,* 70.
228. *Ibid.,* 180.
229. *Congressional Quarterly Almanac 1987,* 495.
230. A constraint communicated in advance from the White House. Marina Weiss, interview by Moore and Smith, May 2, 2003 Also, Rep. Henry Waxman, interview by Moore and Smith, January 25, 2005.
231. At the time, Speaker Wright was proposing a premium set at 25% of the cost of the Part B premium.
232. The original Sec. 301 was short and simple, the ultimate Sec. 303 much more elaborate, substantially increasing the amount of income and assets that could be retained by individuals with spouses, whether institutionalized or living at home.
233. *Congressional Quarterly Almanac 1989,* 149.
234. *Ibid.,* 150.
235. Henry Waxman, interview by Moore and Smith, January 25, 2005.
236. Medicare beneficiaries had SNFs but these were expensive and covered a limited number of days. They could qualify by "spending down" but that involved complex rules, including the attribution of income and resources to one spouse or

the other. Also, the "spending down" often seemed harsh, especially to formerly middle-class sensibilities and sometimes did not make sense: for instance, taking away the resources that might have enabled an individual to continue residing and receiving treatment in the community or to hold a job.

237. *Medicare Catastrophic Coverage Act.* House of Representatives, Rpt. 100-106, Pt. 2. 100th Congress, 1st Session. 1987. 29.

238. For a succinct account, see *Deficit Reduction Act of 1984.* House of Representatives, Rpt. 861. 98th Congress, 2d Session. 1366-68. Prior to 1981, states with medically needy programs had used less restrictive income and resource standards than those required by AFDC. Apparently HCFA misinterpreted the intent of Congress in OBRA '81 and an attempted correction in TEFRA of 1982 and sought to impose on states the more restrictive standards for AFDC and SSI. This led to a "DEFRA moratorium," in which Congress prohibited HCFA for 18 months from imposing penalties on the states based on its earlier misinterpretation. The 1902 (r)(2) provision of the MCCA allowed the "less restrictive methodologies" for aged and disabled and extended this same concession to families and children, except for the mandatory AFDC eligibility; but meanwhile, the Waxman mandates, which severed the link with AFDC, were becoming increasingly important. A regulation dealing with this issue was not finally published until January, 2001. With thanks to Andy Schneider and Marinos Svolos for help in attempting to understand this nest of puzzles.

239. People we have interviewed who are acquainted with the history of 1902(r)(2) hesitate to speculate about aggregate numbers. States differ in their response and estimating growth or totals would require estimates and summing of state-specific data. One experienced official, who doubted that totals could even be determined, said he thought almost all states made use of this option and that it was significant for the Medicaid program as a whole and especially for the aged and disabled, but that it was more like a stream than a torrent.

240. Jennifer Ryan and Nora Super, *Dually Eligible for Medicare and Medicaid: Two for One or Double Jeopardy?* (Washington, D.C.: National Health Policy Forum, September 30, 2003).

241. Henry Waxman wanted the federal government to pay for the QMBs and the SLMBs, but Sen. Bentsen objected—probably correctly—that the measure would never pass.

242. HCFA ruling of 1985. Mechanic Robert E., *Medicaid's Disproportionate Share Hospital Program: Complex Structure, Critical Payments* (Washington, D.C.: National Health Policy Forum, September 14, 2004).

243. House Rpt. 247, 101st Congress, 1st session, 1989, 478-479.

244. Coughlin, Teresa A. and David Liska, *The Medicaid Disproportionate Share Hospital Payment Program: Background and Issues,* (Washington, D.C.: Urban Institute, 1998), 3.

245. Illustration from Coughlin and Liska, *Ibid.*, 3, 4.

246. *Congressional Quarterly Almanac 1991,* p. 357. For background, Alicia Pelrine, "The Art of the Deal: Health Policy Making on the Fly," *Journal of American Health Policy*, May/June 1992, 23-28.

247. PL 102-234; cf. Pelrine, *op. cit.*

248. *Congressional Quarterly Almanac 1991,* 361.

249. Coughlin and Liska, *The Medicaid Disproportionate Share Hospital Payment Program,* 5.

250. *Ibid.,* 5.

251. Mechanic, *Medicaid's Disproportionate Share Hospital Program,* 6.

252. *New York Times,* April 12, 2005, A-15.
253. Schneider, interview by Moore and Smith, May 22, 2003.
254. Thompson and DiIulio, Jr., *Medicaid and Devolution,* 19.

6

A Critical Phase

A critical phase for Medicaid began in 1990 and continues unresolved to the present day. During the 1980s several big and many small steps transformed Medicaid into a "mature" or developed system with new service delivery options, broadened eligibility, a vigorous capacity for growth, and numerous federal mandates. Whether or not this Medicaid expansion and nationalization went "too far," the reality was that a number of state and federal officials and legislators thought so. Rising health care costs and the economic recession of 1991-92 deepened fiscal distress within the states. Because of divided government, ideology, partisan differences, and lack of will to seek common ground, little was done to redress these grievances.

In the first two years of the Clinton administration, Democrats controlled both houses of Congress and the presidency, but Medicaid was ignored as attention centered on larger items on the domestic agenda, especially national health insurance. As for national health insurance, most of the proposals either abolished Medicaid or incorporated it as one element of the larger scheme without significant attention to its reform.

A defining event for the decade, much like the budget reconciliation of 1981, was the election of November 1994, which gave the Republicans control of both houses of Congress—for the first time in 52 years—and brought to power a generation of partisan and ideologically-minded Republicans led by Newt Gingrich, the new speaker of the House. This political upheaval encouraged near revolutionary demands for change. A rallying cry, popular then, was to complete the revolution that President Ronald Reagan had begun—including the dismantling of entitlements such as welfare, Medicare, and Medicaid.

The election added legitimacy and fervor to a highly mobilized and intensely partisan style of politics that carried over into domestic policy, making it part of a continuing campaign for new successes and additional support. Republican attacks upon Medicare and Medicaid began soon in the Balanced Budget Act of 1995, and made even incremental gains—anything beyond staving off eminent disaster—seem dangerously optimistic. Nevertheless, the Medicaid entitlement was preserved, even strengthened. The program was further separated from its historic welfare linkage and some gains made for the working poor. The State Children's Health Insurance Program (SCHIP), enacted in 1997, was the biggest single expansion of eligibility for poor children since the beginning of the Medicaid program. Quality standards, managed care regulation, and additional protections for persons with disabilities were legislated; and. regular and substantial savings from Medicaid achieved along the way.

This experience is worth examining, since it shows how the Medicaid program survived a major political storm largely intact and moved ahead despite the tempest. Yet the same style of highly mobilized and intensely partisan politics exists today and little has happened to resolve the fundamental problems of fiscal federalism, cost containment, and administrative flexibility that helped create the confrontations of the nineties that continued into the next decade. Learning what the fighting is about may help to deal with it.

Balanced Budget Act of 1995

Medicaid was a small part of the huge Balanced Budget Act of 1995, the centerpiece of the Republican domestic program in that year. Yet the fight over Medicaid was a strategic battle and the outcome had major consequences in succeeding years, both for the Medicaid program and for domestic politics more broadly.

An antecedent to BBA '95 was the inglorious effort of the Clinton administration and the congressional Democrats to agree upon and enact a NHI scheme, preferably one with universal coverage. This effort was badly executed and was an egregious misstep that high-level Republicans decided could be their ticket to electoral success in 1994. The degree to which the electoral outcome in 1994 was attributable to the failure of health care reform or Democratic ineptitude is debatable; but the Republicans treated the election as a plebiscite on "big government," taxes, and the "failed" domestic policies of Democrats,[1] of which NHI was made into a leading example.[2]

In the election, Republicans won decisively in every region except the Northeast—a victory that could be seen as a mandate similar to the

New Deal election of 1932 or the Great Society election of 1964. They took the House for the first time in 40 years, gaining 53 seats. In the Senate, Republicans won all the open seats and defeated two incumbent Democrats for a gain of eight seats. In the popular vote, Republicans won nine million more than their 1990 vote, while Democrats lost one million. One could quibble about what the message was, but certainly there was a message being sent.

Whether or not the election of 1994 was a mandate for fundamental change, the House Republicans began organizing as though it were. Meeting in advance of the new Congress on December 7-9 in Washington, the Republican conference took a number of votes intended to centralize and strengthen party leadership within the House. Newt Gingrich was elected the new speaker, with Dick Armey (Tex.) as majority leader and Tom DeLay (Tex.) as chief whip. Seniority was overridden to appoint conservative Republicans as chairmen of several key committees: Robert Livingstone (La.) for Appropriations; Thomas Bliley for Commerce; and Henry Hyde for Judiciary. Incoming freshmen, full of revolutionary fervor, were given seats on the strategic Budget and Rules committees, and some even named sub-committee chairmen. When Congress first met on January 4, 1995, the new speaker held them in session for fourteen and a half hours while the House ratified these appointments, amended procedures, changed committee jurisdictions, abolished a number of committees and sub-committees, and cut committee staffs by one-third. At 2:00 a.m. the next morning, the House adjourned after passing more than 200 resolutions. Not a single Republican voted against any of the resolutions.

For the next 100 days the House debated and passed the ten articles and scores of provisions comprising the Contract with America. At the 100-day deadline, the House had passed all the major items except for term limits. Yet few of the Contract's provisions ever became law. The most important—such as the Balanced Budget Amendment, a middle-class tax cut, product liability reform, welfare block grants, and the missile defense—either lost in the Senate or because of presidential opposition. The biggest procedural change, the line-item veto, eventually became law, but was of little use either to Republicans or Democrats.

To evaluate the Contract with America as a legislative accomplishment, though, is to miss the point. It served its main purpose well, which was to mobilize and unify the House Republicans in support of their new leadership, its campaign style politics, and its agenda for change.

The original reason for the Contract, according to Newt Gingrich, was to nationalize the mid-term elections and turn them into a plebiscite on the Clinton administration. The particular Contract items were chosen primarily for their popularity and their unambiguous appeal to conservatives and disaffected voters. After the election, it had strong appeal to the large cohort of House freshmen Republicans. And for a party long in opposition, it served as an initial agenda, a socializing and educative experience, and a morale-building opportunity for small legislative victories while proposals were being developed for the major engagement—the Balanced Budget Act of 1995.

The Balanced Budget Act of 1995 was central to the continuing revolution set in motion by the House Republicans. Both deficit reduction and tax cuts were prominent parts of the Contract with America, which included a "Balanced Budget Amendment" to the U.S. Constitution. On March 2, 1995, the latter failed by one vote to pass the Senate; but without waiting for the Senate, the House had already begun a campaign of rescissions,[3] adopted a goal of balancing the budget by 2002, and enacted some substantial tax cuts. A major objective, as with the Reagan administration that preceded them was to shrink the size of the federal government and eliminate or devolve many of its programs and activities.

The Senate agreed in principle on this agenda, but with restrained enthusiasm for the ambitious deficit reduction goal and almost none for tax cuts or program reductions. A few conservative senators fully supported the House agenda and more were in favor of deficit reduction, but many went along largely because of partisan loyalty and solidarity with House colleagues who were doing the heavy lifting and taking the political heat.[4]

Republican leaders in both House and Senate agreed early on that entitlements would be considered for the savings needed to reduce the deficit and eventually balance the budget, but did not disclose many particulars. A large amount of "restructuring" was assumed with Medicare expected to contribute the largest savings and undergo the most drastic structural changes. At the same time, Newt Gingrich had a healthy respect for the Medicare entitlement and created a special Medicare task force and allowed an extra two months for this part of the reconciliation.

Medicaid received nothing like this flattering attention. Neither Medicare nor Medicaid had been mentioned in the Contract with America.[5] Prior to the convening of the new Congress, Republicans were considering only incremental changes and $10 billion in savings without any restructuring. But the election of 1994 not only changed the Congress: Republicans captured thirty of the governorships, for a gain of eleven. Some of the more active and vocal governors attending the Republican governors annual conference in December 1994 lobbied to change the welfare program into a block grant, saying that they would accept less money in exchange for greater freedom to manage "their own" programs. Newt Gingrich agreed to this agenda with alacrity and the same concept—already familiar to Republicans—became a leading proposal for Medicaid as well.[6] The National Governors' Association, which met in the following January, was not of one mind, and recommended against any "unilateral" caps on federal spending, but a task force of Republican governors and high level Republicans from Congress was appointed to work on this and other proposals for "reforming" or "restructuring" Medicaid.[7]

Much of the critical discussion about Medicaid occurred in February and March as the House was debating and passing the Contract with America. By mid-February, House Republican leaders and the RGA task force of governors had agreed on a basic formula for Medicaid: a capped entitlement with reduced annual increments—five percent being the figure most commonly mentioned.[8] A "capped entitlement" left Medicaid in the entitlement column since those duly enrolled could claim the benefit; but the federal obligation was "capped," which put a lid on aggregate federal matching which would in turn push states to curb their spending and revise their programs.

The budget resolution set a four-month deadline for the authorizing committees to report out Medicare changes, but less than two months for Medicaid. At the time, Newt Gingrich remarked that the hard work was just beginning, and John Kasich, the House Budget Committee chairman, urged the authorizing committees to be especially "creative" in meeting their global targets. Despite the exhorting, Medicaid took over two months longer, neither the House Commerce Committee nor Senate Finance reporting until late September.

Although Medicare was more important than Medicaid both for budget savings and as part of the larger Republican strategy, the House leadership chose to go first with Medicaid and start early. Part of the reason was logistics: more time was needed for staff work and policy discussions on Medicare. Talks with the Republican governors seemed to be moving in a good direction and had created substantial momentum. Medicaid was perceived as an easy target, both because it seemed less complex and because it lacked the kind of middle class support enjoyed by Medicare.[9] And to go with Medicaid first might also be a way to "steal a march" on Democrats and win a quick victory that would help when attention shifted to Medicare.[10]

Cautionary observations at the time indicated the lack of understanding these views reflected, especially about the human and political costs and the fiscal and federal complexities involved. Howard Cohen, the lead Republican Commerce Committee staffer for Medicaid said that when he heard $184 billion in Medicaid savings, he "wanted to quit" and went to John Kasich, the Budget Committee chairman to plead that "we can't do it."[11] Karen Nelson, an experienced aide to Rep. Henry Waxman, said she knew from the beginning that the numbers were too high and that the savings would get harder as the reconciliation progressed.[12] Raymond Sheppach, the executive director of the National Governors' Association, observed that the NGA was too pluralistic for a "block grant" to be attractive with savings of that magnitude.[13] No matter that the Republican schemes for Medicaid might be imprudent or difficult, few doubted the earnestness of their intentions and Democrats feared that the Medicaid program, as they knew it, might be lost.

The BBA of 1995 was eventually passed by both House and Senate but vetoed by President Clinton and not revived after the historic "shutdown" of the federal government in December and January of 1995-96.[14] Therefore, the details of the "Medicaid Transformation Act of 1995," which was the Orwellian title given to the Medicaid part, are not important for this account, but how and why the Medicaid program could be defended successfully is of lasting significance.

Conventional wisdom at the time, accepted by Republicans and Democrats alike, was that Medicaid would not be strongly defended. Single mothers and dependent children, persons with disabilities, and the elderly poor were not an articulate or united constituency and, except for the elderly, not politically effective. At the time, moreover, welfare reform seemed a near certainty and Medicaid was regarded by many governors and members of Congress as another "welfare" entitlement and hard to defend. Following their resounding defeat over health care reform and their losses in the election of 1994, Democrats were disorganized and without a comprehensive strategy, and political momentum was with the Republicans. For all of these reasons, many Democrats and Republicans alike thought that Medicaid would be significantly reduced in funding, either "block granted" or drastically restructured, and its status as an entitlement ended.

A successful defense of Medicaid owed much to the unity and defensive tactics of the Democrats. The nature of the Medicaid program was also important: both its complexity and its increasingly "mainstream" characteristics. Institutional checks on the majority traditionally associated with federalism and bicameralism and the special role of the Senate and a few senators were a third element, and especially significant because of the weakness of traditional political support for the Medicaid program. Even though the Balanced Budget Act was eventually defeated, an account of how Medicaid was defended illustrates ways in which the Medicaid program is tougher and more resilient than sometimes realized.

A strategic move by President Clinton in his February budget message was to offer the barest of "placeholder" budgets and invite the Republicans to "go first." In effect, by refusing to "come to the table" his move tended to foreclose compromise, but it gave Republicans less opportunity to target their cuts. It also put upon them most of the onus for the pain and collateral damage inflicted and helped Democrats identify who would get hurt and plan how to mobilize the most effective protest.

At the time, Democrats were dazed and demoralized and lacked a message of their own, so there was little they could do except "counterpunch," that is, attack particular budget reductions or program changes as unnecessary, too drastic, or unfeeling. This defensive tactic had worked well on a small scale when Republicans sought to cut funds for school lunches and public broadcasting opening them to a Democratic attack for letting school children go hungry and taking away popular programs like Big Bird and Barney. Especially notable with respect to Medicaid was the speed, skill, and effectiveness with which the Democrats were able to organize this defense.

An important resource was an informal Democratic task force that had developed during the 1993-94 struggle over national health insurance care and that resumed meeting after the 1994 election. Most of its members had been prominent actors in "health care reform," knew each other, and had wide networks of communication and allegiance both in the administration and on the Hill. They brought together a formidable technical and political expertise and had ready access to in-depth resources. The task force could also get a quick response from the White House through Chris Jennings, who as health policy adviser to the President coordinated health policy at that level.

The task force had a major role in the president's June budget and in developing policy options for both Medicare and Medicaid, but most immediately its task was to counter the Republican threat to Medicaid. One tactic was to take the global figures in the budget resolution[15] and translate them—drawing upon agency expertise, OMB options papers, and CBO numbers—into projections of the damage that would be done to existing programs and who would get hurt. This information could then be turned into credible and politically effective talking points for officials or committee members, press releases when political issues were hot, and "message" amendments to delay legislation or put legislators on the spot and lower their comfort levels.

The critical stage was the reconciliation itself, during which the authorizing committees had to translate the reconciliation instructions and numbers into program changes and specific authorizations. Important resources for the Democrats in the House were Henry Waxman, chairman of the Health Subcommittee and John Dingell, chairman of the parent Commerce Committee, both of them iconic figures in health affairs. Although reduced in numbers, their staffs were repositories of institutional memory, policy expertise, and specific knowledge about who had what interests at stake. They also had important connections to advocacy groups and the local "grass tops." Not least, they were familiar with the political terrain and able to spot and take advantage of tactical opportunities.

Democratic effectiveness within the Committee was severely limited, though, by a Republican decision to dispense with subcommittee hearings and keep legislative details secret until immediately before the markup.[16] Democrats were able to stretch out the markup itself and score rhetorical points with a number of "message" amendments that forced Republicans to go on record on issues that could cost them votes. Despite this kind of pain, Republicans maintained a rock-solid discipline and voted out the recommendations by a 27-18 vote. The only partisan defector was a Democrat.

The effectiveness of this kind of counterpunching defense is hard to estimate. During the markup, the majority seemed little deterred and some participants dismissed the Democratic efforts as annoying but of small consequence. Other comments provide some insight into Medicaid politics and the legislative process. One veteran believed that the talking points and message amendments were useful for raising the morale of Democrats and of Medicaid advocacy groups.[17] A member of the Republican staff said they helped educate Republican members, especially freshmen, about Medicaid and the people who depended on it. They also made some members aware that they might need political cover.[18] Several Democrats spoke about the effects their press releases and message amendments were having on governors who were increasingly concerned for the poor, for the nursing homes and the middle class families of their residents, and for the hospitals and other health care providers with high numbers of Medicaid patients.[19] They also speculated that a credible defense for Medicaid in the House may have influenced the president: gotten him to care more about Medicaid, kept him from wavering, or helped convince him there was enough support to sustain a veto.[20]

Although BBA '95 was the gravest threat to the Medicaid program in its history, it occasioned little public outcry or strong interest group protest.[21] Some advocates that were active, such as Families, USA, the National Council on the Aging, and the Catholic Health Association were relatively small, spread thin, or marginally interested. One important exception to this pattern was the hospitals, especially those serving Medicaid patients: providing a historic example of "virtual representation" of the poor by their Medicaid providers.

Part of the strategy of Newt Gingrich and the House Republicans to assure passage of the BBA was to reach out in advance to major interest groups—such as the American Medical Association, the American Hospital Association, the Health Insurance Association of America, and the American Association of Retired Persons—and seek to associate them with their "transformational" schemes and give them a part in the process or, at the least, minimize their opposition. From the beginning, the response of the hospitals was mixed: interested in being part of the future, but concerned about the size of the projected budget savings. Late in January, the AHA appointed a task force to report on the likely impact of the reductions being considered.[22] Although most of the money was in Medicare, the AHA leadership was even more concerned about Medicaid and the regional swings in payment that a block grant could produce.[23] Another issue for the AHA and for hospitals treating the poor was reductions in hospital subsidies such as the Medicaid DSH allowances and the direct and indirect medical education payments.

Hospitals generally, and the "safety-net" institutions in particular, saw these payments, especially the Medicaid DSH allowances, as part of the subsidies and cross-subsidies that enabled them to treat poor and no-pay patients and stay in business. With the local variations and intricacies of this system anything more than a cautious incrementalism risked serious dislocation or financial collapse. This was a dire threat to the poor and afflicted as well as to most local and specialty hospitals, related enterprises, local governments, state hospital associations, and all who represent them politically. As one AHA official put it, "There are some breezes that set all the wind-chimes tinkling," and this was one of them.[24]

The House budget reconciliation of early May called for a five-year reduction in Medicaid of $270 billion and a cap on Medicaid annual growth that would phase down from 10% to 4% in three years. The proposal set off sharp exchanges between the AHA and the House Republican leadership and a flurry of negative advertisements in the media. This was followed, immediately before the Memorial Day recess, by a major national campaign, led by the AHA and joined by other hospital groups and state associations, that was replete with national TV ads, videos and information kits for individual hospitals, and local visitations upon congressional members.[25] House Republicans responded in kind, with action kits for their members, advice on how to counter the "Astro-Turf" (phony grass-roots) assaults, and warnings about what such activities might cost the hospitals if they provoked an angry retaliation.

The hospital alliance won a victory to the extent of getting Medicaid DSH allowances incorporated in the baseline for future calculations and, possibly, in raising the percentage caps. No other provider group mounted a full-scale national campaign, although the American Medical Association and the American Academy of Pediatrics passed resolutions against block-granting Medicaid and a long-term care alliance lobbied Congress on behalf of the middle-class Americans whose parents might need a nursing home, long-term care, or a safety-net provider.

It would be fanciful to see in this single episode the beginnings of a broadly based or robust "virtual representation" of Medicaid recipients and the poor by their providers and middle-class "patrons." In this particular example, only the AHA coalition acted strongly and effectively; and such a gesture was not soon repeated. But interests of this kind often get represented more readily at the state and local levels: for instance, through local providers and their associations, such as hospital and nursing homes or parents' associations speaking out for their children. Some of their concerns can then stir local communities and percolate upward through congressional delegations, governors, and national advocacy groups.

The idea of a 5% cap on Medicaid growth dates back to the Nixon administration and was a prominent inclusion in OBRA '81 early in the

Reagan administration. As frequently pointed out by its defenders, this proposal was not an unvarnished "block grant," but rather a "capped entitlement": the individual Medicaid beneficiary had a right to the benefit and the state and federal governments were obligated to pay, except that the federal share was capped at a 5% annual growth rate.

With the recent history of federal mandates and DSH squabbles, the prospect of greater administrative freedom and, presumably fewer mandates, was attractive to a number of governors, some of whom said that they could take a "hit" of $10 billion if they could have, in exchange, more freedom from mandates and regulations.[26] Newt Gingrich pre-shopped this idea with the RGA and the NGA and increased its visibility. Even at this early stage, many of the governors were wary of a "one-size-fits-all" approach and about the potential impact of a 5% cap if the Medicaid growth rate rebounded to 8-10% or more. As the debate matured, the governors became tangibly aware of what such a cap might mean for their own state's economy and fiscal position and for local authorities, health care providers, Medicaid beneficiaries and their families.

Early on, Carl Volpe, the legislative director for the NGA, warned that a 5% cap would be onerous and likely to provoke a huge "formula fight" among the states.[27] Despite such prophecies and portents of their fulfillment,[28] the Republican leadership in both House and Senate—with a budget resolution to pass—continued to push for the 5% cap. Once that was voted, committing the authorizing committees to the savings targets, attention turned to devising a more responsive formula that would take better account of poverty rates and projected Medicaid growth within the states. But a formula fight was already under way, compounded by the severity of the 5% cap and the difficulty of devising a new distribution equation.

Formula fights occur over the legislative formulas used to distribute federal funds to the states in support of such programs as highway construction, water pollution control, public welfare, and health services. Such fights are common and often hard fought and protracted. For Medicaid, both the amount of money at stake and the complexities of revising the distribution formula made this one especially tough. Raymond Sheppach, the executive director of the NGA, said that he had seen huge formula fights over a $15 billion highway bill. He estimated that there was $50 billion or more in the Medicaid variations that would be involved.[29] Moreover, the 5% cap would mean a drastic reduction over time, so that less and less would be available to apportion, inevitably setting one state against another and making compromise ever more painful.

Fixing the formula was a task that fell, in the first instance, to the House Commerce Committee, and especially the Health Subcommittee staff, since they had the resources, the experience, and the established relations with the Congressional Research Service and the House Legislative Counsel needed to do much of the technical work.

The basic approach was to set a global cap for the next seven fiscal years that would meet the reconciliation target,[30] then devise a set of indices to allocate the money among the individual states[31] and modify the matching rate for a specific state according to the new formula taking account of such factors as poverty population and taxable resources.[32] For the first seven fiscal years, the global updates worked out to be slightly *less* than 4%. Moreover, the allocation formula had to be budget neutral and was significantly redistributive among the states so that it was a zero-sum game in which the indexes and the numbers assigned to a specific state would have enormous consequences and inevitably make the business of allocating the pain among fifty semi-sovereign jurisdictions, the District of Columbia, Puerto Rico, and the territories, a matter of innumerable iterations and endless haggling.

A sense for the difficulties of devising a distribution formula can be gotten by considering some of the differences in history and circumstance of specific states. New York, for instance, had historically spent more for Medicaid recipients than any other state and was proud of its record of beneficence and meant to keep it. Poor states, such as Alabama, Arkansas, Louisiana, and Mississippi, needed recognition both of their poverty numbers and their limited fiscal capacities. Seventeen high growth states in the "sunbelt" region feared a low cap on growth. Texas and California, hard pressed by unpaid care and illegal aliens, thought they deserved help on these accounts. Florida had, in addition to aliens, a continuing influx of elderly, many of them likely to become Medicaid eligible. High DSH states had a good thing going, and wanted to keep the funds flowing. States with big waivers, like Oregon and Tennessee, opposed a distribution formula that would penalize them for their foresight and efficiency. And recession sensitive states feared the cumulative impact of an economic downturn and a capped federal contribution.

At a practical level, the distribution formula had to "work." This meant programming and computer runs with fourteen different rules in the distribution formula and seeing what kinds of swings these produced regionally and for particular states, for providers, and for the protected "set-asides," and then "back-rigging" the formula again and again to improve the outcomes. The subjective and political part was sitting around the table with ten governors, discussing hardship, the needed " fixes," and the trade-offs.[33]

Even veteran staffers were awed by the state and regional variations, the intricate workings of their distributions rules, and the difficulty of finding common ground. The staff worked for six months on the distribution formula, the negotiations alone taking over four months and entailing an estimated 1400-2000 computer runs, mostly done by the General Accounting Office. As the House Commerce Committee prepared to mark up its own version on September 20th, the Republican governors were still unable to agree on a distribution formula.[34] By then, President Clinton had already pledged to veto any bill with Medicaid or Medicare reductions of the size then being proposed by Congress.

The Senate, the Finance Committee, and John Chafee

The Senate, as noted (*supra,* 230) had not undergone a drastic reorganization, had not bought into the Contract with America, and did not share Newt Gingrich's "transformational" enthusiasms. But the Senate did pass a budget resolution with $160 billion in Medicaid savings, supported the block grant concept, and seemed headed toward a Medicaid bill that would be close to the House version, with a few amendments to ease some pinches or address a particular need. That was before the markup and the impact of Sen. John Chafee (R., R.I.) and a few Republican and Democratic health care liberals on the Finance Committee. This episode illustrates again the importance of bicameralism for Medicaid politics and policy, as well as why Republicans complain that the Senate is often more of a problem for them than the Democrats.

To begin with, the Senate Finance Committee is an enormously powerful and prestigious committee, with a considerable amount of autonomy and immunity from the crassest forms of partisan pressure or leadership *diktats.* It is primarily involved with taxes and huge amounts of money. Therefore, it can usually find offsets for expenditures: relatively low-profile Medicaid amendments are not likely to be life-or-death issues and can frequently slip by or be "traded out" with comparative ease. Taxes are serious business and require good sense and give-and-take so that bipartisanship is emphasized, the majority edge is slight, much of the work is done in full committee, and the staff serves both parties.

In 1995, the Finance Committee was often liberal on health issues. The majority, by tradition, was small: eleven Republicans to nine Democrats. The Democratic membership was moderate to liberal, with several senators, especially Rockefeller (W. Va.), Graham (Fla.), and Moynihan, (NY) knowledgeable and deeply concerned about health. On most health issues, the Democrats were unanimous in support of the liberal option. On the Republican side, Bob Packwood (Ore.), who was the committee chairman (until September 7th), was strongly liberal on health issues. Several others—Orrin Hatch (Utah), Charles Grassley (Iowa), Alfonse D'Amato (NY) and Ben Campbell (Colo.)—who might be conservative on most fiscal issues—would sometimes vote with Democrats on health related matters. Especially where Medicare and Medicaid were concerned, 11-9 liberal majorities or 10-10 tie votes were common.

Then, there was John Chafee. A World War II hero, a former Republican governor, and a four-term senator from Rhode Island—an overwhelmingly Democratic state—Chafee came from a patrician family and had a strong sense of responsibility for the poor or handicapped. He was chairman of the Subcommittee on Medicaid and Health Care for Low-Income Families, which he had urged the Finance Committee to establish, despite the Senate's presumption against subcommittees. A skillful negotiator and coalition builder, he could work effectively across party lines and was the leader of a small group of moderate Republicans, mostly from New England and often referred to as "Snow Birds." This group included at the time, aside from Chafee, William Cohen (Me.), Olympia Snowe (Me.), James Jeffords (Vt.), and Arlen Specter (Pa.). With a close numerical balance in the Finance Committee, Chafee's views would often prevail there. And with the narrow Republican majority of 54-46 in the Senate, Chafee and his allies could often win a floor vote. In short, Sen. Chafee was committed, powerful, and a critical figure in most decisions about Medicaid.[35]

The Senate Medicaid bill (S 1357) resembled the House bill (Title II of HR 2491) in broad outlines. It provided for $182 billion in Medicaid savings, a "block grant" (capped entitlement), with a state plan and mandatory set-asides, and more freedom for states to manage on their own. The most significant differences were the use of FY 1995 (instead of FY 1994) for a baseline and revision of the Medicaid DSH formula rather than complete elimination of these payments.[36]

Sen. Chafee was categorically opposed to a block grant or ending the Medicaid entitlement and set about to do what he could within the Finance Committee. One of his first proposals was to require states to provide a minimum benefit package, which would largely vitiate a block grant. This failed to pass by a 10-10 vote, all the Democrats voting with Chafee. An amendment to protect low-income mothers, children, and the uninsured lost in another 10-10 vote.[37] Repealing the ban on federal funding for abortions also lost, 9-11.

These amendments failed but the Finance Committee Republicans were well aware that a tie vote would not get their bill out of committee, so they agreed to accept some of Chafee's amendments in return for his vote to report out a bill. Most important of these was a requirement that states provide benefits for pregnant women, children under 12, and the disabled. Others were an increase in the funding for mandatory populations, and some federal funds for pre-pregnancy planning.[38]

Individual Senate Finance members, some close to Chafee on the issues, added amendments that either reinstated Medicaid provisions or significantly challenged the philosophy of the House's Medicaid Transformation Act. A Hatch amendment required a 1% set-aside for local health care. A Graham addition prohibited states from excluding any otherwise eligible Medicaid recipient because of a pre-existing condition. Amendments by Hatch and Mosely-Brown required states to establish goals and standards for children with special needs. Other amendments restored the protection of spouses against spend-down requirements and prohibited liens against a home or family farm of moderate value. Alfonse D'Amato, facing a re-election campaign, got an amendment to raise the minimum federal match from 50% to 60%.

Chafee and his allies suffered two major defeats in committee. One was the proposal by David Pryor (D., Ark.) to restore federal nursing home standards or, failing that, to have federal review of state standards. This failed twice on 10-10 votes. A second was the defeat of the Chafee-Rockefeller amendments to protect the disabled. Because of the expense, especially for long-term care, the governors were strongly opposed and twenty-four senators wrote to Robert Dole, the majority leader, complaining about this mandate and the restoration of spousal protection. With Dole's intervention and after a floor debate, the Finance Committee agreed to leave it to the states to decide who qualified as "disabled."[39]

On September 26 the Senate Finance Committee reported out S 1357 by a vote of 11-9. The Senate still had to pass the Medicaid Transformation Act as part of the reconciliation bill and, for this, needed the support of Sen. Chafee and his "Snow Birds." Joined by other moderates, including Nancy Kessebaum (R., Kans.), Mark Hatfield (R., Ore.) and Ben Campbell (R., Colo.) this loose coalition negotiated together and separately with Robert Dole and with William Roth for additional modifications. A chairman's (Roth) amendment reinstated most of the federal nursing home standards and added $14 billion to compensate for loss of Medicaid DSH funds. The Senate adopted (66-39) a Chafee amendment that required states to use the SSI definition of "disabled." It also deleted the provision banning use of federal funds to pay for abortions. A motion to recommit the whole bill with instructions to restore the Medicaid entitlement lost by a vote of 48-50. Another to restore the existing Medicaid eligibility for pregnant women and children lost by a vote of 49-50.

As expected, the Medicaid provisions of the reconciliation, adopted on November 16, 1995, followed the House version in most respects. Medicaid was "transformed" into a capped entitlement with mandatory set-asides and detailed state plan requirements. But Chafee and his allies won several victories. The federal nursing home standards were reinstated, largely intact, though enforced by the states with federal oversight. States were required to continue the Medicaid entitlement for poor pregnant women and children under age thirteen, though the states could determine the benefits. States would also be required to spend a specified amount (85% of a three-year historic average) on nursing home residents, seniors, and the disabled. Protection against spousal impoverishment was retained. A set-aside for community health centers and rural health clinics was established. States were also required to cover childhood immunization under a schedule to be established by the states.[40]

One of the late-stage "sweeteners" was to reduce the seven-year savings from the $182 billion in the original budget reconciliation—already down to $170 billion in the reconciliation bills—to $163.4 billion, almost $20 billion below the original target. Mostly, this was to ease the pain for states still distressed by the funding formula. In the House, Newt Gingrich added $12 billion: $6 billion for northeastern states with teaching hospitals and high DSH subsidies, $3 billion to help pay for illegal aliens, and another $3 billion for those pinched by the Medigrant distribution formula.[41] In the Senate, a Roth chairman's amendment added $10 billion, mostly for high-DSH states. To offset these expenditures, the House relied on a lower CBO estimate of seven-year federal Medicaid spending and the Senate cut the Social Security COLA from 3.1% to 2.5%.[42] Ultimately, the formula issues were not so much solved as salved, with enough grease to quiet the most aggrieved, the loudest, and the strongest.

After President Clinton vetoed HR 2491, the Balanced Budget Act of 1995, the "Medicaid Transformation Act" did not so much die as go into a state of suspended animation. In December, the NGA attempted to broker a compromise, based on a modified version of the act. During the edgy negotiations of January 1996, conservative Republicans talked abut a BBA II that would pick up where earlier negotiations left off. As for that theme, the "Medicaid Transformation Act" is still relevant as a model for "restructuring" Medicaid, supported by many Republican governors and members of Congress and might receive serious bipartisan consideration in a calmer political environment.

This episode illustrated especially ways in which Medicaid—a politically weak program without a powerful clientele or strong interest group support—could be defended, mostly because of the stake that powerful groups, other than the recipients, have in Medicaid; the fiscal and institutional complexities of the program; and the opportunities the American system of government gives to determined minorities and well-placed individuals or groups to slow and thwart majoritarian assaults. Whether this is good or bad depends in some measure on the cause: whether it is the Medicaid entitlement that is being defended or racial and other forms of discrimination. Whatever one's persuasion, this episode showed that an effective defense of Medicaid could be mounted and sustained because of latent political strengths and skillful use of institutional resources. To be sure, this was only one episode in a continuing struggle over the Medicaid entitlement. It illustrates defensive strength, not a capacity to reform the program or even change it. Also, more recent attempts to "restructure" Medicaid have relied less on the Congress—even with Republican majorities in both House and Senate—and more on what the administration and economic pressures could accomplish.

Medicaid and Welfare Reform

For Medicaid, the year 1996 was almost a non-event. Many were exhausted by the fierce battles of 1995 and not looking for new fights.[43] There was a lack of fresh, attractive policy options. It was a presidential election year in which rhetoric was important but legislators were risk averse and sought small victories while avoiding unpopular stands or major blunders. Moreover, time was short, because of leftover business from 1995 and the urgent desire to adjourn and get out on the campaign trail.

Economic indicators in 1996 were more favorable. Even in mid-1995 the economy was visibly better. By March 1996, the deficit was reported to be falling for a fourth straight year.[44] Health care costs were moderating, with both Medicare and Medicaid baselines repeatedly revised downward.[45] These developments made deficit reduction or restructuring Medicare or Medicaid less urgent. That also made modest, bipartisan efforts attractive and feasible, such as extending Medicare trust fund solvency, increasing child health benefits, or small-group health insurance reform.

A small and quaintly traditional achievement of the Congress was to pass the Health Insurance Portability and Accountability Act (HIPAA).[46] This legislation was a stand-alone health measure that went through hearings, markups, and reports, passing without benefit of a budget reconciliation or attachment to some larger "must pass" legislation such as Social Security amendments. It was the only significant piece of bipartisan legislation in over two years to make it out of committee and become law. Although of modest importance in itself, it helped legislators and staff get rid of the "bad taste" left by the acrid disputes of 1995. It also gave bipartisan collaboration a lift, "cooled out"[47] some issues, and helped prepare the way for the Balanced Budget Act of 1997.

While there was movement toward bipartisan cooperation, there was still an abundance of partisanship, especially in the House, over matters left unresolved by the demise of BBA '95, such as the deficit, tax cuts, welfare reform, and Medicaid. But how to move forward on these issues was not obvious. Early in the year, House Republicans announced plans to turn their last best offer (during the shutdown crisis) into a "BBA II," and pass that; but few, even among House Republicans, saw the good sense of following one train wreck with another.[48] Meanwhile, Newt Gingrich and John Kasich, the House Budget Committee chairman, had been working on an interim strategy, which was to seek limited savings and concessions on entitlements with separate bills. This approach received some support from an NGA recommendation in February for Medicaid and welfare reform.[49] A major problem, though, was how to get a stand-alone bill on Medicaid or welfare through Congress.[50] The answer was the three-part reconciliation bill of 1996.

With the three-part reconciliation, the plan was to have Medicaid and welfare combined in one reconciliation bill and go first with this bundled option. If it succeeded, it would be followed with Medicare and then with a tax reduction bill. Reconciliation would add some support for three bills that would otherwise have to stand alone, was action forcing, and not subject to a filibuster in the Senate. Also, a tri-partite division would peak issues less, minimize risk, and might get wider support at a time when neither Republicans nor Democrats had the will or resources for a major reconciliation.

An important step was the pairing of welfare and Medicaid. They were combined because the governors wanted it that way and to raise the stakes for President Clinton. The strategy was to link the relatively easy (welfare) with the hard (Medicaid), and keep them linked. If the president vetoed them, he could be pilloried for doing nothing about his campaign promise to "end welfare as we know it." And if the veto were overridden, he would lose on both welfare and Medicaid. Of course, there was also the downside risk for Republicans—that they, too, could lose on both.[51]

Few Republicans thought there was much chance of passing all three bills, but they moved ahead with the reconciliation, linking the two programs, and working in committee to complete the Medicaid and welfare bills.[52] Once these were reported out, both Democrats and Republicans began shifting to a veto strategy, with the president promising to veto the reconciliation bill as it stood, but asking for a "welfare bill he could sign." House Republicans, who had moved closer to agreement on welfare, were increasingly loath to see their gains lost because of a linking to Medicaid reform, which was "going nowhere."[53] In the Senate, the leadership continued to support the linkage,[54] but with diminishing enthusiasm as adjournment approached, deadlock over other issues threatened, and they contemplated the prospect of another go-round with the Finance Committee, a difficult reconciliation conference, and a presidential veto.

This impending stalemate was broken by Senator Dole, who was increasingly frustrated with trying to continue his leadership role in the Senate and run for president. He was also loath to see good efforts come to naught in another partisan bloodletting. On July 11th, Dole sent letters to Speaker Gingrich and to the Senate majority leader, Trent Lott, asking them to pass a welfare bill and urging President Clinton "to sign a real welfare reform that most of our nations' governors can support."[55] Whether these letters were cause or pretext, the Republican leadership released them and announced a de-linking of welfare and Medicaid.

In four weeks time, the Congress completed and passed the Personal Responsibility and Work Opportunity Reconciliation Act of 1996 (PRWORA, P.L. 104-193), a large statute of nine titles and 230 pages that replaced the 61 year old AFDC with "Temporary Assistance to Needy Families" (TANF), a block grant, that set time limits on assistance with work requirements, and gave the states much greater freedom to determine individual eligibility and benefits.

Democrats were distressed at the dismantling of an entitlement, but with some ambivalence. President Clinton had committed himself to welfare reform and saw in this legislation a chance to "change the incentives in the welfare system from dependence to empowerment through work."[56] Unlike the bill he had vetoed in 1996, this legislation kept medical care, food stamps (though modified), and child care assistance. Some members of the administration left or resigned in protest, but many thought that welfare reform was inevitable, were glad that it was welfare rather than Medicaid,[57] and welcomed the final severance of the Medicaid entitlement from welfare eligibility.

One concern, shared by Democrats and Republicans, was to ensure that poor families and children did not lose Medicaid eligibility either in transition to TANF or because of a loss of cash assistance. To this end, during the conference a small bipartisan group of conferees and staff[58] inserted among the Title I conforming amendments a new Sec. 1931. One of its provisions was that the resource and income standards in a state plan as of July 16, 1996 should be used to determine eligibility for Medicaid. Thereafter, a state could lower its income standards, but not below those in effect as of May 7, 1988, and could raise income and resource standards, but not by more than the increase in the urban consumer price index (CPI-U). Sec. 1931(b)(2)(C) further provided that a state could "use income and resource methodologies that are less restrictive" than those under the state plan as of July 16, 1996, pointedly repeating an identical provision already in effect (1902(r)(2).[59] As a further precaution and to emphasize practically and symbolically the severance of the welfare-Medicaid linkage, Sec. 1902(a)(3) was amended to provide for a Medicaid determination of eligibility for any person eligible or seeking to become eligible for medical assistance under Sec. 1931, so that Medicaid and welfare eligibility would be perceived as clearly separate.

The intent of Sec. 1931 on its face was to minimize loss of Medicaid eligibility in the transition to TANF or leaving TANF for work. The flexibility provision would have allowed states to be more liberal with income and resource disregards and thereby qualify people for Medicaid—for instance, by disregarding in-kind child support, a serviceable car needed to get to work, or income above the poverty level. Disregards of this sort were common in welfare eligibility determinations and it made sense to extend them to Medicaid. When Sec. 1931 was drafted, it was intended primarily to prevent *loss* of eligibility not as a hidden agenda to transform Medicaid into a program for the working poor.[60]

But PRWORA was a "work" program: its objective was to get people off welfare and working or seeking work. Medicaid was retained, but people had to apply for it, often to local offices that were overworked and staffed by case-workers accustomed to older eligibility standards. Few were aware of or understood Sec.1931. And poor women who did get jobs frequently lost their Medicaid eligibility, food stamps, and child care. In the first years of PRWORA, Jason deParle estimated that half of the women coming off welfare and 30% of the children were without Medicaid, even as the numbers of uninsured grew because of unemployment.[61]

At this early stage of PRWORA, something like a Medicaid program for the working poor seemed much needed, and some of the more aggressive states began acting on that premise, finding inventive ways to help welfare recipients with additional child care, increasing income and assets disregards, easing eligibility requirements for two-parent families,[62] and extending transitional Medicaid eligibility for adults or continuous eligibility for children leaving TANF. Many of these possibilities were later summarized in a HCFA publication that explained how they could be exploited, identified funds states could draw upon, and exhorted them to reach out to the eligible welfare families and to shorten and expedite the application process. Sec. 1931 would enable states to include many more single and two-parent families than Medicaid has "traditionally covered" and would be

> ...an opportunity for states to recast and market Medicaid as a freestanding health insurance program for low income families, improving the possibility of destigmatizing Medicaid and enhancing the potential of the program to reach families that come into contact with the TANF system.[63]

This vision was more expansive than that of the original Sec. 1931. But the kind of adaptations that grew out of Sec. 1931 made sense given the problems created by transitions back and forth between TANF and work. Historically, Sec. 1931 was also an important step on the way toward SCHIP which, in addition to extending eligibility to a large cohort of uninsured children, also reached the working poor.

The Balanced Budget Act of 1997

The Balanced Budget Act of 1997 (P.L. 105-33) was another huge omnibus budget reconciliation which, like the BBA of '95, cast Medicare and Medicaid in lead roles. Beyond that, the reconciliations differed radically: in political context, in procedures, and in their objectives. One big difference was that BBA '97 was a bipartisan venture that succeeded in large measure because it attempted little. Still, it had important consequences for both programs and, with respect to Medicaid, nudged it in new directions.

The election of 1996 changed little in the number of seats in Congress or in leadership positions, but it affected the political mood and altered the relations between House and Senate and Congress and the president. In the House, Republicans lost nine seats and no longer had a commanding majority. In the Senate, Republicans gained two seats and laid claim to a larger role relative to the House. President Clinton won a convincing victory, widely seen as an endorsement of him and his policies. And the election sent a message that voters were tiring of legislative bickering and rancor and would like to see some constructive legislation. Potentially, at least, the way was more open for pragmatic compromise and bipartisan cooperation.

There had also been some learning in 1995 and thereafter. Republicans learned how difficult it was to restructure entitlements as complex and well established as Medicare and Medicaid. They found that President Clinton was a wily and dangerous opponent who sometimes did not bluff. And they developed more caution about being first with a controversial proposal. Democrats, for their part, learned how to go on the offense as well as make good use of defensive resources. They also learned that the Republican base was solid and committed and that the leadership would do "whatever it takes" to hold that base.

The economy and key indicators were still cooperating. The deficit had declined for the last three years lowering the five-year projection by one-third.[64] Medicare was expected to be $15 billion lower than anticipated.[65] And for Medicaid, the news was especially good. Medicaid spending in 1996, projected to grow 9.7%, had actually grown only 3.3%.[66] In December of that year, the Urban Institute predicted that Medicaid spending would drop by as much as $94 billion without any additional intervention—greater savings that either the Congress or the president had sought.[67] That many numbers going in the right direction tended to move thoughts away from block grants or radical restructuring toward what might be done to take advantage of the promising trends.

Congress and the White House generally assumed that there would be an omnibus budget reconciliation in 1997, though what form it would take was unclear. Major reconciliation bills had failed in 1995 and 1996 so that, aside from negotiating the budget and reducing the deficit, a major reconciliation would be useful as a vehicle for the multitude of legislative amendments—small and large, technical and politically hot—needed to regulate and direct the administrative agencies and to update and modify taxes and subsidies.[68] An omnibus reconciliation would also have high visibility and demonstrate that legislators could accomplish something.

One indication of how the political climate had changed was President Clinton's "pre-shopping" of his 1998 budget with Republican congressional leaders before positions began to harden around specific proposals.[69] He put on the table a figure of $100 billion of Medicare savings that Republicans welcomed as a good basis for talks. He also said that he was "not necessarily opposed to" some Republican proposals, such as higher Medicare premiums for the wealthy or even some reduction in the capital gains tax.[70] At the time, he had not made a final decision about Medicaid, though there was a view within the administration that Medicaid had performed so well that he might not propose any additional savings except, possibly, some DSH cuts.[71]

At the time, the House Republican leadership was pleased, John Kasich agreeing with Clinton's claim that he had moved more than halfway toward the Republicans and that they should be able to pass a budget sooner rather than later.[72] But prospects "too good to be true" usually are, and so it was. Some Republicans were suspicious of Clinton, thought the savings were inadequate, and did not trust the figures of the HCFA actuary. Then, in late February, the CBO reported that Clinton's Medicare proposal would fall $19 billion short of the $100.2 billion savings claimed and that health benefits would cost $4 billion more than projected.

To many Republicans, the CBO numbers sounded like "same old, same old"—Clinton jerking them around once more. John Kasich was especially disappointed and called for a new Clinton budget. To this, Franklin Raines, Clinton's OMB director, responded that if the Republicans didn't like the Clinton budget they were welcome to put forward one of their own—which they would have found hard to do (and Raines knew that).[73] From there the budget process degenerated, stalled out not so much over partisan differences as the risk to either side of going first with a consensus proposal that would serve as the basis for negotiation and get severely mauled in the process.

At this juncture, President Clinton invited Pete Domenici, John Kasich, and the ranking Democratic members of the Budget Committees to meet with him at the White House to negotiate a way out of the impasse. The group was then broadened to include chairmen and ranking members of the House Ways and Means and the Senate Finance committees and top-level members of the White House staff.[74] On the first day, as a gesture of good faith, Clinton offered $18 billion more in Medicare cuts to make up for the shortfall earlier noted by CBO.[75] Even so, little progress was made, and pressure on the Republicans grew as they fretted over whether to continue with the negotiations or break off the talks and develop their own budget.

Two more rounds of talks and three weeks later, the budget "summit" seemed likely to end as the initial talks had, with neither party budging. Help came on April 28th—two weeks after the April 15th deadline for the budget resolution—from a CBO report that the five-year deficit would be $114 billion less than previously estimated.[76] This windfall unsettled a number of deals already negotiated but helped make the whole package acceptable, especially to conservative Republicans and liberal Democrats. About $64 billion more was allocated to deficit reduction. Another $24 billion went to eliminate an "adjustment" to the consumer price index (CPI), an unpopular measure no longer needed. Per capita caps for Medicaid went out. And small amounts were earmarked for child health, transportation, and Clinton's welfare-to-work amendments.[77] With minor changes, this summit agreement then became the basis for the budget resolution that was passed with large majorities in both House and Senate on May 21st and 23rd.[78]

As a process, apart from its substantive provisions, the budget resolution was remarkable in several ways. Unlike other budget resolutions, it was not primarily negotiated between Democrats and Republicans in the Congress but between the president and Republicans in the House and Senate. In was a remarkably successful example of "triangulation," in which the president associated himself with a number of Republican objectives but in ways that protected Democratic priorities and got some substantive concessions in exchange.[79] It was also important for what it decided *not* to decide: a block grant or global cap for Medicaid; a "defined contribution" or a privatizing option for Medicare. Especially important for the ultimate success of the reconciliation, this restraint reduced the scope of conflict and gave each side some of what it had to have.

An important consequence was that the Medicaid debate did not bog down over "restructuring." President Clinton's initial budget had included a proposal for Medicaid per capita caps but that was dropped because of its unpopularity with the governors—who saw it as either a nightmare or a booby trap, and perhaps both.[80] As a result, debate centered more on flexibility versus beneficiary protection within the existing program. The Clinton budget also included a child health initiative that would at least acknowledge the estimated five million poor children without insurance. This began as a modest proposal: $8.6 billion over five years, of which only $3.7 billion would be for Medicaid.[81] This initial child health commitment grew to $16 billion in the budget resolution and $24 billion in the final reconciliation, but that is another story (*infra,* 263-264). The budget resolution called for $17.5 billion in five-year savings from Medicaid, most of it to come from the DSH subsidy.[82] The amount was comparatively low, in part, because the Medicaid baseline was low; but the DSH cuts were high because only minor savings were expected from the flexibility amendments.

Medicaid and SCHIP

An important result of the favorable economic and political environment of 1997 and of the unusual, if not eccentric, budget reconciliation of that year was constructive debate and the enactment of some moderate, bipartisan reforms that are broadly important for the future of Medicaid. The actual changes in the Medicaid program were relatively modest: some flexibility amendments and some managed care regulation that brought new perspective to the debates over flexibility versus protectiveness. SCHIP, the major new initiative, was a huge expansion in coverage, that also sharpened the issue of how much and how Medicaid eligibility should grow.

Medicaid in the House

For Medicaid, the approach agreed upon was increased flexibility for the states compensated for or softened by additional beneficiary protections. This formula represented in part the wisdom of experience, acquired in the budget struggles of 1995 and 1996. There was a widely shared view that nothing else would work. This approach was also endorsed by the NGA, part of the budget summit, and incorporated in the budget resolutions of the House and the Senate. At the same time, the changes proposed for Medicaid amounted to a partial restructuring of the program and a shift toward a new philosophy. Partisans disagreed about how much flexibility was a good thing and what protections were needed, but they were at least talking about an issue that lent itself to constructive compromise.[83]

In the Commerce bill, "State Flexibility" was the first and longest chapter, providing broadly for greater freedom with respect to managed care, payment methodologies, eligibility and benefits, and dropping or easing a number of administrative requirements.

A high priority for the NGA and Republicans was repeal of the Boren Amendment (*supra,* 131). This amendment, which set legislative standards for determining hospital and nursing home rates largely enforced by lawsuits, was replaced with a public notice and comment procedure. There were objections on behalf of providers, the elderly, and the mentally retarded, but governors disliked being sued and having their budgets upset. Moreover, Boren Amendment repeal had acquired strong emotive and symbolic content, especially among Republican governors, and was supported by the Clinton administration.

One of the most important flexibility amendments was to allow states, without a waiver, to restrict provision of Medicaid benefits to managed care plans, including primary care case management (PCCMs), so long as there were at least two plans available. Related to this provision was repeal of the 75/25 restriction on risk contracts, which required plans to limit Medicaid recipients to 75% of the total enrolled. In addition, the threshold amount for managed care contracts requiring the secretary's approval was raised from $100,000 to $1 million.[84]

These amendments illustrated a central problem with the House bill. Eliminating the 1915(b) waiver requirement gave states more freedom to manage—not just managed care plans but also the Medicaid recipients. Repealing the Boren Amendment removed an irritant for the governors, but took away an enforceable protection for providers and, indirectly, for vulnerable population, such as the elderly and persons with disabilities. Categories such as these—the institutionalized, persons with severe disabilities, the frail elderly, and the chronically and severely ill were, and continue to be, a "problem" population. They were expensive, in 1997 making up a third of the Medicaid population, but accounting for two-thirds of Medicaid expenses. They were also difficult to treat and often without resources, so that some state agencies or at-risk managed care plans would like to avoid them. Both the House and Senate bills sought to balance flexibility with essential protections for this population, but Democrats and Republicans disputed what was essential and what protections would be effective.

An underlying presumption of this legislation was that an increasing amount of care under Medicaid would be provided by PCCMs and managed care plans. Therefore, much of the protection for beneficiaries would have to be provided by regulation or other measures affecting the behavior of these plans, which posed two second-order problems. One was that the federal government did not contract with or pay these plans, the states did. Therefore, regulations or incentives had to take an appropriate account of this mediated relationship. The other second-order problem was that Medicare and Medicaid managed care plans were different, so that experience relevant for the one was not necessarily applicable to the other.

What was needed along with this devolution of operational activities was a workable method for monitoring them and assuring their quality. Fortunately, state Medicaid officials, private accrediting bodies, and HCFA had begun in 1992 to work on a Quality Assurance Reform Initiative (QARI), a project specifically designed to improve state quality measures and help implement systems of quality assurance and improvement. This project was sufficiently well developed that it was proposed by John Dingell (D., Mich.) for inclusion as part of the Medicaid amendments in BBA '95. By 1997, there was a broad consensus that quality standards for Medicaid HMOs were needed. It was also understood to be part of the budget summit agreement on Medicaid. The NGA did not endorse it, but expressed no objection, and was mostly concerned that it be included in the planning.[85]

A notable feature of the quality improvement provision was its adaptation to the realities and constraints of the federal system and the Medicaid program—structuring and encouraging a process but leaving much to the discretion of the states and their Medicaid agencies. The standards were intended to be about midway in scope and prescriptiveness between Medicare and the child health plans.[86] State agencies were to develop and implement a "quality assurance and improvement strategy" consistent with standards that the Secretary would "establish and monitor" (Sec. 3461). The state efforts must include standards of access to care, and procedures for "monitoring the quality and appropriateness of care" for a "full spectrum" of the population enrolled under the managed care contract, "regular and periodic" examinations of the quality improvement strategy, and "other aspects of care and service directly relating to the improvement of quality of care (including grievance procedures and marketing and information standards." Compliance with these requirements could be "deemed" when an MCO met the standards of, and was approved by, an accepted private accrediting body such as NCQA or JCAHO. Implied in this approach was, of course, an encouragement for states to act on their own initiative and to go farther than the secretary's prescriptions.

The emphasis is upon a "strategy" and a process, rather than a specific CQI methodology in contrast, for example, to the House Medicare amendments of 1995 (Sec. 1852(e)) and 1997 (also Sec. 1852(e)). In part, that was because quality improvement was seen as central to a largely "devolutional" objective. It could help improve the organizational culture and aspirations in Medicaid managed care and in state agencies, establish a basis for delegation of responsibilities, and move away from federal micro-management, replacing a command and control approach to administration with internalized standards. A number of the leadership states were already heading in this direction and clamoring for more "flexibility." Assuming that these states would increasingly buy into this approach, the movement could encourage emulation and help bring other states closer to a common standard and to "mainstream" provider behavior.[87] Politically, the initiative looked good, had widespread provider acceptance, and was being pushed by the administration.

"Professionalism" in Medicaid administration might be a misdirected and fatuous hope, but pride in and loyalty to state programs and a striving for steady improvement characterized many Medicaid programs and these attitudes should be acknowledged and used. The quality improvement initiative was one attempt to invest in and capitalize on these resources.

Improving quality of care, though, does not necessarily protect patients' or consumers' rights, especially against those not concerned about quality or who arbitrarily exclude from or terminate care. "Managed care reform" and patients' bills of rights was one of those poorly examined ideas whose time had apparently come, with bills aimed at HMOs sprouting in a number of states and in the House and Senate. At first, much of the animus was anti-HMO and aimed at MCOs serving the public generally, but the movement was blocked by ERISA[88] and by opposition in the Senate, mostly from Republicans. Nevertheless, some of the ideas seemed sensible and had strong bipartisan support, especially in the House, and several of the "patients'" and provider rights proposals found their way into the Medicare and Medicaid provisions of BBA '97.

The "prudent layperson" standard for access to emergency care was popular at the time and not especially controversial since most managed care plans saw its adoption as inevitable. In the Commerce version, a Medicaid managed care plan would be required to provide emergency medical services, without regard to prior authorization, in the case of "acute symptoms of sufficient severity" such that "a prudent layperson ... could reasonably expect the absence of immediate medical attention to result in (1) placing the health of the individual (including a mother and unborn child) in serious jeopardy; (2) serious impairment of bodily functioning; or (3) serious dysfunction of any bodily part or organ." Also included was responsibility for post-stabilization care that would conform to guidelines established for Medicare Plus plans under Part C of Title XVIII.

A second patient protection was a ban on "gag rules," which were MCO protocols prohibiting plan providers from advocating courses of treatment, devices, or prescriptions that might be appropriate for the patient but would be contrary to or undermine a policy of the MCO—such as recommending drugs more expensive than those in the MCO formulary. Included with this provision was an exception for an HMO that had "moral or religious grounds" against covering such a service, *e.g.,* abortions or reproductive services.[89] This was one illustration of a Medicaid issue that does not go away. The Hyde Amendment,[90] first passed in 1976, came up repeatedly in the Medicaid debates of 1997 and was again included in the DHEW appropriations for that year.

Another patient protection, included in the flexibility provisions, would have required that the length of a hospital stay be determined by the attending physician and not, as Rep. Tom Coburn of Oklahoma put it, by an "insurance clerk 600 miles away."[91] This provision was pushed by three House Republicans who were health care professionals: Tom Coburn (Okla.) and Gregg Ganske (Iowa) who were physicians, and Charlie Norwood (Ga.) who was a dentist. Within the House, they were lead supporters of Norwood's bill, the Patients' Access and Responsible Care Act (PARCA), and they and many Republicans were prepared to vote for this bill against their own leadership.

An important addition to patient protections was to mandate an appeals process. The Commerce bill included practices of some of the better HMOs with several popular additions and some weighty legal language. There had to be a "meaningful and expedited" procedure for resolving "grievances" that would meet "notice and hearing" requirements. And plans were required to establish a board of appeals that would include plan representatives, consumers who were not plan enrollees, and providers expert in the relevant field of medicine. Filed complaints were to be resolved within thirty days. External review or appeal to the courts was not included, but there was legal language about "notice and hearing" and consumer and provider representation on the board that seemed calculated to give the enrollee a timely and fair hearing without disrupting plans or driving providers away.

This approach seemed to seek a realistic balance between beneficiary protection and the interests of Medicaid managed care plans. But writing legislation for a grievance procedure is not easy, and the Senate essentially passed on this one, specifying only that Medicaid MCOs had to establish an "internal grievance procedure" under which a member could "challenge the denial of coverage ... or payment..." of plan services.[92] This was the version adopted by the conference, leaving most of the issues to be resolved in the managed care implementing regulations (*infra,* 267-269).[93]

Associating Medicaid with the quality improvement movement was one way to internalize standards and improve performance. There were other ways in which the Commerce bill sought to raise quality. One approach was to raise entry requirement for new HMOs, for instance, by requiring Medicaid HMOs to meet the same solvency standards set by a state for private HMOs or certification by the state as a risk bearing entity.[94] Regulating of marketing materials and practices would have a similar effect.

The marketing requirements were tough and highly prescriptive, similar to those required for Medicare HMOs. Under these provisions, all managed care marketing materials had to be approved by the state—consulting with a medical advisory board—before they could be used. The secretary would prescribe "procedures and conditions" necessary to insure enrollees "accurate oral and written" information sufficient to make an informed decision. HMOs found guilty of distributing false or misleading materials would be barred from the program.[95] Targeting specifically some objectionable practices, HMOs were required to market the entire service area and refrain from "directly or indirectly" conducting "door-to-door, telephonic, or other 'cold call' approaches." [96]

The House bill included several[97] provisions extending coverage for Medicaid beneficiaries. Children under 18 years of age were allowed a year of continuous coverage once eligibility had been established. The capitated Program of All-Inclusive Care of the Aged (PACE) was made a permanent option of Medicaid as it already was for Medicare. The requirement of a prior institutionalization in order to receive habilitation services from a home health agency was abolished. But in some respects, the beneficiaries did not make out so well. The Boren Amendment was repealed and states could mandate enrollment in managed care plans. Contrary to the Democrats' understanding of the budget summit, only $500 million, not $1.5 billion was included to pay for the premiums of low-income Medicaid beneficiaries.[98] And another measure that seemed gratuitously stingy to Democrats was the phasing down of cost reimbursement for Federally Qualified Health Centers (FQHCs) and Rural Health Centers (RHCs)[99]

An important task for the Commerce Committee was to get Medicaid savings of $17 billion, as agreed by the budget summit. Initially, this was thought to be an easy task since the flexibility provisions were expected to produce $8 billion in savings and the rest could come from DSH payments. But CBO scored flexibility savings at a mere $2.9 billion and later lowered that to $1.8 billion. It also added a 25% "offset" to the DSH savings on the reasonable assumption that DSH gambits such as provider taxes and IGTs would continue in existing or new forms.[100] One response of the Commerce Committee was to reduce by $1 billion the $10 billion that had been allotted for low-income Medicaid beneficiaries.[101] Beyond that, the Committee stubbornly refused to accept the CBO scoring and reported out savings based on its own estimate. The staff also devised a complicated formula for DSH savings that hit high-DSH states the hardest, especially New York, Florida, Louisiana, and Texas, all represented on the Senate Finance Committee. Included in the committee report was an essay on the plight of the safety-net hospitals and the pernicious effects of relying on DSH funds for Medicaid savings.[102]

Medicaid in the Senate

In 1997, child health was occupying center stage in the Senate, with less attention directed to Medicaid. On many items, the Senate went along with the House. But there were fundamental differences relating to "flexibility" and how much and what kind of beneficiary protections needed to accompany these amendments. These differences continue to this day and have much to do with the two-tiered approach of Medicaid and SCHIP that was established then.

The flexibility provisions of the Senate bill resembled those of the House, up to a point. The Boren Amendment was repealed and a public notice and comment procedure substituted. States no longer needed a waiver to enroll beneficiaries in a PCCM or a managed care plan. But when it came to underlying philosophy and the limits to flexibility, the similarities ended. Sen. Chafee and a bipartisan coalition of health care liberals and moderates put together a new Sec. 1932,[103] of some 16 pages and lengthy, detailed paragraphs designed to ensure that enhanced protection went along with increased flexibility and to extend to Medicaid many of the standards and protections that existed for Medicare beneficiaries.[104]

Unlike the House bill, in which much of the emphasis was upon "flexibility," the Senate bill put first the new Sec. 1932, which was primarily about beneficiary protection, and had flexibility amendments in the next chapter. This new section went with particularity into the enrollment process, setting up requirements similar to those for Medicare managed care plans.[105] Violations were included under a new section on "fraud and abuse" and penalties strengthened by requiring that states contracting with MCOs have in place "intermediate sanctions" other than contract termination for these and other violations. While not as detailed as the Sec. 1847 Medicare+Choice marketing and enrollment procedures, the Medicaid requirements were similar in general principles and stringency and notable for the fraud and abuse provisions.

The Senate also required managed care quality standards: in theory a substitute for the 75/25 formula, as well as a complement to or constraint upon the flexibility provisions. Again, Sen. Chafee's initiative was important. He had long supported both legal protections for patients' rights and managed care quality standards. In 1995, he introduced an earlier version of quality standards that failed to pass.[106] The Breaux-Chafee bill of 1997 built on this earlier initiative and was adopted almost word-for-word in BBA '97.

In the final legislation, states were required to develop a "quality assessment and improvement strategy" in which the emphasis was not upon "strategy' or process but upon specific standards. Under "quality" the Senate version also included—in addition to quality and appropriateness of care—access standards, patients' rights and grievance procedures, and "marketing and information" standards. The access standards came from Sen. Chafee's concern over Medicaid managed care plans that promised but did not deliver. They were quite prescriptive, including ratios of primary care practitioners to enrollees, access and appropriate referral to specialists, services for children with special needs and, finally, delivery of services on a 24/7 basis. Also included under quality assurance were data requirements, external independent review of quality outcomes and timeliness and access to services.[107]

Sec. 1932 incorporated a heading on "Increased Beneficiary Protections" (Sec. 4704 in the BBA) that took notice that managed care posed special problems of beneficiary protection. Given the rising storm over patients' rights and "managed care reform," the provisions were remarkable for their restraint. They start with a requirement that each contract with a managed care entity shall "specify the benefits the provision (or arrangement) for which the entity is responsible." Assured coverage of emergency services is included with a "prudent layperson" standard and "severe pain" as one of the criteria. Gag rules were outlawed.[108] An internal grievance procedure was mandated. MCOs had to provide "adequate assurances" both to the state and to the secretary of their capacity to serve the expected enrollment.[109] Enrollees were also protected against debts or payment defaults by the MCO or balance billing by its sub-contractors. In retrospect, this modest effort seems prudent, especially in light of later unproductive fights over patients' rights.

The Medicaid fraud and abuse protections were originally part of a comprehensive approach developed by Sen. Bob Graham (D., Fla.) and his staff that included both Medicare and Medicaid. Sen. Graham, who had been a state legislator and a governor, was familiar with Medicaid, with HMOs, and with fraud and abuse. The Medicaid fraud and abuse provisions dealt with Medicaid managed care under Sec. 1932 and with other providers and practices under Sec. 4724 of BBA '97 as amendments to Secs. 1902 and 1903 of the Medicaid act.

These amendments aimed especially at moderate and usable measures to deter or prevent fraud and abuse rather than increase the penalties for offenses. Directors of MCO boards could not have more than a 5% proprietary interest in the plan. Surety bonds of not less than $50,000 were required for home health agencies or suppliers of durable medical equipment.[110] States could terminate contracts or refuse to contract with any person or entity convicted of a felony determined to be "inconsistent with the best interests of the beneficiaries" under the state plan (Sec. 4724(d)). And Medicaid brokers had to be independent of any plan or provider in the state, have no financial interest in participating MCO, and not previously excluded from participating in any Medicare or Medicaid plan, debarred from any federal agency, or subjected to a civil monetary penalty under a Medicaid statute.

These Medicaid fraud and abuse amendments both supported and were supported by the provisions dealing with quality and with marketing and enrollment, both of which strengthened the proactive and preventive approach: the first by tending to screen out shoddier plans and the second by preventing shady marketing practices.

The conference was not especially important for Medicaid, largely because there was little left to resolve. Benefits for the SLMBs,[111] disabled legal immigrants,[112] and the "SSI kids"[113] had already been largely settled and occasioned little difficulty in conference. However, the conferees continued to tussle over Medicaid DSH until the end and provided another example of how Congress is likely to deal with complex distributive issues. Neither the House nor the Senate had resolved this matter, leaving it to the conference. Initially, the conference would let the individual state decide: pick whichever formula—House or Senate—it preferred. But twelve of the high-DSH states disliked both formulas and lobbied the conference for a better one. Meanwhile, the CBO was persuaded to reduce its offset from 25% to 15%, the DSH cuts were readjusted so that no state would lose more than 3.5% of its total funding, and $600 million was allotted to help out four states—Texas, New York, New Jersey, and Missouri—each with large numbers of low-income uninsured beneficiaries. Congress then wrote into law the lesser of the House or Senate DSH cuts for each state.[114]

In one of those vagaries of the legislative process, the Senate restrictions on payments to Institutions for Mental Diseases (IMDs) and other mental institutions remained but the conference extended mental health parity to Medicaid managed care and to SCHIP by prohibiting the use of lower annual caps or lifetime limits for mental health coverage than for physical illnesses or injuries. The conference report made the Hyde Amendment permanent for Medicaid and extended it to SCHIP funding.[115]

An oddity in both House and Senate bills that survived the conference was language that "a person who, for a fee, assists an individual to dispose of assets" to qualify for a nursing home would be liable to a fine and/or imprisonment. This replaced an earlier version in HIPAA known as the "Granny Goes to Jail" law that made the elderly person directly liable. Most people thought that "Granny's Lawyer Goes to Jail" was equally ridiculous and probably unconstitutional on its face. Janet Reno, then the attorney general, said she would not allocate any funds to defend the provision should it be challenged in court.

State Children's Health Program

A widely shared presumption in 1997 was that *something* would be done about the ten million or more uninsured children in the United States. There was less agreement about the size of the problem, its sources, or what to do about it. Much of the concern grew from a recognition that despite continuing prosperity and years of effort by government the number of uninsured children had remained about the same since 1989 with an increasing percentage failing to get critically needed attention.[116] One reason for this state of affairs was that employers were providing less insurance or none at all. In 1996, according to a GAO report, 18 million people worked for corporations that provided no health insurance and another five million that covered employees but not their families.[117] Among the estimated 10.5 million uninsured children, 3.5 million were not enrolled by their parents because of transience, the stigma attached, lack of motivation or ignorance about the program. Down the list but especially distressing were the "SSI kids," of whom 308,000 would lose their eligibility over the next five years because of welfare reform.[118]

The various proposals being floated early in 1997 illustrated different aspects of the problem and demonstrated that it was not only, or even primarily, a health problem and that the solutions proposed depended upon who was speaking, their jurisdiction, and the resources they controlled. The earliest initiative came from President Clinton, who needed to repair some of the political damage left by welfare reform. In his February budget he put $9.8 billion on the table to help pay for insurance for temporarily unemployed workers—not a huge sum, but it indicated serious intentions. For children, he proposed mainly enrolling eligibles and extending coverage for one year for children losing coverage because of welfare reform or other reasons.[119] Senators Hatch and Kennedy were first with a major child health initiative, proposing early in March a block grant to be paid for by an increase in the tobacco tax. Phil Gramm (R., Tex.), chairman of the Senate Republican healthcare task force, proposed the addition of $3.75 billion to the Maternal and Child Health block grant, a minimal and inexpensive alternative that would be paid for by reducing the Earned Income Tax Credit (EITC). Tom Daschle, the Senate minority leader, and Bill Thomas (R., Calif.), chairman of the Health Subcommittee of Ways and Means, both favored tax credits to help the working poor pay for coverage. There were others, including Sen. Specter's proposal for health care vouchers. There were in fact, so many bills that progress was impeded by inability to agree on any one.[120] Moreover, these were stand-alone bills, without broad authorizations to draw upon, and "new taxes" that were not popular. They failed to win support.[121]

On April 24th, as negotiations over the budget resolution were nearing a conclusion, Sens. Chafee and Rockefeller announced a different approach that was clean and simple, though controversial. It would expand Medicaid to cover children in families up to 150% of the FPL, an increase from 133% of FPL. States that chose this option would receive a bonus of 30% increase in their matching rate for the children enrolled. Like the president's bill, it included continuous Medicaid coverage for a year and $25 million for outreach. Costs were estimated at $15 billion over five years, but nothing was said about how that sum would be raised.

As was common in the Senate, much support had been secured in advance and it was apparent that this bill would be a major contender. It was bipartisan, and had been endorsed by both Hatch and Kennedy and by nine Democrats and six Republicans. Six of this group were on the Senate Finance Committee, so this bill quickly became the main alternative to Gramm's proposal. It also had the support of a number of Democrats on the House Commerce Committee, including John Dingell and Henry Waxman.

Despite this strong support, the Chafee-Rockefeller Medicaid expansion was by no means an easy winner in the Senate. It was opposed by the chairman and conservative Republicans as well as several key Democrats on the Senate Finance Committee and in direct competition with the Gramm proposal. A compromise between the two major bills was cobbled together by Trent Lott (R., Miss.), the majority leader, but that satisfied neither side.

Meanwhile, seething discontent within the NGA because of the meager concessions they were getting on Medicaid issues came to a boil over the Chafee-Rockefeller proposal, which they categorically rejected.[122] Following this action by the governors, four members of the Finance Committee withdrew their support, and the administration began looking for a viable compromise.

Within the House, a Medicaid approach had been debated, but Republicans generally— including Commerce Committee Republicans—were strongly, even passionately, opposed to a straight Medicaid expansion, both as policy and as principle, or ideology. None of the early initiatives had begun in the House, except for a tax credit proposed by Bill Thomas. Newt Gingrich had appointed a task force to consider the issue, but mostly in order to have a counter-proposal to Hatch-Kennedy. Meanwhile, child health was a popular cause, for which money was being found in various ways,[123] and in the House budget resolution grew to $16 billion. The $16 billion was allocated to both Commerce and Ways and Means without specifying how much each committee got. This led to a brief jurisdictional dispute or "turf war" between Commerce chairman Thomas Bliley—who wanted to use the money for grants to the states, and Bill Thomas, chairman of the health subcommittee of Ways and Means, who wanted it for tax incentives to purchase insurance. When Thomas eventually receded, the way was open for the Commerce Committee to develop a major proposal.

The Child Health Assistance Program (CHAP) was the Commerce Committee's five year, $14.4 billion program of health grants to the states. This bill was the basis for SCHIP. In structure and general policy, it resembled closely the block grant proposal of 1995, though adapted for child health. A separate paragraph stated that "nothing in this title" should be construed as creating an entitlement under a "State child health plan." But a number of state plan requirements were set forth, including approval by the secretary, laying out of strategic objectives, performance goals and measures, and methods for monitoring results, with extensive reporting requirement to the secretary.

Beneficiaries were protected in several standard ways under the state plans. Eligibility had to be spelled out. Outreach activities and enrollment assistance were mandated. Pre-existing conditions could not be invoked to exclude an otherwise eligible person. Child health assistance must make available including, as a minimum, inpatient and outpatient hospital care, physician and laboratory services, and well-baby and well-child health care with preventive care and primary dental care. Premiums and cost sharing could be used, but must take a fair account of family income. Access to specialty care for children with chronic or life-threatening conditions also had to be assured.

A state that qualified could receive 80% funding of its program—with a 20% match required—up to the limit of its allotment, which was based on the number of low-income children and a "state cost-factor" that reflected average wages within the state. The allotment could be spent for Medicaid expansion, group health plans or private insurers, direct services from providers, outreach or other health related activities set forth in the state plan. The allotment could also be used for Medicaid expansion, and a small fund of $2 million with a different matching rate was set aside for that purpose. Administrative and non-assistance activities were also allowable, with a cap of 15% of the CHAP expenditures.

The child health provision was settled in conference, in large measure through the prospective contributions of the tobacco industry and cigarette smokers. After the mid-June NGA rejection, Breaux-Chafee was dropped, leaving the House Commerce CHAP proposal as the only plausible alternative. With Medicaid expansion blocked, the White House was even more committed to an increased authorization for child health and a robust benefit package. But early in the conference, the momentum was going the other way, with the conferees moving back toward a $16 billion proposal with a flexible benefits package.[124]

In connection with the Hatch-Kennedy proposal, though, the Finance Committee had agreed to a 20¢ increase in the cigarette tax and to earmark $8 billion of the revenues for child health. This decision by Finance did not bind the conference, but President Clinton took a strong position on $24 billion and increased benefits for child health and congressional Democrats weighed in, with Sen. Daschle threatening that the August recess might have to be postponed. The solution, first put forward by the White House and some lead conference negotiators, was to reduce the cigarette tax somewhat and move it from the tax side of the reconciliation to the spending side, which would leave the net tax reduction the same, add $8 billion to the child health authorization, and make it immediately available.[125] This formula was discussed at the top level by White House negotiators and the Senate Republican leadership, after which, as Sen. Nickles put it, "We started letting them know where we feel we could compromise and they did the same."[126]

Often a good predictor of durable bargains is that both sides walk away claiming victory. That was true for SCHIP, the child health legislation.[127] But another good test is that no one is too satisfied. SCHIP also passed that test. The grand compromise over basic structure was that each state would be free to use the funds in three different ways. It could choose to use all of its allotment for Medicaid expansion, or for SCHIP, or for both. This was contrary to the Senate version, which would have required states to choose one or the other, in part to avoid confusion but also to prevent slow encroachment upon state Medicaid programs. The act contained a proviso that children found to be eligible for Medicaid had to be enrolled in that program. But allowing both Medicaid and SCHIP was an important concession to flexibility (Sec. 2102(b)(3)(B)).

The benefits package had been from the beginning a major source of disagreement. The House version had a minimal list of services with additions of well baby and well child care, immunizations, and a prohibition against discrimination.[128] The Senate version called for health services equivalent to Blue Cross-Blue Shield PPO coverage under the FEHBP. These differences gave rise to considerable negotiation with the result that two other "benchmark" plans were added: 1) any state employees' health plan; or (2) the health plan of the HMO with the largest commercial enrollment.[129] Also, three existng state child health programs were "grandfathered" into SCHIP: New York, Florida, and Pennsylvania.

The use of SCHIP funds for direct purchase of services was a major issue. This was only one of several opportunities for cost shifting created by the new program and that would not be apparent to the inexperienced. It helps illustrate why Medicaid financing is an insiders' game in which often the moves are understood only if their objective is known. For instance, under Sec. 2105 (Payment for the States), subsection (d) (Maintenance of Effort) strictly prohibits any state from adopting Medicaid eligibility standards more restrictive than those in force as of June 1, 1997—this, of course, to prevent a state from evading the requirement that children found to be eligible for Medicaid would be enrolled in that program—which had a lower federal match. Subsection (d) then goes on to say that the state could count in-kind, county, or other federal funds for matching.[130] In other words, take from Peter to pay Paul. The direct purchase was another cost-shifting device: in this instance, by targeting payments either to favored contractors or DSH hospitals and safety-net providers. The Republicans wanted 15% of the total allotment for direct purchases and the Democrats none. Eventually they compromised on 10% but then created a waiver authority allowing direct payments for cost-effective "community based" hospitals.[131] To the cynical, this would seem like an opportunity for the ingenious to evade the DSH limitations and possibly help some friends as well. Still, as one Republican staff aide observed, the Medicaid infrastructure needs support, especially in poor states—an observation illustrating the moral complexities of these issues.

Regulatory Implementation

Developing the implementing regulations for the Medicare and Medicaid titles of BBA '97 involved more than 300 identifiable tasks and projects. Neither program was fundamentally "restructured" by the legislation or its implementation, but both were modified in detail and recast in important ways and both programs became *more* regulative, especially with respect to managed care, quality standards, fraud and abuse, and cost containment.

Producing these regulations was significantly more difficult because of HCFA reorganization which was gathering momentum as this regulatory process began. While reorganization may have worked in the long run toward greater effectiveness, in the short run it did not, since it separated experienced work groups, dispersed expertise, and disrupted communications—important particularly in the early stages of rulemaking when understanding the issues, identifying the problems and tasks, and agreeing about policies are essential preliminaries to writing the regulatory texts and "preambles." This situation was made worse by the resignation of Bruce Vladeck, a popular and effective leader who had been the administrator since January 1993. People worked around these difficulties, but they cost much in time, energy, and stress.

The "Y2K" problem[132] was a gratuitous and additional complicating factor that affected Medicaid rulemaking at two levels. At the federal level, the impact was mostly indirect, slowing their efforts when the Medicaid task forces needed computer time, numbers or expertise, or a decision from Medicare policy people or technicians. More troublesome was a second part, assuring that the states and Medicaid managed care providers were also Y2K compliant so that they could continue to participate in the program. This was not strictly a part of rulemaking, but it was essential for initial implementation, and kept HCFA officials busy "jawboning" laggards until the end of 1999.

Developing regulations of great scope and complexity within acceptable time limits was another major challenge.[133] The Medicaid staff's primary experience was with state plans and waivers and negotiating with state agencies, not with the nuances of legislation, developing the operative concepts and language for new programs or making clear to regulation writing staff what the preamble and text of a regulation should communicate. Nevertheless, the draft regulations for Medicaid managed and for SCHIP were published in less than fifteen months—a testimony to hard work and adaptiveness.[134]

The SCHIP regulation began with the convening of a large task force co-chaired by Deborah Chang from HCFA and Earl Fox from HRSA.[135] The "HHS CHIP Steering Committee,"[136] as it was known, had over 100 representatives from some 40 organizations within the DHHS. It met twice a week over the next year and a half, to sort out priorities, get people to "take ownership" of projects, and monitor progress.

Almost immediately, state plans and waiver requests began trickling in, without criteria or standards to guide decisions on approval. As a result, most of the policy decisions for the SCHIP regulation were made on an *ad hoc* basis, much like case law. Each plan had, within HCFA, a point person and a review team, with representatives from the steering committee, OMB, and the White House. Larger issues or task priorities that arose from this process would be dealt with as occasion demanded: by a task force, or developing policy papers and reviewing options. Failing agreement, final appeal was to Kevin Thurm, the deputy secretary of DHHS. Issues once settled were not to be re-opened except under extreme circumstances.[137]

The steering committee recast its emerging policies, with comments, into a growing list of "Questions and Answers," some quite elaborate, publishing them in installments both in print and on the internet, for the guidance of regional and state officials, providers, consumer groups, and interested parties. As they learned from this iterative process, members of the steering committee formulated policy guidelines to be communicated through "Dear Director" letters. They also worked with the National Academy for State Health Policy to draft a model state plan for SCHIP. As this work moved forward, smaller, specialized task forces were formed to develop recommendations and policies on waivers, "crowd out,"[138] cost sharing and direct expenditures; to collect data on eligibility and enrollment; create a monitoring instrument; and prepare state and regional officials for "going live." Meanwhile, working from these materials and collaborating with regulation writers in Baltimore, a small task force developed most of the proposed regulation. One dividend of the steering committee procedure was that most of the difficult issues of policy or procedure had been resolved along the way, so that the regulation was largely a codification of this experience and, according to several HCFA officials, almost "wrote itself." The proposed rule was published on November 9, 1998, fourteen months after the passage of BBA '97, allowing time for a full "roll out" and OMB clearance.

The steering committee approach was especially useful in working with the states. Officials in each state knew the membership of their review teams and were in frequent communication with them. HCFA officials would allow the states to file "placeholder" state plans and would work with them to achieve approval on technical or difficult matters, such as enrollment procedures, maintenance of effort, or "crowding out."[139]

The managed care regulation was much more difficult and perplexing, especially for Medicaid people with little or no experience in regulative policy development or writing. As with Medicare regulations, the managed care regulation was aimed at health care delivery and changing managed care behavior, for which legal precision was important. But its operation, like Medicaid directives generally, would be indirect, addressed in the first instance to state agencies and beyond that, to their relations with HMOs and other managed care entities—a task sometimes calling for studied ambiguity or pregnant silence. Despite the conference agreement, moreover, there remained major differences between House and Senate as to how regulative or prescriptive to be and often a lack of clarity with respect to such open textured notions as quality improvement, access, or grievance. And the White House had its point of view and strong commitments on a number of items, most importantly in the present context, the "Consumer Bill of Rights and Responsibilities," which had been mandated for all federal agencies.[140] All that was needed was a preamble and text that would effectively regulate managed care entities, be adapted to the layered complexity of the Medicaid program, meet legal constraints (both the clear and the unclear) and be acceptable to the Congress, the White House, the states, the NGA, and the Medicaid constituency.[141] The regulation was not entirely successful, though it was a solid achievement, given such constraints.

The 385-page managed care proposed regulation was completed within the deadline and published in the Federal Register on August 28, 1998. It generated a huge number of comments, all of which had to be answered over the next fifteen months, some in great detail. The final regulation was published on the last day of the Clinton administration; and one of the first acts of the incoming Bush administration was to withdraw it from consideration.[142] The regulation was denounced by the NGA during its winter meeting in Washington, D.C. The Medicaid state directors, in response to a solicitation from the Bush administration, criticized almost every paragraph, singling out for special attention the quality provisions and the grievance procedures as "too detailed and prescriptive" and "over the top."[143] They criticized the SCHIP regulation as prescriptive and lacking flexibility as well, but with less hostility. Following three additional six-month delays, HCFA (CMS) postponed the regulation for another year, during which it published its own new and superseding regulation. The original managed care regulation never went into force.

This rising of the critical spirit was in part encouraged by the change of administration. It also represented increased partisanship within the Medicaid constituency, which included the NGA. But there were factors contributing to this development and evolutionary stages to be noted. Even before the passage of BBA '97, the governors expressed their disappointment over how little additional flexibility they were getting, especially with respect to benefits and services. Later, when the regulatory impact of the new legislation became clearer, they and the state directors complained of that as well, adding force to their earlier objections. The persistence of these objections is important, suggesting that whatever else the governors and state directors would like, they put a high priority on flexibility, fewer mandates, and less regulation. In this respect, BBA '97 and its implementing regulations upgraded the traditional Medicaid program, secured additional rights for he beneficiaries, and made Medicaid itself more like Medicare—but it may also have made it less attractive in comparison with SCHIP as a vehicle for expanding eligibility or coverage.

Other than getting BBA '97 implemented, little was done about either Medicare or Medicaid in the last years of the Clinton Administration. BBA '97 had called for a "Bipartisan Commission" on Medicare,[144] which proved, despite its title, to be highly partisan and failed to agree, but helped spawn the Medicare Advantage Act of 2003.[145] Patients' rights, *aka* "managed care reform," heated up in 1997 and diverted much attention from other health affairs for the next five years. President Clinton proposed a Medicare "buy in" for unemployed workers and a Medicare prescription drug benefit, neither of which passed. Medicaid initiatives included a program for workers with disabilities, optional home and community based coverage up to 300% of FPL, and "Family Care" coverage for families of children enrolled in either Medicaid or SCHIP. Republicans countered with various kinds of tax credits and deductions for the uninsured. In addition, there were several "give back" bills, increasing payments for providers who claimed hardship because of the harsh workings of the BBA '97 payment formulas.[146]

Two Cheers

Supporters of the Medicaid program could find grounds for reassurance and congratulation in the events of the '90s. Despite the successive disasters of health care reform and the election of 1994, the Medicaid entitlement was stoutly defended, the welfare link severed, SCHIP passed, and substantial progress made on quality standards, managed care regulation, and protections for persons with disabilities. Millions more were insured under Medicaid and SCHIP and billions of dollars saved through waivers and other methods of cost containment.

Some less visible achievements went along with the more obvious ones. Managed care was rehabilitated and became a major part of Medicaid service delivery. An important shift was begun from a "command and control" approach to regulation to a process oriented emphasis upon quality improvement. The SCHIP option provided a less constraining alternate way to cover higher income families and some of the working poor. And despite the mobilized and intensely partisan politics of the time most of these changes were made with bipartisan support in the House and Senate and among the Medicaid constituency.

In taking stock, though, it is important not to read too much into a particular victory. The failed assaults on the Medicaid entitlement in 1995-96 showed that Medicaid had more latent support than expected and that it could be successfully defended. But how much of that outcome should be attributed to institutional factors such as separation of powers, federalism, and the layered complexity of the Medicaid program, and how much to favoring circumstances, such as economic prosperity? How much should be attributed to the particular roles of President Clinton, key figures such as Henry Waxman and John Chafee, and to experienced and policy savvy staff? However these questions might be resolved, it is worth noting these defenses of Medicaid involved *both* institutional factors that worked well at the level of committees in the Congress *and* a strong presidential commitment and mobilization of the administration. Under the following Bush administration, the situation was quite different: a campaign to modify the Medicaid entitlement largely carried on independently of the Congress—leaving a question of how much, if any, of the past experience is relevant.

Progress was made over the decade, especially in exploiting the potential of program modifications made in the 1980s, such as incremental expansions of eligibility, flexibility amendments and waiver authority, and improved benefits and protections for persons with disabilities. But little was done to resolve differences over the entitlement status of Medicaid or "restructuring" of Medicaid, long-term cost increases, responsibility for the "dual eligibles," or the continuing demands for flexibility and devolution. Partisan mobilization, ideology, and underlying distrust made genuine collaboration on these larger issues impossible except occasionally or on tangential issues. These basic differences were walled off, resolved through pragmatic compromise, or finessed when that could be done without too much outcry or damage to principles.

One legacy of this period, in addition to eligibility expansion and numerous incremental modifications, was to leave behind a large amount of stored up frustration and demand for change. Two precedents from the past were also important. One was SCHIP, which got wide acceptance and was soon widely promoted, especially by those in the devolution camp, as a model for the Medicaid program itself. The other was the Sec. 1115 waiver (*Infra*, Ch. 8). Democrats had pioneered its use to expand Medicaid coverage during the 1990s, often with huge managed care systems. There seemed no reason, in principle, why it could not be used to provide greater freedom for the states, restructure state Medicaid programs more along the lines of SCHIP, and/or reduce them in size and scope. This was an ironic sequel, and a reminder about the danger of precedents.[147]

Notes

1.   Prior to the election, over 300 Republican incumbents and new candidates signed a "Contract with America" on the Capitol grounds to "change the nation." It contained a number of "hot button" issues well suited to mobilize the Republican base and ideological conservatives. Other important purposes were to nationalize the campaign and pre-select the issues, thereby adding to the plebiscitary nature of the election.
2.   Behind the Republican victory of 1994 was a long history—reaching back at least to 1964—of developing a message, cultivating attractive candidates, and nursing key constituencies. By 1994, a number of issues favored Republicans, such as crime and taxes, and Democrats had lost some core supporters over NAFTA and the tax legislation of 1993. Also, Republicans mobilized their own base effectively, while Democratic turnout was low. Interview with Christopher C. Jennings, June 23, 2005; *Congressional Quarterly Almanac* 1994, 561.
3.   "Rescinding" or canceling appropriations already made.
4.   Smith, *Entitlement Politics,* 50 ff.
5.   Medicare especially was postponed as too tough to take on at that time.
6.   Smith, *Entitlement Politics,* 47.
7.   *Ibid.,* 47.
8.   *Health Care Policy Report,* February 20, 1995, 269-270.
9.   Republicans had Medicaid grouped with welfare and food stamps, distinguishing it from "middle class" or "main street" entitlements such as Social Security and Medicare. Interview with Jennings, June 23, 2005.
10.   Howard Cohen, interview, January 13, 1999. Prospects for "stealing a march" were considerably improved by the low morale and disorganization of the House Democrats; also by the reduction of minority committee staffs.
11.   *Ibid.*
12.   Karen Nelson, interview by Smith, August 19, 1999.
13.   *Ibid.,* June 16, 1999.
14.   For a detailed account, see Smith, *Entitlement Politics,* ch. 3; also Elizabeth Drew, *Shutdown: The Struggle Between the Gingrich Congress and the Clinton White House.* New York: Simon & Schuster, 1996.
15.   the budget resolution figures are aggregated or global, not broken down into specific items or programs.
16.   Smith, *Entitlement Politics,* 73.
17.   Schneider, interview by Smith, June 5, 1999.
18.   Cohen, interview by Smith, May 19, 1999.

19. One issue that polled strongly was the repeal of the 1987 nursing home standards. This egregious misstep aroused a powerful bipartisan constituency that had been working for over twenty years on nursing home reform and it enabled Democrats to revive horrific images of grannies with untreated bedsores, strapped to gurneys, or dumped on the sidewalks. It played so well that Dick Armey, the formidable Republican chairman of the House Appropriations Committee, complained to a bipartisan gathering that he was getting telephone calls from his own mother asking why Congress was "being so mean" to the elderly. Jennings, interview by Moore and Smith, June 23, 2005.

20. According to Jennings, President Clinton was always a strong supporter of Medicaid—it was HCFA he didn't like. Whether any of these speculations is true, it seems plausible that the absence of a spirited defense might have been quite important.

21. The closest to an exception was the repeal of the nursing home standards, but that did not produce an organized or sustained public response. Notable for its absence was the AARP, a powerful lobby and advocacy group, that for reasons of its own was sitting this one out. Also, by then the Children's Defense Fund had shifted from Medicaid advocacy.

22. Since early in the 1980s, the AHA had functioned as an informally constituted leadership group for the not-for-profit hospitals, representing their interests collectively, especially in legislative activities and encouraged to do so by Congress

23. Herbert Kuhn, vice president for federal relations, AHA (Currently Deputy Administrator of CMS). Interview by Smith, January 13, 1999.

24. *Ibid.*

25. *Ibid.*

26. *Health Care Policy Report,* January 23, 1995, 205.

27. *Health Care Policy Report,* March 13, 1994, 412.

28. Mostly indications that "anything but" the 5% cap would be preferable, such as per capita caps, federal-state program swaps, and three block grants rather than one.

29. Interview by Smith, June 16, 1999.

30. The updates for the first seven years were specific dollar amounts. After that, the update would be the lesser of 4% or the growth in the Urban Consumer Price Index (CPI-U).

31. The state's "aggregate need" would be determined by four factors or indexes: the number of residents in poverty; a case-mix index taking account of aged, disabled, and other Medicaid recipients; an input (provider) cost index; and the ratio of the state's expected spending per recipient to the national average. "House Commerce Committee Staff Memo to Transform the Medicaid Program" September 18, 1995, as reprinted in *Health Care Policy Report,* September 25, 1995, 1545. The baseline for calculating an individual state's allocation was the state's expenditure in FY 1994. To this was to be added 14.3% (more precisely, 14.3193649139%) as a replacement for DSH payments. However, this add-on did not increase the total, it only redistributed the allocated amounts. *Ibid.,* 1545.

32. The FMAP would be the greater of the older FMAP or a new one based on the ratio of "total taxable resources" to population in poverty, this ratio to be multiplied by a factor to achieve budget neutrality. Payments under the existing FMAP varied from 50% to 83%. Under the new system, the FMAP would vary from 40% to 80%, *Ibid.,* 1545.

33. Cohen, interview by Smith, March 2, 2003.

34. *Health Care Policy Report,* September 18, 1995, p. 1438.

35. He died of a heart attack in October, 1999. His son, Lincoln Chafee, was elected to his Senate seat.
36. *Congressional Quarterly*, September 28, 1995, 2998.
37. *Congressional Quarterly Almanac,* 1995, 7-21.
38. *Ibid.*
39. *Ibid.*
40. Chafee lost on the issue of requiring the SSI definition of "disability." For a summary, see *Congressional Quarterly Almanac, 1995,* 7-19.
41. *E.g.,* California, Florida, Texas, and Nevada with low per capita expenditures. *Health Care Policy Report,* October 30, 2005, 1803.
42. Cost of living adjustment. *Health Care Policy Report,* November 6, 1995, 1840.
43. Not just the partisan battles, but also the enormous work, long hours, and stress involved in a major "policy effort," such as the BBA. For the useful concept, "policy effort," we are indebted to Gail Wilensky.
44. CBO projected the deficit (for the year) at $140 billion, the lowest (as percentage of GDP) in twenty years. *Congressional Quarterly*, March 29, 1996, 752.
45. *Health Care Policy Report,* February 12, 1996, 265.
46. P.L. 104-191, 1996.
47. Especially in the House, HIPAA acquired some add-ons intended either to increase support or to use the bill as a legislative vehicle. Some of these were left over from the vetoed BBA of '95, such as Medicare Savings Accounts, malpractice liability, and fraud and abuse. The medical malpractice section was stripped in the Senate and MSAs put on a trial basis. One short-term effect—important for the Balanced Budget Act of 1997—was to "cool out" these hot issues and reduce the scope of conflict for BBA '97.
48. *Health Care Policy Report,* January 29, 1996, 127.
49. *Health Care Policy Report,* February 12, 1996, 229.
50. In the initial Gingrich-Kasich version, and while the government was still running on continuing resolutions and debt limit extensions, the strategy was to condition debt limit extensions on White House support for these bills. This was tried with the NGA proposal but failed for a number of reasons: because the governors took too long to resolve their differences and their plan was unworkable; because the debt linkage probably would not survive a Senate filibuster; and because the House Republicans were bluffing and more afraid of another shutdown than were the Democrats. Cf. Smith, *Entitlement Politics*, 150.
51. *Ibid.,* 213.
52. The Medicaid bill relied heavily upon a draft recommended by the NGA, that was later repudiated by the Democratic governors. It was similar to the bill vetoed in 1995, and strongly opposed by President Clinton.
53. Smith, *Entitlement Politics,* 154.
54. In a presidential election year, to keep Clinton from getting credit for brokering a welfare bill.
55. *Health Care Policy Report,* July 15, 1996, 1044.
56. William J. Clinton, *My Life.* New York: Vintage, 2005, p. 720.
57. Christopher Jennings, health adviser to President Clinton, made an interesting distinction between welfare and health care: that not working was volitional, while illness or disability was not. Most people, he observed, did not blame a person for needing health care and were often willing to help those without insurance or struggling with disabilities. On the other hand, they thought people should work and would help the handicapped to work, but not without efforts on their part. Interview by Moore and Smith, June 23, 2005.

58.   Child advocates and staff from Congress and HCFA were aware there would be loss of Medicaid eligibility with people cycling in and out of TANF and began working on the Sec. 1931 legislation, especially with Sens. Chafee and Breaux and Rep. Nancy Johnson and their staffs. Sec. 1931 was included by the conference without being considered in committee or on the floor of either house. In addition to preventing loss of eligibility, another major concern was to promote some measure of uniformity in state rules covering Medicaid eligibility in relation to TANF. Cindy Mann, telephone interview by Smith, October 14, 2005; also Cohen, interview by Smith, July 21, 2005; and Schneider, interview by Smith, July 18, 2005.

59.   According to Schneider, the "less restrictive" income and resource methodologies concept followed the earlier 1902(r)(2) provision. But this language was patently expansive in its reach and OMB and HCFA had sought to limit it. Therefore, including 1931(b)(2)(C) was an emphatic way of saying that Congress wanted it clear that the earlier flexibility applied to TANF as well.

60.   At the same time, PRWORA was doing away with categorical eligibility, and some of those drafting Sec. 1931 saw it as opening the possibility for states to increase coverage of the working poor if they wished. Cindy Mann, Interview by Smith, October 14, 2005.

61.   Jason deParle, *American Dream.* New York: Viking, 2005, 213.

62.   Earlier regulations barred Medicaid eligibility for two-parent families if the principle wage-earner worked more than 100 hours per month. A 1998 regulation repealed this "100 hour" rule, allowed states to use an income test, and to ignore the distinction between one and two parent families. Cf. Schneider *et al. The Medicaid Resource Book,* 15.

63.   *Supporting Families in Transition: A Guide to Expanding Health Coverage in the Post-Welfare Reform World,* (Health Care Financing Administration, N.D.).

64.   *Congressional Quarterly*, February 1, 1997, 25.

65.   *Health Care Policy Report,* January 27, 2977, 138.

66.   *Ibid.,* January 13, 1997, 67.

67.   *Ibid.*

68.   Vladeck, interview by Smith, February 8, 1999.

69.   *Congressional Quarterly,* February 1, 1997, 275.

70.   *Health Care Policy Report*, January 27, 1997, 138.

71.   *Health Care Policy Report,* January 13, 1997, 66, 67.

72.   *Congressional Quarterly,* February 1, 1997, 275.

73.   Part of the White House strategy was *not* to push the Republicans to the point they developed their own budget since that would have mobilized them around an alternate budget rather than negotiating over the Clinton proposal.

74.   Chief of Staff Erskine Bowles, Office of Management and Budget director Franklin Raines, National Economic Council chairman Gene Sperling, and Legislative Affairs director, John Hilley.

75.   At the time, large sums of money were available because of the booming economy, high tax revenues, Medicare and Medicaid savings from waivers, the Prospective Payment System and Medicare physician fee schedule, and DSH reductions, so that the difference between $100 billion and $118 billion was not that important. Jennings, interview by Moore and Smith, June 23, 2005.

76.   *Congressional Quarterly,* May 3, 1997, 993.

77.   *Ibid.,* May 10, 1997, 1052.

78.   The large majorities—331-99 in the House and 78-22 in the Senate—did not indicate so much approval of the substantive provisions of the budget resolution

as the importance to both parties of having a deal at all. *Congressional Quarterly,* May 24, 1997, 1185.

79. Smith, *Entitlement Politics,* 182-185.
80. A nightmare because of interstate migration and the difficulties of tracking and monitoring individual accounts; a booby trap because governors would be stuck with expenses beyond the caps.
81. *Health Care Policy Report,* February 10, 1997, 218.
82. The net Medicaid savings would be only $13.6 billion, but there would be additional outlays of $4.2 billion that would need to be offset. This made the total $17.8 billion. After the budget resolution was adopted, CBO added a "behavioral" offset of 25%, to compensate for "adaptive" behavior by the states. This made a total of $21.6 billion in DSH savings, a number that caused great distress among the safety-net hospitals. *Health Care Policy Report,* May 26, 1997, 616-617.
83. Smith, *Entitlement Politics,* 115.
84. *Ibid.,* 202.
85. *Ibid.,* 122.
86. *Ibid.,* 123.
87. *Ibid.,* 124.
88. The Employee Retirement Income Security Act (ERISA) was enacted in 1974 primarily to protect pension benefits but was later extended to health plans. Under the so-called "ERISA pre-emption," large, self-insured "ERISA" health plans are largely exempt from state regulation and from most lawsuits, especially those for denial of benefits or malpractice that originate in a state. Large "Fortune 500" corporations have a big stake in keeping this immunity and trial attorneys would like to see it go. It is an understatement to say that the legal and policy issues were and are complicated.
89. The plan had to notify members of such a policy before or during enrollment or within 90 days of adopting such a policy.
90. Cf. P.L. 96-123 (1976). Rep. Henry Hyde (R., Ill.) submitted an amendment to a DHEW appropriations bill, which was passed in 1976 and renewed each year after that, providing that no federal Medicaid funds could be used to pay for abortions except where the mother's life is endangered or pregnancy results from rape or incest, promptly reported.
91. *Congressional Quarterly Almanac 1997,* 219.
92. "Special Supplement—Conference Managers Explanation of Medicaid, Child Health Agreements," *Sen. Rpt. S211,* August 4, 1997.
93. P.L. 105-33, Sec. 4794(b)(4), "Increased Beneficiary Protection."
94. This provision became part of the law. Sec. 4706, "Solvency Standards." One effect of such legislation, aside from raising the entry bar for Medicaid HMOs, would be to bring them under state insurance standards.
95. States participating in the program could not contract with them.
96. Sec. 4707(d)(2) of P.L. 105-33. A small but interesting point: these provisions were part of the Fraud and Abuse section.
97. Important because they and their parents would frequently lose eligibility with changes in income.
98. Democrats thought the summit agreement was to pay their Medicare premiums; Republicans that it was only to pay the *increments* in their premiums. Smith, *Entitlement Politics,* 115.
99. A category of special concern to Democrats. *Ibid.,* 202.
100. Ironically, this estimate was based on one of the Committee's own amendments reinstating provider taxes.

101. This was strenuously objected to by OMB director Franklin Raines and was restored in conference.
102. The Senate did come to the aid of the big states. But it also specified the allowable DSH savings for each state over the next five years and capped future DSH payments at no more than 12% of total Medicaid expenditures.
103. Senators Chafee, Graham, and Breaux were the primary figures, with Sen. Chafee the leader. The various provisions were combined in a Chafee-Breaux amendment based on an earlier Chafee bill dealing with quality and access standards for managed care and comprehensive fraud and abuse legislation initiated by Sen. Bob Graham (D. Fla.). Sen. Breaux and his staff assembled the parts and developed much of the language for the amendment.
104. It is interesting to note that the statute uses the term "beneficiary" rather than "recipient." According to a legislative aide, Sen. Chafee would have preferred to proceed incrementally and pragmatically, but also shared with Sen. Graham a desire to get as much as they could of the Medicare-type protections. Bruce Lesley, formerly staff aide to Sen. Chafee as well as Sen. Breaux. Interview by Smith, July 13, 2000.
105. In general, the Senate bill allowed restricting of Medicaid enrollment to MCOs, but exempted Native Americans, special needs children, and QMBs. It then goes with particularity into the enrollment process: requiring at least two plans to choose from; priority and default mechanisms; continuous enrollment for a year; opportunities to disenroll; and a long list of required information, including coverage, particulars about contracting providers, grievances and appeals procedures, and comparative information in "chart-like" form with quality and performance indicators.
106. S839, "The Medicaid Managed Care Act," included federal quality standards, curbs on marketing abuses and operating with inadequate staffing or facilities. It was intended for adoption in BBA '95. *Health Care Policy Report,* May 29, 1995, 875.
107. Most of this to be approved by or consistent with standards established by the secretary.
108. With an exception for objections on moral grounds, requiring the organization to make the policy known to enrollees.
109. With an "appropriate range of services ... for the expected population" and "a sufficient number, mix, and geographic distribution of providers..." Sec. 1932(b)(5).
110. The surety bond was pushed by Sen. Graham, who had success with a surety bond of $10,000, the point of which was not insurance as such but to have a way to register and check the credentials of operators or suppliers. Through the vagaries of drafting, the $10,000 became $50, 000, an amount which changed the emphasis and that was said by the National Association of Home Care to be onerous. Bryant Hall, staff of Sen. Graham, interview by Smith, September 2, 1998.
111. Specified Low-Income Medicare Beneficiaries. A Medicare beneficiary with income or assets too high to qualify as a dual eligible but not over 120% of FPL or $4,000 in assets. Medicaid will pay the Medicare premium but not the cost-sharing obligations. Cf. Schneider, et. al., *The Medicaid Resource Book.,* 172.
112. The president and the House conferees were in disagreement over whether legal immigrants who became disabled in the future would be eligible for Medicaid or only those who had lost eligibility as a result of welfare reform (PRWORA). The president regarded this as covered by the summit agreement and seemed prepared to veto the bill over this dispute, but the House receded on the point at issue.

113. The "SSI kids" were children who had lost their Medicaid eligibility because of welfare reform. During earlier negotiation, the House and Senate had gone part of the way, allowing but not requiring the states to cover these children. In the conference, they mandated coverage. They also dropped a provision that would have allowed states to discontinue SSI benefits entirely, which would have affected as many as 345,000 aged and disabled persons. Smith, *Entitlement Politics*, 217, 230.

114. *Ibid.*, 230-231 for a fuller account. The Conference also let stand the Senate's reaffirmation of the historic ban on payments to IMDs.

115. Sec. 2105(a)(7); also *Health Care Policy Report,* August 4, 1997, 1206.

116. *Congressional Quarterly* , April 12, 1997, 851.

117. *Health Care Policy Report,* March 3, 1997, 371.

118. *National Journal,* March 22, 1997, 568.

119. The administration's bill had a small grant program of $25 million to facilitate state efforts to develop small business health insurance pools.

120. *Health Care Policy Report,* February 3, 1997, 202.

121. Hatch-Kennedy was unpopular with southern states because of the tobacco tax and with large, populous states because it did not do enough. The administration proposal had a per capita cap and was strongly opposed by the NGA. Gramm's proposal was popular with conservatives and within the Finance Committee, but was seen as too minimalist. Specter's voucher scheme, whatever its merits, was not taken seriously. Funding was especially difficult because deficit reduction still had high priority and new taxes were pretty much off the table, except for something like the cigarette tax, which could be seen as a "sin" tax.

122. Matthew Salo, National Governors' Association, interview by Smith, Sept. 17, 2005.

123. The windfall from a lower deficit projection, lowered estimate of the Medicaid baseline, and expectations of more tobacco tax money.

124. Smith, *Entitlement Politics,* 213.

125. *Health Care Policy Report,* July 28, 1997, 1165.

126. *Ibid.,* 165. The negotiators for the White House were the Chief of Staff, Erskine Bowles, Treasury Secretary Robert Rubin, and John Hilley, the director of Legislative Affairs. Republicans included Trent Lott, the majority leader, Don Nickles, the majority whip, and several other members of the Senate Republican leadership. A remarkable feature was negotiation directly with the president without Democrats or House members.

127. SCHIP—the states insisted that the "state" be added. Medicaid advocates of long standing preferred the original language and for years afterward, have continued to refer to the program as "CHIP."

128. This list was adopted as a minimum for all plans in the final legislation. Plans could not "discriminate" meaning, here, they could not deny eligibility because of a pre-existing condition nor favor children from higher income families in cost sharing. Cf. Sec. 2103(f)(1)(A); 2103(e)(1)(B).

129. This concession might seem to open up a major loophole, but according to Chris Jennings, White House health adviser, the benchmark plans were carefully screened to be sure that they provided acceptable coverage in these categories. *Health Care Policy Report,* August 4, 1997, 1205.

130. *Ibid.* p. 1205.

131. Sec. 2105(c)(2)(B). The statute says to community-based delivery systems "such as … health centers receiving funds under Sec. 330 of the Public Health Service Act" or hospitals "such as those that receive disproportionate share payment adjustments."

132. Y2K, "Year 2000," referred to the computer dating problem that would arise on January 1, 2000 at 00.00 01 in the morning because most computers had only two spaces for the year date. In that situation, dates would be incomplete or incorrect and programs would begin "crashing" with unpredictable and even catastrophic results. Within HCFA, this meant that whole programs and data files had to be walled off while technicians worked to make them "Y2K compliant," with the result that others needing computer time would wait, go elsewhere, or find ways to "trick" the computer or work around the "firewalls" that had been set up to protect various program and data files.

133. BBA '97 did not impose specific deadlines for either the SCHIP or Medicaid managed care regulations; but HCFA and Nancy-Ann Min (DeParle) was especially concerned to demonstrate to a Republican Congress that the agency could complete regulations expeditiously.

134. Publication in the Federal Register for the managed care regulation was September 29, 1998; for SCHIP, November 9, 1998.

135. HRSA had jurisdiction over the Title V Maternal and Child Health Block Grant.

136. Not yet accepting the "S" in SCHIP.

137. For a fuller account, see Smith, *Entitlement Politics,* 202 ff.

138. Displacing private insurance.

139. Smith, *Entitlement Politics,* 300. For SCHIP, though not for Medicaid.

140. *Ibid.,* 213.

141. For additional details, 302 ff.

142. An established procedure for a new administration is to delay any new regulations not yet in effect. The SCHIP regulation was also delayed, though subsequently treated more gently.

143. *Health Care Policy Report,* March 5, 2001, 330.

144. The National Bipartisan Commission on the Future of Medicare (Sec. 4021) met from January 1998 to March 1999 and deadlocked in a final vote on March 16, 1999.

145. The Medicare Prescription Drug, Improvement, and Modernization Act of 2003 (P.L. 108-173).

146. The Balanced Budget Refinement Act of 1999 (BBRA, P.L. 106-113) provided $16 billion of targeted relief for providers and health plans for hardships or inequities occasioned by expenditure reductions in BBA '97. The next year, the Medicare/ Medicaid and SCHIP Benefits and Improvement Act (BIPA, P.L. 106-554) gave back $35.3 billion. Some of these "givebacks" reflected complaint levels and political clout but there were real inequities and hardships occasioned largely by underestimating the impact of the savings formulas. Also it was a time when the projected budget surplus was big and getting bigger, so there was money to ease the pain.

147. The allusion to the common law is intended. Like the common law, Medicaid policy tends to build upon past precedent but allows freedom for adaptation, especially incremental ones. Therefore it is important to think about uses that "bad men," or the next administration can make of the change. Cf. Oliver Wendell Holmes, Jr.'s famous lecture to entering law students on "The Path of the Law."

7

Medicaid Under Siege

From 2001 to the present, Medicaid policy has been shaped less by programmatic issues than by extraneous factors: economic and demographic trends, the 9/11 terrorist attacks, narrow legislative majorities, and unfinished business from the past. A worrisome development has been the shifting of Medicaid policy initiatives away from the Congress and the administration's deftness in reshaping policies without out legislative authorization. As noted, one effect of BBA '97 was to "improve" Medicaid more than some governors or states liked, making a program like SCHIP seem even more attractive, especially with its matching bonus. And much of Republican policy toward Medicaid could be described as pretty much that: to move toward the SCHIP model for Medicaid itself, doing so by legislation if possible but, failing that, by means of waivers, negotiation, and incremental changes. These developments may not amount, as yet, to a coherent alternative to either Medicaid or a block grant, but they are developing infrastructure and policy options and could move discussions about the future of Medicaid to a new level.

The closeness of the election in 2000 was important both for the administration and the Congress. George Bush's victory was disputed and finally resolved by the U.S. Supreme Court.[1] At the time, there was talk about a "national" government, but President Bush made it clear that doubts about his mandate would not affect his priorities or how he would govern. Yet the Republican margin in the House was narrow: 221 to 211 with several recounts under way; and the Senate was tied at 50-50. In June, 2001, Sen. James Jeffords (Vt.), a moderate Republican, defected and declared himself an independent, though saying that he would vote with the Democrats in organizing the Senate.[2]

This precarious balance of power was critical in the early years of the Bush administration since it tended to restrict its domestic agenda to top priority items and exclude those not in need of immediate attention or likely to turn into a protracted and inconclusive bloodletting—such as a Medicaid formula fight or managed care reform.[3] In this context, one legacy of the Clinton era struggles over Medicaid was that both the Congress and the Bush administration tended to avoid language such as "block grant" or even "capped entitlement" and to devise new terminology and non-legislative strategies to restructure or "modernize" the program.

The economic environment significantly affected the initial ordering of domestic priorities. From a decade of economic prosperity and sustained deficit reduction, the Bush administration inherited a huge budget surplus.[4] Other indicators were also favorable: the Social Security trust fund with a 10-year $2.6 trillion surplus, Medicare solvency assured through 2015, and the Medicaid baseline continuing to decline.[5] These trends strengthened President Bush and congressional Republicans in their demands for a tax cut of historic proportions and shifted the policy debate, for a time, away from deficit reduction and restructuring Medicare and/or Medicaid toward using the surplus savings being generated: distributing them with tax breaks, swelling the trust funds, or adding a Medicare pharmaceutical benefit. During the first two years, Medicaid was almost invisible, except for such perennials as increased flexibility, closing DSH loopholes, improving quality, and childhood immunizations.

The September 11, 2001 terrorist attacks profoundly affected foreign and domestic policy but in different ways and some areas more than others. There was a great rallying of support for the commander-in-chief and, for a time, a resurgence of national unity. But any bipartisanship over domestic policy was quickly dispelled, primarily over how to respond to the deepening economic recession: by another tax cut or by spending on unemployment benefits, health insurance for laid-off workers, and infrastructure projects.[6] National unity remained strong with respect to foreign policy, but partisanship returned for most domestic policy issues, although neither Congress nor the administration pushed for new Medicaid legislation.

Several factors contributed to this dearth of new initiatives. Medicaid programs were still doing fairly well in the first year of the recession.[7] After the Jeffords defection in June 2001, any strongly partisan Republican initiative would have been unlikely to pass in the Senate unless attached to a major reconciliation bill and Congress wasn't doing those at the time. And Medicaid, unlike Medicare and a pharmaceutical benefit, had not figured in the campaign. In essence, a legislative Medicaid initiative would have been difficult and there was little incentive to venture on that path.

In November of 2002 Republicans regained their majority in the Senate and strengthened their hold on the House. Meanwhile, rising health care costs and a weakened economy were pushing state Medicaid programs toward fiscal crisis. Against this background, two of the most significant Medicaid initiatives of the decade emerged—not from the Congress, but from the administration—in the form of a new waiver, the "Health Insurance Flexibility and Accountability Demonstration Waiver" (HIFA) and the administration's "New Freedom Initiative," both of which came about opportunely and somewhat inadvertently, yet were of critical importance for the future of Medicaid policy.

The Governors' Proposal and HIFA

In a broad sense, the governors' proposal of 2001 originated with BBA '95 when a number of governors, mostly Republican, worked with the Republican Congress on a scheme to block grant Medicaid in exchange for greater program flexibility.[8] That initiative failed although it emerged again in a modified form in the summer prior to the election of 2000 and was adopted as a policy position by the National Governors' Association in February 2001.[9] It might seem egregious for the governors to complain before they experienced real pain, but they were already being financially squeezed and saw more trouble ahead. Medicaid expenditures continued to grow faster than state per capita incomes or tax resources and the disparity was increasing with states losing the capacity to close the gap.[10] Prescription drugs, increased numbers of the aged and disabled, and federal mandates drove costs upward as savings from managed care declined, states lost DSH money, and had other lucrative loopholes closed. All but a few states had constitutional prohibitions against budget deficits; and raising taxes was difficult because of such factors as interstate competition, a slowing economy, a traditionally regressive tax base, and fiscally conservative legislatures. In 2000 or 2001, governors could foresee the multiple and growing pressures of recession and whatever their differences, they tended to unite over Medicaid, especially when needing help.

Their proposal reflected the agendas of two groups within the NGA. One of these, represented by Howard Dean (D., Vt.) wanted more money and greater flexibility to enroll the uninsured. The other, led by Donald Sundquist (R., Tenn.), wanted freedom to alter benefits and reduce the existing Medicaid requirements. This is a common difference that has tended to become increasingly associated with partisan differences.

Whatever their ultimate purposes, both sides wanted more money and greater flexibility.

In broad outline, the governor's prescription was simple: make Medicaid more like SCHIP and add money. A second part included a number of specific recommendations that give a lively sense for their grievances and some of the federal-state issues. Some of the most salient of these were:

- States should be partners, not just "stakeholders."
- Letters to directors or regulations that undermine flexibility or relate to managed care should receive special scrutiny.
- There should be wide latitude for plan amendments and adoption of innovative options without requiring a waiver.
- Initial waivers should all be for five years and thereafter become part of the state plan:
  1) Waiver applications or amendments should receive automatic approval if HCF does not act upon them within 60 days.
  2) "Budget neutrality" should be changed to count savings from additional federal programs.

The more substantive part of the plan modified the "all-or-nothing" approach of Medicaid, largely along the lines of SCHIP. To begin with, it recognized a special obligation to "core vulnerable" populations and the "safety-net" providers and the need to maintain federally established "minimum standards" for these groups. The plan would do away with categorical eligibility, allowing states to expand coverage up to a percentage of the federal poverty level. The only categories remaining would deal with levels of coverage or benefits. In Category I would be the current "mandatory" populations, those required by the Medicaid statute to be covered. They would receive the current mandatory benefits with no cost sharing but could—with a few exceptions—be subject to co-pays on optional benefits. States would continue to receive their current federal match for this group. The second category would include optional populations (such as the "medically needy" or children above the FPL) and optional benefits (such as dental care or prosthetic devices). For optional populations, states could provide a reduced benefit package, such as that required for SCHIP or an actuarial equivalent. And for optional services, they could require premiums, co-pays, and deductibles up to 5% of family income. For optional populations and/or optional services states would receive a bonus—similar to that under SCHIP—of a 30% reduction in their state match (up to a limit of an 85% FMAP). Category

III would allow states to target specific groups, define the benefit package, and require cost-sharing with no restrictions. For this category the regular Medicaid matching percentage would apply.

The emphasis in the governors' proposal was upon innovation and expansion of coverage. Both new groups and additional benefits would have an enhanced match. Cost-sharing could be used to offset program benefits. States that had already "significantly expanded" coverage through a Sec. 1115 waiver could terminate the waiver and implement expansions through Categories II or III, regardless of existing maintenance-of-effort requirements, so long as the original eligibility standards and mandated benefits were maintained. Coordination of insurance with the private sector for high-income groups was strongly encouraged. Also, under Category III, "full flexibility expansions," states could expand coverage to any population or target services to at-risk individuals "as defined by the States" up to an established level of income, with maximum flexibility to determine the level of benefits and amount of cost-sharing, for which the would receive the Medicaid level of matching funds.

There was much that was appealing and good in the governors' proposal. Extending the SCHIP approach to childless adults would reach a large uninsured population. The enhanced match would provide an incentive to reach out to this population, expand benefits for the existing Medicaid beneficiaries, help pay for the vulnerable, high-cost groups, ease the fiscal pinch for the states, and enable them to manage more efficiently and experiment with new programs. The dominant theme was expansion of benefits and eligibility, not reducing them; and the importance of a safety net for vulnerable populations was acknowledged, along with a guarantee of federal minimum requirements for benefits.

There was another side. The governors' plan would help the states, but with a major shifting of costs to the federal government and increased risks for existing Medicaid beneficiaries, especially the most vulnerable. For example, states would get a higher match for enrolling the near poor than they would for the poor or the traditional Medicaid beneficiaries. And since two-thirds of Medicaid benefits were currently optional,[11] states would be paid a handsome bonus for services they were already providing and some of the neediest and most vulnerable could be worse off. In addition, Category III, with no "strings" attached and a great opportunity to target expenditures might be used for all sorts of "Medicaid maximizing" schemes with money even finding its way, as in the past, to football stadiums and highways. In a word, the NGA proposal could be used for good, but like many expansive schemes, it had little protection against its misuse.

An outstanding feature of the governors' plan, according to John Holahan of the Urban Institute,[12] was its potential for shifting costs to the federal government with no change in coverage or benefits. At 200% of FPL, he calculated, coverage for children and all adults would cost the federal government $39 billion, while the states would save $6.5 billion. One simulation by Holahan showed that if states required cost-sharing and reduced optional benefits 40% for the optional category and 10% for the mandatory category, they could increase their savings to $18.1 billion or 21.3% of their program costs. Of this amount, only $2.4 billion would come from "flexibility" savings, while $15.7 billion or 87% would be from increased federal support. The budget-neutral requirement would, of course, provide some protection against any such "worst case" scenario, but the hypotheticals make a point about the underlying fiscal tendencies of this scheme and the importance of how "budget-neutrality" would be defined and administered.

The governors' proposal, if successful, would have accomplished much of what the NGA sought in 1995 in flexibility gains and would have stuck the federal government with the bill. Even before the budget surplus vanished, informed sources including the NGA itself doubted that Congress—especially the Senate—would be so indulgent.[13] But there was another way to secure some of the same objectives.

The new secretary of DHHS, Tommy Thompson, had been one of the leading Republican governors working through the NGA in 1995 and espousing more flexibility for Medicaid and its conversion to a block grant. As governor of Wisconsin, he had worked over the summer of 2000 to develop the NGA proposal. After he was appointed secretary, he began putting into effect the administrative components of this plan by expediting waivers and initiating the Health Insurance Flexibility and Accountability Demonstration Waiver (HIFA).

HIFA was announced on August 4, 2001. In form, it was another Sec. 1115 waiver, but it was also seen as the administrative component of a three-pronged initiative supported by both the White House and the NGA. The basic conception of HIFA was simple: states could apply for a Sec. 1115 waiver to increase health insurance coverage for low-income individuals and receive, in turn, program flexibility to modify health care delivery and existing benefit packages and impose cost-sharing requirements on the beneficiaries. HCFA—now CMS—promised a priority review for state programs within the project guidelines. On the same date, it also published an application template that simplified the application process and the information requirements.

The HIFA waiver closely tracked the governors' proposal. Most important, it authorized modification of benefits for current Medicaid optional populations in line with SCHIP provisions. But it differed from SCHIP in two important ways. It did not provide for the SCHIP enhanced match nor did it include the governors' recommendation on budget-neutrality, which would have allowed states to count savings from and apply them to any program under the Social Security Act. Either of these would have required action by the Congress. The NGA addressed these changes in lobbying efforts directed at the Congress, DHHS, and OMB, but without success.

Meanwhile, CMS and the DHHS continued to implement the HIFA initiative but ran into trouble: rumblings of protest within the Finance Committee and an adverse report by the GAO.[14] The GAO found especially questionable the use of reallocated SCHIP funds to cover childless adults; use of waiver authority to supersede the Title XXI (SCHIP) cost-effectiveness requirement for coverage of parents or guardians of SCHIP eligible children; and counting improbable "savings" to achieve budget-neutrality. The GAO criticized the lack of adequate notice and comment at the state level and the haste with which waivers were approved by CMS and drew attention to the impropriety of using the demonstration authority not just to test innovations but for continuing support and "to waive statutory provisions that the states found objectionable."[15] In any event, HIFA produced relatively modest results: only eight HIFA waivers in 2001 and few, if any, transformative effects, possibly because of the budget-neutral requirement and the lack of an enhanced match. Yet the larger purpose—of turning Medicaid into a version of SCHIP—grew even more salient with the deepening of the Medicaid fiscal crisis and the approach of the national election of 2002.

The New Freedom Initiative and Related Programs

The "New Freedom Initiative" was one of the first substantive health measures of the Bush administration and may, in time, prove to be one of the most important. Ostensibly, the moving cause was a Supreme Court decision, *Olmstead v. L.E. ex rel. Zimring* (1999),[16] which held that "unnecessary institutionalization of persons with mental disabilities" against their will violated the Americans with Disabilities Act (ADA) and that states could be required to provide community-based care where institutional care is inappropriate and community-based services are a reasonable accommodation and do not require the state to "fundamentally alter" its public programs. The decision held less than many would like to believe. It applied only to the ADA, not Medicaid. Also, it dealt with statutory construction, not with constitutional law, although it contained *dicta* about "discrimination *per se*" that invoke weighty constitutional authority. It covered only "mental disabilities" not disabilities generally. And it left much discretion to the states, in meeting the "community-based services" mandate.[17]

One of the first acts of President Bush upon assuming office was to announce the "New Freedom Initiative," which would respond to *Olmstead*; help carry out the purposes of the American with Disabilities Act of 1990 and the Ticket To Work and Work Incentives Improvement Act of 1999; and integrate persons with disabilities more fully into the community and improve their lives with the help of assistive technology, transportation, and services.[18] It was one of the items chosen by President Bush to head his social agenda, the others being better education for poor children and faith-based approaches to social and welfare services.[19] All of these related to the overall campaign theme of "compassionate conservatism" and had varying amounts of bipartisan support. Another appeal of the New Freedom Initiative was that it could build upon the ADA which had been sponsored by the first George Bush. It was also supported by Tommy Thompson, the new secretary of DHHS, who had some experience with a similar program in Wisconsin.

Along with this announcement, the president called for a task force with representatives from six different departments and agencies[20] to inventory existing and developing initiatives and future opportunities to remove barriers to independent community living for persons with disabilities. The task force responded in May 2001 with a three-volume report. Much of the intellectual content of the report came from the Clinton administration. The proposals were incremental in nature,[21] and dealt largely with physical disabilities rather than mental or emotional disorders.

An important next step, in June of 2001, was Executive Order (EO) 13217, entitled "Community Based Alternatives for Individuals with Disabilities," which made a strong commitment to the community-based principle and to swift implementation and enforcement of the *Olmstead* decision. It directed federal agencies to work cooperatively with each other and with the states to remove barriers to community living and to provide services to persons with disabilities "in the most integrated settings." It also assigned HHS a lead role in this effort and directed a list of seven agencies to evaluate their policies, programs, statutory provisions and regulations to see what changes should be made to further the objectives set forth in EO 13217.

Of the nine reports eventually issued under the heading of "Delivering on the Promise,"[22] that of the Department of Health and Human Services was the most comprehensive and detailed. The assessment and proposals had little immediate effect; but they provided an opportunity to add new options and endorse some old ones, including a number of holdovers from the Clinton administration.[23] Eventually, a number of these proposals were sponsored by the Bush administration or found their way into the Deficit Reduction Act of 2005.

At this stage of the New Freedom Initiative, mental health advocates were concerned about the scant attention given by the task force to mental health and the lack of thrust or consequence that the initiative seemed to generate, at least for the emotionally disturbed and mentally ill. When these objections were made known, President Bush said that he would appoint a commission: a move that is sometimes a prelude to significant action but often a substitute for it.

The New Freedom Commission on Mental Health was formally initiated by EO 13263[24] with a charge to conduct a "comprehensive study" of the "mental health service delivery system" and advise the president on "improvements to enable adults with serious mental illness and children with serious emotional disturbances to live, work, learn, and participate fully in the community." The commission of fifteen members was broadly representative of providers, payers, administrators, and consumers with *ex officio* members that included representatives of HHS, the Departments of Labor and Education, and the Veterans Administration. The commission was put on a fast track, with an interim report to be submitted in six months and a final report by April 2003, one year from the date of the executive order. The final report, *Achieving the Promise: Transforming Mental Health Care in America*[25] was submitted to the president on July 22, 2003.

The report emphasized especially preventive services, consumer and family involvement, and maintaining individuals in the community. It comprehensively related mental health care to the family and community, to schools and employment, to alcohol and drug abuse, and to the criminal and juvenile justice systems. The Vision Statement pointed toward "a future when everyone with a mental illness will recover … mental illness can be prevented or cured and … everyone with a mental illness at any stage of life has access to effective treatment and support—essentials for living, working, learning, and participating fully in the community." Like a strategic plan, the report set forth six major goals for pursuing this vision, with explanations and justifications of these goals, obstacles to achieving them, and a number of reforms needed in the existing system of mental health care.

The single most important concept in the report was "recovery," defined as "the process in which [*sic*] people are able to live, work, learn, and participate fully in their communities."[26] Implied in this definition was a practical optimism along with a therapeutic realism, even pessimism. With serious mental illness, cures are rare, which is one reason why screening and early intervention are especially important. For the major psychoses, with the benefit of contemporary and improved psychotropic drugs and strong community support, "recovery" was still a realistic objective: the ability to function in a community setting and to have, at least, "a job, a home, and a date on Saturday night." The report was optimistic in the confidence put in scientific research and the increasing efficacy of medication and in setting a goal of "recovery" for everyone, though pessimistic in the view that severe mental illness or emotional disturbance, much like alcoholism, was likely to be permanent and had to be managed.

Comprehensive in scope and revolutionary in implication, the Report was reminiscent of that extraordinary paragraph in Sec. 1903 (*supra,* 50) of the original Medicaid statute and the 1978 President's Commission on Mental Health.[27] Fully implemented, it would require many large and small changes in mental health administration, in housing, employment, and education. Indeed, the Report tended to cover everything, without an ordering of priorities—of what steps should be taken first. That was one reason for the formation of a national Campaign for Mental Health: to push for some specific policy initiatives.[28] Despite its "New Freedom" title, neither the president nor the Congress have, as yet, taken any significant measures to implement its recommendations or put a serious amount of money on the table. Still, the Report did establish a direction and an objective with steps that should be taken and may, like the 1978 commission establish a template to guide future action.[29]

The mental health commission was only one of many DHHS programs gathered under the New Freedom tent that shared several prominent characteristics. Most of them had a previous existence, were given new and exciting titles, but never got high priority or strong support.[30] They began earlier in Congress or the Clinton administration, some prior to *Olmstead* reaching back to the 1970s. The common themes were treatment in the community, normalization, autonomy or empowerment, and cost containment. There was much agreement about ends combined with disagreement about means or methods for reaching them—which could lead either to creative compromises or to mystifying and protracted struggles over credit claiming and blame shifting.

One of the broadest initiatives was the Medicaid Community Attendant Services and Supports Act (MiCASSA) first introduced in 1997 by House Speaker Newt Gingrich and in each succeeding year by others such as Sen. Tom Harkin (D., Ia.) of the Senate Finance Committee and Arlen Specter (R., Pa.) of the Senate Appropriations Committee. This proposal would amend Title XIX to create a new Medicaid benefit of home and community-based services; give states a short-term enhanced match to pay for these services; and provide financial assistance for "real system change," that moved Medicaid programs in the community based direction. MiCASSA quickly became a national movement, but has failed to gain enough support at the committee and sub-committee level to pass either house.

Experiments with "money-follows-the-patient" date back to the 1970s. This was an effort to assure access to and payment for community-based services for Medicaid beneficiaries leaving nursing homes and other long-term care institutions by developing individual treatment plans, informal supports, and adaptable funding sources. This approach was popular at the state level and in the Congress. It was also included by the Bush administration as part of the New Freedom Initiative, with special emphasis upon "rebalancing," that is, redressing the institutional bias of Medicaid.

"Cash and Counseling" is a Sec. 1115 waiver established in 1996 by the Clinton administration in collaboration with the Robert Wood Johnson Foundation that provided technical assistance and financial support to the states. Under this program—which was first developed in the Netherlands and Germany—persons with disabilities would have their needs assessed and then get a cost allotment along with counseling on the development of a treatment strategy and its implementation and, as needed, help with purchasing and paperwork, but would otherwise be largely free to purchase their own personal services or assistance technology. The program has been popular, has demonstrably encouraged Medicaid beneficiaries to become prudent purchasers, and has saved money.[31] It was also a successful example of consumer directed health care and has been strongly supported under the Bush administration.

Another significant initiative during the Clinton administration was the Ticket to Work Act,[32] designed to remove some of the barriers and disincentives that prevented persons with disabilities from getting and keeping jobs. Primarily, the act provided vouchers for support, counseling, and services and expanded Medicare and Medicaid benefits so that workers could keep their health insurance as their income or condition(s) of disability improved.[33] At high income levels, states could "buy in"—pay all or part of the Medicaid premium—for workers who wished to keep their Medicaid coverage, which was often better than either Medicare or employer supported insurance because of the added coverage and lack of cost-sharing. An innovative and potentially far-reaching provision of Ticket to Work was Sec. 203, which authorized eleven years of Medicaid Infrastructure Grants to encourage states to strengthen administrative linkages with Medicaid and promote the development of job-related supports for persons with disabilities. The authorizations were small, but infrastructure development was of importance for the Ticket to Work program to succeed and, by extension, for home and community based services.

The *Olmstead* decision of 1999 was an important catalyst in part because interest in community services for disabilities was already high[34] and because the Clinton administration, approaching its end, was seeking ways to enhance its legacy. Within days of the *Olmstead* decision, the HHS Office of Civil Rights and HCFA began working on regulations and issued five joint State Medicaid Directors' Letters on compliance with *Olmstead* prior to January 1, 2001. The Clinton administration also successfully sponsored legislation establishing the "Real Choice System Change Grants," that would support states in their efforts to create the infrastructure and service options needed for unified systems of long-term community-based care. Again, the authorizations were small, but the program was important for including children, adults, and the elderly along with the disabled and for broadening supports for infrastructure.

The Aging and Disability Resource Centers was a related program that developed late in the Clinton administration under unusual circumstances.

In October 2000, members of ADAPT,[35] a direct action group and strong supporters of MiCASSA, chained themselves to the gates at the White House and demanded an audience with President Clinton—which was granted. One result was a final push by the administration to get a number of disability related initiatives enacted, one of which was the Aging and Disability Resource Centers. Aside from the "one-stop" features, this legislation was another investment in infrastructure, helpful to the elderly and/or disabled in need of information about providers, prescription drugs, and assistive devices and important to them as consumers and prudent purchasers. As a joint effort of DHHS and the state agencies on aging to promote integrated service delivery at the local level this program added another linkage to the politically powerful older Americans constituency.

The New Freedom Initiative was more of a continuation and re-naming of Clinton administration initiatives than contemporary CMS program descriptions suggest.[36] But that fact should not obscure nor detract from its significance or from some of the Bush administration's contributions, one of which was to give priority to implementing the *Olmstead* decision and direct the relevant administrative departments and agencies not only to come up with ideas for implementing the decision, but to set about collaborating among themselves and working with the states to enforce it.[37]

An Independence Plus Initiative, announced in May 2002, went beyond "Money Follows the Person" and "Cash and Counseling" to allow consumer direction of a much wider range of long-term services and supports. Under a 1915(c) waiver the list was restricted to home and community based services; but under a Sec. 1115 waiver, consumer direction could be extended to any long-term Medicaid service or support. Beyond the obvious purpose of delaying or preventing institutional placement, and encouraging self-direction and cost containment, Independence Plus also sought to encourage family involvement in planning or purchasing health care and allowed direct payments to family members. Moreover, under a Sec. 1115 waiver it would apply to a much broader range of services or assistive devices than Cash and Counseling. Some of the potential risks are lack of consumer information, unpredictable costs, inadequate budget allotments, counseling, or other supports, and lack of evaluation.[38]

A follow-on to Independence Plus was the LIFE[39] Accounts Program, first announced in 2004, under which persons with disabilities who choose to direct all of their Medicaid community-based long-term care supports could put up to 50% of their self-directed care into a LIFE account and use this account and employment earnings plus limited contributions by others for purchases to improve their independence and productivity. This program, also first developed in the Netherlands and Germany, resembles Independence Plus except for the addition of a personal health savings account.[40] It is of more than passing interest since it illustrates some of the underlying political issues at stake. Personal accounts could greatly encourage independence and self-confidence, especially among the more capable and self-directing who could, in turn, be an example and inspirations for others.[41] It could also be one more maneuver in the persistent campaign to diminish and privatize the Medicaid entitlement so that Medicaid supporters might regard the LIFE program as suspect for strategic reasons.

As for building infrastructure, the Bush administration continued measures begun under the Clinton administration, such as the Real Choice Systems Change Grants, the Ticket to Work Medicaid Infrastructure Grants, and the Aged and Disability Resource Center Grants with modest financial support and included them as part of the New Freedom Initiative. Of course, credit claiming and blame shifting are normal practice in Washington politics as currently practiced, but the important point is that the Bush administration *did* continue these initiatives because they advanced objectives shared with a Democratic administration.[42] The funding was minimal, but it was money that local Medicaid programs had not previously had and welcome as rain upon parched land. These infrastructure initiatives did not thrive in the succeeding years of fiscal stringency—but they survived, established precedents, and developed know-how that could be useful in more favorable times.

Medicaid Under Siege

Early in 2002, trends and events indicated that health care would likely be a major domestic priority in 2003. Health care inflation was moving strongly upward, with insurance premiums rising 15-16% a year, employers cutting back on insurance, and Medicaid expenditures eating up ever larger shares of state budgets.[43] Pundits were likening the situation to the health care crisis of the late 1980s that created a groundswell of support for national health insurance. Neither Republicans nor Democrats made bold to take on these issues in an election year, but November 2002 changed that, restoring control of the Senate to the Republicans, adding to their margin in the House, and giving President Bush an unambiguous mandate of his own. In the new year, the Bush administration and the Republican Congress picked up where they had left off prior to the defection of Sen. Jim Jeffords, with proposals to restructure the big entitlements, Social Security, Medicare, and Medicaid.[44]

By 2003, state Medicaid programs were in serious financial trouble. Many states had expanded their programs, established reserves, and cut taxes when times were good. But after two years of recession or minimal growth, state tax revenues were down and budgets were tight, while the numbers of uninsured continued to grow and medical and pharmaceutical costs increased sharply. Meanwhile, state savings from managed care, pharmaceutical purchasing plans, and DSH payments were flattening or declining. Caught in this squeeze, states used up their "rainy day" funds and tobacco settlement proceeds, reduced payments to providers and laid off staff, and by year three were increasingly cutting optional benefits and facing prospects of tightening eligibility or raising taxes.[45]

Facing an even bleaker future, governors began seeking ways in which the federal government might help them and reviewing proposals for NGA position statements at the winter meeting in Washington, D.C. One popular suggestion—both in the NGA and among Democrats in Congress—was a temporary increase of 2% in the FMAP which would be one-time, cease with the easing of the fiscal crunch, and not require repayment. More fundamental in nature was redressing the "imbalance" between Medicare and Medicaid by shifting more of the financial responsibility for the dual eligibles, at least the pharmaceutical costs, to the federal government. This was a burden upon the states, increased by the MCCA, (*supra,* 206), steadily becoming more onerous, and probably unsupportable over the long term.[46]

The administration's position was that it made no sense to pour more money into an outdated system without attempting to "modernize" it, especially when SCHIP and welfare reform had shown how states could save money if given increased flexibility.[47] Its proposal was $12.7 billion over seven years to raise the FMAP for those states that would agree to merge Medicaid with SCHIP into a new program resembling SCHIP in its essentials. This initiative was similar to the governors' proposal of 2001, though with much less favorable financing. Under the administration proposal, states would be required to continue coverage of mandatory populations and benefits but would have(as with SCHIP) "complete flexibility" [48] with respect to optional populations and benefits. Funds for Medicaid and SCHIP along with DSH payments would be continued and paid out according to an allocation formula in two block grants, one for long-term care and the other for acute care. The supplement would be "front-loaded" with $3.75 billion available in the first year, but it would also be budget-neutral and had to be paid back by reduced matching in years eight through ten.[49]

The secretary's announcement was intended as a prelude to legislation that would be proposed by the administration, so it was discreet in wording and silent about some details. For instance, the term "block grant" was not used, nor did the secretary discuss what would happen after year ten had elapsed. Also, his message was specifically directed to the NGA with the thought that its support would be essential to overcome the intense opposition of Democrats within the Congress.[50] The administration initiative was an audacious move that would have accomplished—through an alliance with a quasi-official outside body—a more sweeping transformation of Medicaid than the proposal of the House Republicans in 1995 under Newt Gingrich's regime. It might also have had a lasting effect in establishing for the NGA a kind of "advise and consent" role in matters of Medicaid fiscal policy.

The response of the NGA and of congressional leaders was somewhere between non-committal and dismissive, much to the chagrin of Secretary Thompson. On all sides, the administration was praised for putting Medicaid on the agenda and recognizing the complexities of the program. But Sen. Charles Grassley (R., Iowa), chairman of the Finance Committee, said he "needed time to study it" and the Commerce Committee chairman, W. J. (Billy) Tauzin (R., La.) said he would consult with the governor of Louisiana.[51] Members of the NGA complained not only that they had to pay back the "loan," but would lose money on the deal. The governors sought a straight subsidy with no payback, assumption by the federal government of the entire costs for elderly dual eligibles, and more flexibility to make program changes.[52] Declining to accept the basic thrust of the proposal, the NGA adopted its own guidelines and proceeded to set up a bipartisan taskforce of ten members to negotiate their differences with the administration.[53]

Some progress was made. As part of a $350 billion tax reduction bill, Congress allocated $10 billion for increases in federal Medicaid payments over a term of 18 months. The NGA task force committed in principle to a Medicaid spending cap if the federal government would assume the costs for low-income seniors and cede the states more program flexibility.[54] But that was as far as it went. As for the senior dual eligibles, whatever the merits of the proposal, it was politically unrealistic in 2003 with both the administration and Republicans in Congress struggling to sustain their own Medicare reform initiative, that included an expensive and contrived pharmaceutical benefit. The Finance Committee, the governors' best hope, intended to leave drug benefits with Medicaid, although with a federal contribution of some undetermined amount to help the states.[55] Shortly thereafter, the task force split along partisan lines, the Republicans saying that the task force should recede on the dual eligible switch and Democrats objecting to the potential impact of capped funding for the Medicaid program. No agreement was reached, though the issue was resolved, in a fashion, by Medicare legislation, then under consideration.

The "reform" of Medicare and the addition of a pharmaceutical benefit were concerns that have been around but not active since the Bipartisan Commission of 1998-99. In 2003, they became top priorities for the Bush administration and the Congress largely to get them out of the way before the election of 2004 and not leave them around to become Democratic campaign issues in 2004. Finally passed in December 2003 at the end of session, the "Medicare Prescription Drug, Improvement and Modernization Act of 2003" (P.L. 108-173) was a remarkable example of arm-twisting, legislative manipulation, and coalition-building accompanied by exceptions, concessions, and subsidies that left its main constituency—senior citizens—struggling to understand the legislation and tell whether they were better off or not.

The NGA and state Medicaid officials were especially disappointed. The legislation provided a drug benefit for elderly dual eligibles, to be implemented in 2006. But there was a "clawback" feature which required the states to pay back most of their savings: 90% in the first year, declining to 70% in the tenth year and thereafter (Sec. 1935(a)(5)). The states would probably lose substantial amounts of money if they sought to hold their beneficiaries harmless by maintaining their existing "wrap around" benefits and picking up the increased co-pays. The new law would cut the Medicaid market share for prescription drugs by about half, reducing the program's leverage for negotiating reduced prices.[56] In addition to all of this, the states had to make the eligibility determinations, screen for cost-sharing, and provide information as needed by the secretary. These were not especially onerous requirements, but they added to the tenor of the legislation as a whole which an exasperated NGA official described as a "reverse block grant," noting that the states would have nothing to say about how the federal government used the states' "clawback" payments.[57]

Another feature that Medicaid officials found of dubious merit was the "specialized Medical Assistance for special needs individuals."[58] These special needs plans or SNPs ("snips" as they were dubbed), were Medicare demonstrations available for Medicare Advantage or for dually eligible beneficiaries who required a SNF/NF level of care or suffered from a severe and chronic disabling condition.[59] The benefit for Medicaid was that the dual eligibles were included. But some Medicaid officials objected that they were already doing well under PACE and their existing waivers and that this new program, by requiring Medicare Advantage quality criteria and administrative procedures and involving them in the Medicare drug benefit, was complicating matters and might be a disservice to the dual eligibles.[60] They also, and especially, deplored the implementation of the new program without benefit of consultation with experienced state officials or evaluation of existing Medicaid experience.

A weighty reason for passing the Medicare bill in 2003 was to avoid dealing with it in an election year; and for much the same reason, 2004 was a relatively quite time for Medicaid. Also in 2004, the Senate passed the Family Opportunity Act (S622) under which states could permit families with children who met the SSI definition of disability to buy into the Medicaid program at income levels above the FPL; but the House version stalled in committee over how to offset the additional expense.[61]

A dearth of legislation did not indicate that nothing happened in 2004, only that events of importance for Medicaid were less visible or public because they were centered largely on oversight of administration. In fact, 2004 was a good year to make improved oversight a priority. State Medicaid programs had been under enormous stress and, of necessity, adapted in many ways, some of them questionable. In 2003, the GAO had, for the first time, listed Medicaid as a high risk program for fraud, abuse, waste, and mismanagement.[62] An election year can be a good time to emphasize fraud and abuse since legislating is difficult or dangerous, and fraud and abuse gets bipartisan support and makes good press copy. So, early in the year, saving dollars by rooting out fraud and abuse was endorsed by the administration and both houses of Congress, though with selective emphasis upon the Medicaid drug rebate program, abuse of upper payment limits, and Sec. 1115 and HIFA waivers—important topics, but not what most would regard as the darkest examples of fraud and abuse. Apart from fraud and abuse, much of the oversight was about the administration or CMS not doing enough or overstepping and making policy on its own, especially with waivers.

Both the Senate Finance and the House Commerce Committee undertook extensive investigations relating to the Medicaid drug rebate[63] program. With the House Commerce Committee,[64] the concern was whether "average manufacturer's price," (AMP) would work better than the conventional "average wholesale price" (AWP).[65] For the Senate, it was the narrow question of whether drug companies were systematically cheating on the "nominal price exception," which exempted certain drugs already deeply discounted with "charitable intent" from further reductions to benefit low-income or other groups.[66] These are good topics for congressional oversight, but they are arcane, with asymmetries of information between congressional staff and the drug companies' experts, and require enormous amounts of data, much of doubtful reliability—not unlike the situations that earlier gave rise to the Prospective Payment Assessment Commission and the Physician Payment Review Commission to deal with hospital and physician charges.

Upper payment limits were a chronic problem, most recently addressed by Congress in 2000 in BIPA,[67] which directed HCFA/CMS to issue a final regulation restricting UPL arrangements and to establish transitional periods and procedures for phasing out excessive UPL payments. While these directives were being implemented, the GAO published its report citing Medicaid as at risk[68] and followed this with another in February 2004[69] expressing discontent with CMS transitions—especially the eight-year program established for some nursing homes—strongly suggesting that Congress consider proactive measures such as eliminating transitions of such length and payments to government-owned facilities that exceeded costs.[70] Early in the year, there was strong bipartisan support in both houses of Congress and the administration for more effective preventive action. This consensus was soon dispelled by a Federal Register notice on January 7th (69 FR 923) that CMS would seek a change in the state budget reporting form (CMS-37) to capture "up front documentation" about potential funding, ostensibly to help identify improper payments in advance rather than let them drag on and cumulate as in the past.[71]

Although this suggestion seemed reasonable, especially in the light of the GAO recommendations, neither the states nor the Medicaid providers were comfortable with giving this kind of power to CMS. A former

CMS official, who noted the difficulty of trying to recover money after the event and was generally sympathetic with the approach, observed that it might have been better if CMS had consulted and collaborated with some of the Medicaid stakeholders in advance rather than seeking emergency clearance from OMB to implement a change of this magnitude.[72] The NGA quickly picked up on this theme, objecting to the emergency clearance procedure and the 24-hour comment period. In response, Secretary Thompson said that he would consult with Medicaid stakeholders and opened a new 60-day comment period. According to a report in *Medicine & Health*, though, CMS continued to move ahead, hiring people to perform the budget reviews.[73]

CMS behavior and the proposal itself raised fears in the Medicaid constituency that the ultimate intent was to establish *de facto* caps or negotiate concessions with respect to legitimate IGTs or provider payments and even unrelated budget items. House and Senate Democrats went one step farther, complaining (correctly) that CMS had never specifically defined the impermissible financial "gamesmanship," raising a concern that the ultimate purpose of the new policy was to strangle the states with bureaucratic requirements and denial of federal funds and coerce them into accepting capped federal payments in exchange for regulatory relief.[74] Yet another attack, by the National Association of Public Hospitals, took a legal form, arguing that obtaining "voluntary" cooperation in resolving questionable IGTs through threatened denials of state plan amendments and/or denials of legitimate IGTs/CPEs was coercive and illegal [75] Leaving aside the factual or legal aspects of these various charges and denials, such events reveal a level of distrust in federal-state relations that can thwart constructive and well-intentioned reforms.

Another approach, espoused by CMS, sought to draw a line between legitimate IGTs—in which states would share their Medicaid costs with local institutions through tax revenues or "certified public expenditures" (CPEs)—and illegitimate "recycling" schemes in which excess payments were returned to the state. This approach could be strengthened, as recommended by the GAO, by prohibiting Medicaid payments to public facilities that exceeded costs.

This proposal, which seemed reasonable on its face, brought forth two kinds of objections: one procedural and the other substantive. As to the first, NAPH president, Larry S. Gage objected that such a change in policy required a "notice and comment" rulemaking procedure, not just a CMS letter, and was technically illegal. The process, he complained, would compel providers to negotiate with CMS officials over permissible and impermissible IGTs "without any coherent standards for states to distinguish between [them]."[76] This omission could presumably be fixed by rulemaking; but the substantive issue went deeper. The formula itself seemed too procrustean. Democrats complained that it could be used as a Medicaid capping device; and providers said that it would destroy too many safety-net institutions. Whether true or not, the complaints show how far there is yet to go: the first, illustrating the distrust between the political parties in Congress and, the second, raising the issue of what happens to the safety-net providers in a new, "reformed" dispensation.

Another Time Around

With the election of 2004, Republicans gained control of both houses of Congress and the presidency for the first time in over fifty years. Moreover, it was a convincing victory. President Bush was elected with a clear electoral majority of 286 and with 3.5 million more votes than his opponent, John Kerry. Republicans gained four seats in the Senate, raising their numbers to 55; and in the House, they increased their majority to 232, more than they had after the House turnover in 1994. Moreover, they had campaigned on conservative themes of tax cuts, family values, and defense of homeland security and American interests abroad.[77] Both the re-elected president and Republicans of the 109th Congress brought to their work in 2005 a renewed sense of popular mandate.

From the Republican perspective, especially the conservatives, 2005 was a good time to take on entitlements again. The welfare legislation had expired and needed to be renewed. Medicare legislation passed in 2003 had gotten only part of the way. Medicaid was in serious trouble. And debate had already opened over Social Security, the biggest prize of all.

Past experience had shown that taking on a major entitlement is hard and dangerous work, requiring both a sound strategy and effective mobilization of energy and resources. It is also helpful to create a sense of impending victory and to "shock and awe" the opposition. With these observations in mind, it is useful to view the early moves in this renewed assault on entitlements as behavior that is theatrical and rhetorical as well as practical and instrumental.

An important bit of rhetoric was George W. Bush's campaign pledge to cut the deficit in half by 2006, which was preposterous on its face and remotely plausible only because it excluded future military action in Iraq and Afghanistan, the cost of modifying the alternate minimum tax (AMT), and a hugely expensive Social Security restructuring to add private accounts.[78] The president's budget—which translated this agenda into domestic program reductions—was then soberly blessed by Senate Budget chairman, Judd Gregg (R., NH) as a good job "because everyone's ox gets gored ... including defense..." even though the budget cuts were almost entirely from domestic spending. Meanwhile, Senate majority leader Bill Frist sent his supporters an e-mail urging them to "remain calm," saying that this was "just the beginning of the process, not the final product."[79] All of this is not to say that the senators' behavior was egregious, only that much of the budget and reconciliation process is theatre and rhetoric.

Another early move that was also instrumental and symbolic was to plan both a tax and a deficit reduction reconciliation. Twice since 2001 there had been reconciliations on taxes, but this would be the first budget reconciliation since BBA '97. A budget reconciliation made sense because of President Bush's promises about deficit reduction and because of the rule that it is not subject to filibuster in the Senate. Notice that a budget reconciliation was coming was also a good way to stress the gravity of the coming engagement and warn members that serious budget cutting was in prospect.[80]

The nomination of Michael O. Leavitt to be the new secretary of DHHS had symbolic importance. Leavitt was a widely respected Republican who had been for eleven years the governor of Utah and a past chairman of the NGA. The symbolic or "message" significance of this appointment lay in the fact that—like former Secretary Tommy Thompson—he was chosen in large measure because of views on health policy that coincided with the president's agenda. He had gotten a HIFA waiver in 2002 which helped finance an expansion of Medicaid coverage of primary and preventive care for working class parents with incomes up to 150% of the FPL by reducing benefits and imposing cost sharing on Medicaid recipients at or below the FPL.[81] In 2003, President Bush had singled out the Utah waiver as a show-case example of the kind of Medicaid flexibility he had in mind and again emphasized his approval when "Mike" Leavitt was nominated in December 2004, shortly after the election.

Secretary Leavitt's first speech left no daylight between himself and the administration and seemed to confirm some of the worst fears about this next phase in the ongoing entitlement struggles. He called for $60 billion[82] in Medicaid savings over the following decade to be achieved by tightening restrictions on IGTs ($40 billion), rebasing the Medicaid drug rebate ($15 billion) and closing the loopholes that allowed nursing home applicants to hide or transfer assets in order to qualify for Medicaid long-term care ($4.5 billion).[83] Along with these reductions would come additional flexibility to reduce coverage for optional populations and benefits, although still under budget-neutral restrictions applicable to 1115 waivers.

The secretary denied that his proposal was another attempt, like that of 1995, to "block grant" the program or that it was a repeat of 2003, in which the Bush administration offered the states $12.7 billion over seven years[84] to opt out of Medicaid in exchange for a non-entitlement program resembling SCHIP. Yet for the Democrats and liberal Medicaid advocacy groups, this looked like the same thing in a different form, this time, a squeezing device intended to move them in the direction of a block grant without calling it that.

Early in the new year, scores of advocacy groups began protesting the proposed Medicaid cuts. Notable among these, aside from the NGA, were the American Hospital Association, concerned about their safety-net institutions, and the American Association of Retired Persons, speaking out for senior citizens—both of these indications of the growing popular support for and concern about Medicaid.

As in 2003, the NGA was the one external body significantly involved in the development of a compromise proposal, intensively discussed in the winter meeting that began in February 2005. The governors had no trouble with the basic premise that reforms were needed, especially of the flexibility sort. They accepted rebasing the drug rebate and closing the assets loophole. They approved of greater flexibility with respect to benefits, cost-sharing, and routine waivers. But they disagreed strongly with the proposal to curtail IGTs by $40 billion—both because of its likely fallout and because it would hurt most those states bearing the greatest burdens. There was also a fault line opening between those who supported the administration's approach and those who thought Medicaid restructuring should be about "covering more people with the same money."[85]

Action in the Congress

It was not a good year for deficit reduction. Congress had grown unaccustomed to the budget reconciliation discipline. Social Security was off the table and Medicare—the perennial "cookie jar"—had been recently "reformed" and was not deemed good for any substantial savings.[86] The economy may have been in recovery but it was hard to tell and many groups were hurting. In a word, savings were hard to get and Medicaid was expected to be an important contributor to the total.

As for Medicaid, there was strong sentiment against any cuts at all. State Medicaid programs were beginning a fourth year of hardship that, as state officials saw it, was more because of the recession, loss of private insurance, increased complexity of their cases, and rising medical costs—than their own extravagance. All of this in addition to the federal government's refusal to help with the dual eligibles.[87] In the Congress there was deep concern about Medicaid recipients and their providers and uneasiness that the reconciliation process could hurt many people "while not putting us on the path to comprehensive reform and improvement that the program needs."[88] It was a hard sell.

The House passed its budget resolution on March 17th, with $69 billion in mandatory spending cuts over the next five years, $20 billion of which would come from the Energy and Commerce Committee, and almost all of that from Medicaid. Once again, it was an impressive display of Republican unity and party discipline, but the savings were far below the White House figure and the vote was close (218-214). House Republicans were also painfully aware of the possibility that the Senate would take Medicaid off the table.[89]

Once again, the Senate played its traditional role of cooling out—or thwarting—House designs.[90] The Senate was usually less unified or disciplined in a budget reconciliation, and this time was no exception, despite the accession of a new chairman, Judd Gregg (NH), who was charged with enthusiasm over the president's agenda of cutting the budget deficit in half.[91] In addition to the independence of the senators, many were less enthusiastic about this particular effort since calculations showed that, taking the tax reconciliation into account, the deficit would actually increase. With this in mind, moderate Republicans and Democrats insisted that deficit reduction precede the tax bill. They also sought to restore budget rules that required pay-as-you-go offsets for tax cuts or new entitlement spending.[92]

Critically important in deflecting the budget reconciliation was the junior senator from Oregon, Gordon H. Smith, and his impromptu following of several moderate to liberal Republicans who were defenders of Medicaid.[93] Smith first ventured into politics in 1992 when he ran for and was elected to the Oregon State Senate. He so impressed his Republican colleagues that they elected him their minority leader in his first term.

Elected to the U.S. Senate in 1996, he was a Bush supporter and served as deputy whip, but he was known for his independence and ability to work across the aisle. He also had strong interests in substantive policy, was chairman of the Senate Special Committee on Aging, and served on four major committees including the Finance Committee. Education and health were among his strongest interests and he had helped develop the innovative Oregon Health Plan.

Early in February, before the Medicaid reductions were officially announced, Sen. Smith led a pre-emptive strike, joined by Senate Democrats, with a bill to put a one-year hold on Medicaid reform and establish a "Bipartisan Commission on Medicaid" to study long-term Medicaid goals, fiscal sustainability of the program, and the relations of Medicaid to Medicare.[94] Heather Wilson (R., NM) introduced a similar bill in the House, also co-sponsored by Democrats. Proposals for commissions are, of course, often regarded as diversionary tactics that seldom produce anything timely and relevant; but the proposal drew attention to a major failing of the reconciliation approach: that it was not focused on systemic change or consequences.

The decisive moment came with passage of the Senate budget resolution on March 17th.[95] Even before the resolution came to the floor it was in deep trouble. Initially, Sen. Gregg, the Senate Budget Committee chairman, had hoped to produce a resolution close to the $69 billion target; but as negotiations proceeded, he reported to his House counterpart, Jim Nussle, that he would be doing well to reach $43 billion—$26 billion less than projected.[96] Some more wrestling with the big authorizing committees and the figure dropped to $32 billion, almost half of that expected to come from Medicaid, largely on the dubious premise that $14 billion could easily be reached by eliminating "accounting gimmicks," such as illegitimate IGTs.[97]

In the March 17th floor debate on the budget resolution, Gordon Smith spoke with emotion about his distress at going against his budget chairman and the president, but said that it was a matter of principle and conscience not to abandon the neediest in our society. He didn't know whether the Medicaid cut was too large or too small, but he did know that another 60,000 Oregonians might lose their health care.[98] He then moved that the Medicaid reductions be stripped from the resolution. The amendment was adopted, 52-48, with seven Republicans voting in favor. Also carried was Smith's proposal for a bipartisan Medicaid commission. With the Medicaid cuts removed from the bill, the five-year savings dropped to an embarrassing $17 billion.

The matter did not end there. Talks continued variously between Sen. Smith, the Budget Committee, Sen. Frist, Secretary Leavitt, and the NGA leading eventually to lengthy negotiations with Secretary Leavitt and an agreement by Sen. Smith to accept $10 billion in Medicaid reductions over five years. After recalibrating, Sen. Gregg, the budget chairman, agreed to try for $40-$45 billion in reductions, but said that $12 billion would be an absolute limit for Medicaid.[99]

As the budget committees were regrouping, DHHS moved to appoint its own commission, that was to report by September, on how the $10 billion savings could best be achieved and how to assure the "long-term" sustainability of the program. The secretary was to appoint a chairperson and fifteen voting members. Congress was invited to designate eight non-voting policy experts. The initiative seemed calculated to restart the "reform" process and point it in a direction favorable to the administration. Sen. Max Baucus (D., Mont.) opined that it needed to pass a "smell test" and Democrats generally took the position that Congress should decide whether and how much Medicaid should be cut and not an administrative commission. They decline to participate, and so did Sen. Gordon Smith.

The bipartisan Medicaid Commission was charged to come up with *scorable* five-year Medicaid savings of $10 billion by September 1, 2005, which it did—most of it ($8.3 billion) by saving on prescription drugs.[100] It was "scooped" by an NGA release of August 29th, "*Short-run Medicaid Reform,*" that contained most of the same recommendations with several additional "flexibility" amendments, acknowledged the Commission's work, and expressed a desire to "work with" them over the next 16 months.[101]

The Commission labored on for another fourteen months, holding a series of seven 2-3 day sessions during which its members heard from national and state Medicaid officials and experts on a list of topics and issues. The Commission took its work seriously. But it was not bipartisan. The Republican chairman, Donald Sundquist, knew little about Medicaid and prominent Medicaid experts of the Democratic persuasion neither sought nor were sought after as members. Moreover, the Commission lacked the resources to develop weighty option papers and articulate the alternatives. Whatever the substantive merits of the Commission's report, when it appeared shortly after the election, it was dismissed by congressional Democrats as no longer relevant.

Hurricane Katrina

On August 29, 2005, Hurricane Katrina struck the Mississippi and Louisiana coasts and New Orleans, inflicting widespread damage and revealing a lack of preparedness and responsiveness at all levels of government. A dislocation of such proportions interrupted electricity and water supply, forced people to evacuate their homes, and left many without employment, transportation, or money. It also disrupted health care: shutting down hospitals and clinics, and displacing thousands, leaving them to make shift in another county or state, without eligibility or access to care. Much of the domestic agenda was temporarily shoved aside as state and local governments, the federal administration, and the Congress debated how to provide emergency relief, help displaced families, restart local services and economic activity, and pay for it all.

One legislative initiative of significance for Medicaid was the Grassley-Baucus "Emergency Health Care Relief Act of 2005" (S1716)[102] which would have provided five months of non-categorical fully funded Medicaid coverage for low-income hurricane survivors. The legislation is of interest because it illustrated both the deficiencies and the potential of Medicaid as disaster relief. Among the deficiencies were the categorical restrictions on eligibility: for instance, lack of coverage for single males or childless women under 65, or severely injured hurricane victims not technically "disabled." Another was interstate variation: for example, Louisiana's income limit for families was 20% of the FPL. Irksome before Hurricane Katrina, these categorical and income limitations were intolerable with tens of thousands losing health insurance and seeking emergency health care in a different state. Within days, governors were seeking relief and appealing to Washington.

Much of the thinking behind the Grassley-Baucus proposal came from previous experience with the 9/11 terrorist attacks and New York's success in putting together Disaster Relief Medicaid, a temporary program of disaster relief making use of a Medicaid waiver. This episode demonstrated important resources of the Medicaid program, such as an existing infrastructure, a working relationship with the federal government, familiar procedures, adaptability, and acceptance by providers.[103] Not least, of course, was the speed with which it could be adapted and deployed.

The administration objected to the Grassley-Baucus proposal on the grounds that it would increase Medicaid eligibility and expense and prove difficult to rescind once the emergency was over. On September

27th, Secretary Leavitt sent a letter to Senate leaders expressing CMS views and the administration's preference for proceeding under existing waiver authority, which would speed implementation. Critics pointed out that the waivers would, in terms, continue existing Medicaid categories and income standards, so that many evacuees would receive inadequate care or none at all. Also, these waivers would have to be budget-neutral, with no authority to compensate states and safety-net providers for their additional burdens.[104]

In responding to the secretary's letter, Senators Grassley and Baucus expressed dismay, pointing out that the Bush administration had been much more generous in post-9/11 actions, including the New York waiver it had granted then. In view of the largesse bestowed upon New Orleans, Louisiana, Mississippi, and Alabama for other kinds of aid, this response to Grassley-Baucus seemed stingy and pretextual.

Grassley-Baucus was not the only option. Within the Senate there was strong support for another bipartisan initiative backed by Sen. Michael Enzi (R., Wyo.) and Sen. Edward Kennedy (D., Mass.) both members of the Committee on Health, Education, Labor and Pensions. Their proposal would have provided three months of premium support for relocated Katrina survivors—an approach that would be easy to implement as well as highly productive. Disaster Relief Medicaid, as the name strongly suggests, would be taking on one more expansive role for Medicaid, a step much at odds with administration efforts to cap the program. In contrast, the premium support alternative would soon terminate and did not expand the role of Medicaid; but it lacked support in the Senate Finance Committee.

The DRA authorized $2 billion for Medicaid payments to hurricane victims or evacuees under Sec. 1115 waivers, although both the House and Senate bills included full federal funding (FMAP of 100%) for affected individuals living in designated areas of Louisiana, Mississippi, and Alabama.[105] For Medicaid advocates, this outcome was objectionable because the $2 billion was included as part of the Medicaid amendments—reducing the total savings by $2 billion—and because this use of waivers both limited the use of funds and added momentum to the campaign to restructure Medicaid.

Independent of responses to Katrina, comprehensive waivers continued to grow as instruments of federal administrative policy through such initiatives as HIFA, Pharmacy Plus, and the next generation of Sec. 1115 waivers. These developments will be more fully explored in the next chapter, but they were part of the context for debates over responses to Hurricane Katrina.

Deficit Reduction Act: Denouement and Afterthoughts

Congress returned to work after the August recess intending to act quickly on the reconciliation instructions; but the extent and urgency of the Katrina disaster soon led to a five-to-six week postponement of the House and Senate deadlines. More than concern over hurricane victims was at work: the reconciliation process was already endangered in the Senate and Sen. Grassley, for one, said that he doubted that any resolution could pass the Senate Finance Committee if the plight of the hurricane victims was not speedily addressed.

Prior to their postponement, both the House and the Senate had indicated that they would accept the governors' recommendations as a basis for their talks. What that amounted to was a short list of recommendations for the immediate future,[106] not the longer agenda for comprehensive "overhaul." The thrust of this short list was to make Medicaid more like SCHIP and waivers even more effective as devices for restructuring Medicaid. Greater freedom to modify benefits and assess co-payments, deductibles, and premium charges was also a key item. For additional cost savings, the governors recommended changes in the drug rebate formulas and restricting the use of asset transfers to qualify for nursing home admissions or care.[107] The total figure for Medicaid savings was $10 billion, the amount earlier negotiated by Sen. Smith and his allies.

The savings eventually squeezed out of Medicaid by the DRA were modest: reductions in federal Medicaid spending of $11.5 billion over five years and $43.2 billion over ten years. These were offset by various additional expenditures so that the net savings would be a mere $4.5 billion over five years and $26.1 billion over the next decade.[108] These unimpressive numbers were achieved after a fierce struggle that sharpened differences and revealed the political costs of proceeding farther with legislative attacks on Medicaid.

The House and Senate differed fundamentally over who was to bear the burden of cost containment: the Medicaid beneficiary or someone else. In the House bill, the full burden fell on the beneficiary: for co-payments and premiums, reduced benefit packages, and limits on asset transfers to qualify for nursing home admissions. In broad outline, the House bill:

- Allowed co-pays and premium charges up to an aggregate limit of 5% of annual family income. For beneficiaries under the poverty line, co-pays were limited   to $3 per prescription or service, though this limit could be raised by the percentage increase in the Medical CPI.
  a) providers could deny services to beneficiaries who did not meet the co-pays
  b) tiered drug co-pays were permitted and could include pregnant women, children, and nursing home residents, who were otherwise exempt from co-pays
- States could reduce benefits and provide "benchmark equivalent coverage" (similar to SCHIP) for most children, all parents, and persons with disabilities, other than the dual eligibles.[109]
  a) EPSDT coverage for children would no longer be required
  b) amount, duration, and scope requirements would no longer apply
- The "average wholesale price" (AWP) and "retail average manufacturers' price" (RAMP) would be used as a basis for Medicaid drug rebates.
- Extended the "look-back" period for asset transfers from 3 to 5 years, denying exclusion for homes valued at more than $500,000.
- Required U.S. citizens applying for Medicaid to provide evidence of their citizenship status with a passport, birth certificate, or other specified materials.
- $2.5 billion allotted for Katrina survivors; extended coverage for families leaving welfare; a new Medicaid buy-in for children with disabilities and family incomes above the poverty line; demonstrations for "Health Opportunity Accounts" (Medicaid version of MSAs).

The Senate was another story, with some interesting variations. As noted, both House and Senate agreed to use the NGA recommendations as a starting point in seeking to meet their budget reconciliation targets. But the Senate was on a different trajectory: more concerned about the Medicaid beneficiaries and the fiscal status of Medicaid programs in the states and not interested in transforming Medicaid into a version of SCHIP. Initially, there was a strong push, led by Sen. Gordon Smith and his allies,[110] to exempt Medicaid from any budget cuts. That attempt failed, but the reconciliation target was reduced to $10 billion in net savings from *both* Medicare and Medicaid. Along with this reduction went the proposal for a bipartisan commission on Medicaid,[111] reflecting a view that reform of Medicaid ought to be deliberate and bipartisan. In keeping with this view, the Senate went its own way, ignoring the administration's Medicaid task force as well as a last-minute endorsement of flexibility amendments by the National Governors' Association.

The Finance Committee met its Medicare/Medicaid reconciliation target of $10 billion in net savings without the flexibility amendments and without imposing any additional costs on the beneficiaries. Almost all of the savings came from the providers. The largest part of the Medicaid savings ($4.6 billion over 5 years) were from more aggressive and systematic reform of the payment formula for prescription drugs.[112] Another major saving—from Medicare—was to eliminate the Medicare managed care stabilization fund ($5.4 billion in savings), which was seen as unnecessary and/or inappropriate.[113] Other Medicaid savings came from relatively minor and technical changes in the treatment of asset transfers for elderly beneficiaries seeking nursing home placements ($305 million); improving recoupment from claims payments ($512 million) and clarifying definitions for targeted case-management ($750 million).

In addition to holding the beneficiaries harmless, Senate Finance added some benefits. The costliest was $1.8 billion for healthcare coverage (Medicaid and other) for Katrina hurricane victims. The reconciliation package also included money for states that had run out of their SCHIP allotments ($128 million) and for a Family Opportunity Act ($834 million) that would allow low- and middle-income parents of children with severe disabilities to purchase or "buy into" Medicaid for their children ($824 million). This benefit would, in principle, create an additional "pathway" for the severely disabled child as well as another linkage between Medicaid and the working family.

On most issues, the Senate version lost, both in the conference and in the final legislation.[114] Following the House bill, the DRA protected providers.[115] The cost-sharing provisions and the flexibility on benefits survived, with a few amendments. So did the proof of citizenship requirement.[116] In spirit and substance, this legislation was an important step in making Medicaid more like SCHIP. It also bestowed considerable legitimacy on the notion of using increased flexibility to reduce access and shrink the Medicaid program.

Two Senate amendments to the benchmark benefit provisions (Sec. 6044; 1937(a)) may be of critical importance, especially for preserving Medicaid's commitment to children and persons with disabilities. One was the inclusion of the "blind and disabled," along with the dual eligibles, in the exempted categories. The other was some murky language that seems to require at least wrap-around EPSDT coverage or a benchmark equivalent for any child under 19 years of age covered by the state plan.[117] How robust and effective these provisions will be when implemented remains to be seen. Nothing is said about procedural protections of the sort associated with existing EPSDT provisions. It would seem, moreover, that the benchmark, targeting, and cost-sharing provisions could be used in ways prejudicial to vulnerable recipients.[118] Still, the Senate amendments reaffirm a commitment to EPSDT children and persons with disabilities and provide some ground to stand upon in their defense.

Much will depend on administrative interpretation, how the states respond to this new infusion of flexibility, and the impact of the November 2006 elections. But there are indications that Congress may have gone about as far as it wishes, even with the present political balance in the House and the Senate.

One indicator was the narrowness of the majorities and the growing unity of Democrats over Medicaid even as Republicans became less so. The first budget resolution passed the House by a vote of 214-211 and the Senate by 52-47. The reconciliation bill passed the House by 212-206, near dawn on December 19th after an all night session.[119] In the Senate, the vote on the conference report was delayed until the new year and finally passed by a vote of 51-50, with Vice President Cheney breaking the tie. Not a single Democrat voted for either of the budget resolutions or reconciliation bills. For a change, it was Republicans who were experiencing the defections. In the Senate, a coalition of Republican health care liberals and Democrats largely determined the content of the Senate bill. In the House, noted for Republican discipline, nine Republicans defected,[120] some of them specifically objecting to the association of tax breaks with cuts in Medicaid, scholarships for low-income students, and child care payments for welfare mothers.

A controversial budget reconciliation, such as the DRA, consumes a huge amount of time and energy and using this process to shrink or restructure a popular entitlement such as Medicare or Medicaid raises the struggle to a higher level. As for the DRA, the Katrina catastrophe was a supervening event. But the unusual delays in the reconciliation process were symptomatic of underlying difficulty. Initially, the Senate stripped the Medicaid expenditure reductions from the budget resolution. In September, both houses announced five-to-six week delays to allow the authorizing committees to negotiate key changes in the entitlement programs under consideration.[121] Then, in November, the House postponed decision while the leadership sought to round up votes. When the conference reported on December 18th, the Senate delayed final passage over several points of procedure, so that the DRA was not finally passed until February 8, 2006.[122] During these delays, the committee staffs, members and committee chairmen, and the party leadership worked on the development and of program modifications, negotiation and persuasion, and dickering for votes—sometimes into the night and early morning and over weekends. In brief, the transaction and opportunity costs of a partisan and contentious budget reconciliation can be enormous.

A troubled reconciliation, such as the DRA, has a tendency to get into deeper trouble, which threatens the integrity of the whole enterprise as well as putting increased pressure on the political leadership. The DRA associated taxes and entitlement "reform," so that it invited charges of cutting entitlements to benefit the rich. Also, putting together and then holding a majority was difficult, requiring numerous inducements to win over "holdouts" or keep potential defectors. These "sweeteners" in the form of tax and regulatory concessions or indulgences for social welfare or entitlement programs anger the purists of both left and right, make it harder for the reconciliation to pass a "smell test," and often less effective as an instrument of programmatic change. It would seem that the DRA of 2005 was pushing limits of this sort and that small shifts in the political balance in the House and/or the Senate could make a major difference in the future of the Medicaid program.

Yet this optimistic reflection needs to be qualified by an awareness that the administration has already accomplished a considerable amount of "restructuring" of Medicaid through its promotion of HIFA and Sec. 1115 waivers and other means of devolution or increasing flexibility—to be discussed in the following chapter. Moreover, a method of combining both a legislative initiative and administrative action developed early in 2006, that contemplates yet another method of deficit reduction.

As part of its deficit reduction goals in the president's budget for FY 2007, the administration proposed major reductions in federal grants to the states. For Medicaid, this initiative would entail projected savings of $14.5 billion over five years and $35.5 billion over ten—more than those achieved by the DRA of 2005. Most of these savings—85% of them—would be gotten through administrative action rather than legislation. The legislative part would reduce matching percentages and provider payments. The administrative and regulatory changes were about what CMS would or would not match and fell, presumably, within the authority of CMS to change. They involved such issues as payments for uninsured patients treated by state and local public hospitals; transportation and administration costs for children under the Individuals with

Disabilities Education Act (IDEA); coverage for certain rehabilitative services, such as special instruction and therapy for mental illnesses and developmental disabilities; and a reduction of hospital taxes from 6% to 3% of gross provider revenues.[123] The changes attacked mostly practices of questionable origin and legitimacy, but ones that had some sanctity of custom. Much to the point, reducing the flow of funds or terminating it would have shifted a $29.7 billion burden of service provision or administrative expense to the states.[124] Whether by design or not, this scheme could be a squeezing device applied to states already in fiscal distress, forcing them to cut back on eligibility and coverage, and to "restructure," like it or not.

The cries of outrage were loud and immediate, especially from the National Governors' Association and some of the states that would be most affected. Nevertheless, the initiative remained on the administration's agenda and legislative language and implementing regulations were drafted, but held in abeyance to await the outcome of the November 2006 election.[125] Indications are that they are still on the agenda, despite the election, illustrating in a small way the difficulty of translating electoral results into predictions about policy.[126]

As for the historic significance of the election, that will not be known for some time and will depend in large measure upon unfolding events, how Democrats and Republicans respond to foreign and domestic challenges, and the candidates and framing of issues in the next presidential campaign. The election of 2006 may or may not be a turn toward moderation and bipartisanship in domestic policy. Democrats gained heavily among women, suburban voters and independents. The failure of the Republican strategy of energizing the base and concentrating on turnout and the lowered response or "backlash" from "hot button" issues such as gay marriage, abortion, and immigration would seem to support such a view. Yet a number of moderate Republicans lost their seats and many of the rest see little to be gained through bipartisan collaboration. Also, Democrats won largely with Republican tactics: turning the election into a national plebiscite on Iraq and President Bush's policies, mobilizing their own base more skillfully, and exploiting local scandals or failures.[127] Their success says little about long-term trends[128] or how the Democrats might fare in a 2008 re-match. Moreover, the new Congress will start with a hangover of bad feelings and a strong incentive to move into a campaign mode as partisan mobilization begins in anticipation of the next presidential election.

State elections in 2006 were less dramatic but important. Democrats added six governorships, building a majority of 28-22. They also gained six legislatures, controlling both houses in 24 of the states while Republicans fell to 17. Included among the power shifts were leadership states such as New York and Ohio and states that had been deeply "red," such as New Hampshire, Oklahoma, and Wyoming. These changes will be important for national politics in 2008 and for congressional redistricting; but what they signify for Medicaid is hard to say. Democrats will be in a majority in the NGA and may be somewhat more inclined than the recent Republican membership to support the NGA's traditional bipartisanship. Democrats will also control more governorships and state houses, including some important leadership states,[129] but local tradition and conditions are strong where Medicaid is involved, so that the partisan turnover may have small impact. Moreover, the election changed little in those states most bent upon restructuring and privatizing Medicaid.

The election probably ended any prospect for a serious consideration of the Report of the Medicaid Commission.[130] In different circumstances, this Report might have provided a basis for bipartisan discussion.[131] It canvassed a number of policy options, served to add visibility to some and keep others alive, and raised issues that needed serious legislative attention. But the Commission was commonly referred to as "Leavitt's Commission" and was perceived by Democrats as "stacked," and unsympathetic to Medicaid[132] It seemed more suited to mobilize partisans than to bring together a bipartisan majority. From a Democratic perspective using the Report as a basis for discussion would cede to Republicans undue influence over selection of priorities and framing of the issues. Democrats that spoke out declared the Report "dead on arrival" or expressed lukewarm interest or non-committal approval for some of its proposals Among the consequences of the election those most important for Medicaid may be to weaken and divide the Republicans who have been laying siege to the program and increase the resources (if not the unity) of Democrats seeking to defend it. Of course, the election will be seen as an opportunity to raise the issue of national health insurance, which will detract attention from Medicaid, so that there would be time—and possibly the motivation—to think constructively about how to improve the program.

Notes

1.   *Bush v. Gore*, 531 U.S. 98 (2000).
2.   *Congressional Quarterly Almanac,2001*, 1-3,4.
3.   One early success of the Bush administration was to kill off PARCA and managed care reform although, arguably, it may have taken 9/11 to do that. Cf., Smith, *Entitlement Politics,* 331-343.
4.   The original figure reported by OMB was a 10-year surplus of $5.6 trillion. By mid-year it was apparent that this figure was enormously inflated, and with the Bush tax bill, 9/11 related expenses, and the recession, the budget surplus shrank dramatically. FY 2002 ended with a deficit of $151 billion which would have been $317.5 billion without $166.5 billion from the Social Security trust fund.
5.   *Congressional Quarterly Almanac 2001,* 1-4.
6.   *Ibid.,* 1-11.
7.   States could use money from the tobacco settlement reduce provider payments, use co-pays, and eliminate some optional services without much affecting eligibility. By the end of 2002, that situation was much changed, with states experiencing large revenue shortfalls of $60 to $80 billion, representing 13% to 18% of individual state budgets for FY 2004 (*Medicine & Health*, January 6, 2003, 5). Nearly one million beneficiaries, mostly parents and children from working families, were expected to lose coverage, with no relief in sight. (*Health Care Policy Report*, January 6, 2003, 25)
8.   Smith, *Entitlement Politics,* 61.
9.   *NGA Policy Position HR-32*, "Health Care Reform Policy." February 2001.
10.   John Holahan, "Restructuring Medicaid Financing: Implications of the NGA Proposal," paper prepared for the Kaiser Commission on Medicaid and the Uninsured, June 2001, 16-17.
11.   Estimated at 65% in 2002. Schneider, *et. al., The Medicaid Resource Book*, 82.
12.   Cf. Holahan, "Restructuring Medicaid Financing," 14 ff.
13.   Schneider, interview by Moore and Smith, August 17, 2001.
14.   *The Medicaid and SCHIP Recent Approvals of Demonstration Waiver Projects Raise Concerns,* GAO-02-817, (Washington, D.C.: GPO, 2002).
15.   *Ibid.,* p. 18.
16.   527 U.S. 581. "New Freedom" applied initially only to the implementation of the *Olmstead* decision, though it was subsequently broadened to the elderly and to other categories of disability and to the "New Freedom Commission on Mental Health." The title "New Freedom" is itself interesting as is the language in EO 13217, "tear down the barriers to community living." Putting this alongside the ideal articulated by contemporary mental health advocates of "a job, a house, and a date on Saturday night," serves to remind that money, skillful services, community support and effective coordination are important along with freedom and tearing down barriers. Frank Sullivan, SAMHSA. Interview by Smith, April 10, 2003.
17.   The "most integrated setting," requirement was in the implementing regulation for Title II which was drafted in the attorney general's office.
18.   *Congressional Quarterly Weekly,* January 3, 2001, 264.
19.   *Ibid.*
20.   These were Health and Human Services, Justice, Education, Housing and Urban Development, Social Security Administration, and the Veterans Administration.
21.   Incremental as opposed to structural or systemic, which made the recommendations less controversial, fundable with existing authorizations, and avoided major commitments of resources or energy.

22.   Other agencies were included. For the final nine reports, see www.hhs.gov/new-freedom/final.

23.   Thomas Hamilton, telephone interview by Smith, October 26, 2005.

24.   April 29, 2002, 67 FR 22337.

25.   *Achieving the Promise: Transforming Mental Health Care in America,* Report of the President's Commission on Mental Health (Department of Health and Human Services, Substance Abuse and Mental Health Services Administration, 2003.)

26.   *Ibid.,* p. 5.

27.   Which led to the Mental Health Systems Act of 1980.

28.   Such as parity for mental health or changes in Medicaid funding. Chris Koyanagi, telephone interview by Smith, August 23, 2005.

29.   Cf. Chris Koyanagi and Howard H. Goldman, "The Quiet Success of the National Plan for the Chronically Mentally Ill," *Hospital and Community Psychiatry,* Vol. 42 (9), Sept. 1991, 899-905.

30.   Jason deParle observed that Governor Thompson approached welfare demonstrations in Wisconsin in a similar way: one or more exciting experiments each year but little follow-through. *American Dream.* New York: Viking, 2004, 76-77. One official observed that the New Freedom Initiative suited the new secretary well because it had lots of grants but no system change.

31.   Christine Kent, "Cover Story—Cash and Counseling, the Way of the Future," *State Health Notes,* Vol. 26, Issue 450, August 8, 2005. In the evaluation of a trial group, Mathematica found that the first year expenses were higher than pre-test years, but that by the end of the second year costs were declining in Arkansas and increasingly constrained in Florida and New Jersey. *Ibid.,* 1.

32.   Ticket to Work and Work Incentives Improvement Act, P.L. 106-170, Dec. 17, 1999.

33.   For Medicaid, states could set whatever level they liked for income or assets, but over $75,000 income they had to "buy in" or charge the worker a premium equivalent to Medicaid coverage. Under SSI or SSDI, workers had to have a severe, medically determined impairment but lost eligibility if that condition improved. Under Ticket to Work, improvement alone would not disqualify so long as the worker remained severely impaired.

34.   MiCASSA was being pushed and consumer choice and community based options were receiving foundation support in the private sector. Cf. "Consumer Choices and Control: Personal Attendant Services and Supports in America," *Report of the RWJ Blue Ribbon Panel of August 1999.*

35.   Americans Disabled for Attendant Programs Today, a direct action group established to demonstrate for better public access for persons with disabilities.

36.   Most of these programs are described as part of or in support of the Bush administration's New Freedom Initiative, which makes them seem elements of a new and original design rather than an assemblage of earlier starts with a new names.

37.   Even so, the language of EO 13217 does not expand on *Olmstead* (beyond *mental* or *developmental* disabilities) nor does it adopt the "most integrated" language.

38.   Jeffrey S. Crowley, *An Overview of the Independence Plus Initiative to Promote Consumer Direction of Services in Medicaid.* Washington, D.C.: Kaiser Family Foundation, 2003, 2.

39.   Living with Independence, Freedom, and Equality = LIFE.

40.   This program was initiated with grants to Wisconsin and New Hampshire and has yet to be evaluated or implemented more widely.

41.   Hamilton, telephone interview by Smith, September 12, 2005.

42.   One modest but potentially significant new Bush Administration grant, established in 2003, was for demonstrations testing ways to recruit or retain direct service workers aiding persons with reduced "activities of daily living" (ADLs).

43.   *Congressional Quarterly,* March 23, 2002, 1 ff.

44.   *New York Times,* February 24, 2003, A1.

45.   *Health Care Policy Report,* January 6, 2003, 25.

46.   Cf. Leighton Ku, *The Medicare/Medicaid Link: State Medicaid Programs are Shouldering a Greater Share of the Costs of Care for the Dual Eligibles."* Washington, D.C.: Center on Budget and Policy Priorities," February 25, 2003, 1.

47.   "HHS Secretary Tommy G. Thompson Announces Medicaid Reform Plan." Kaisernetwork.org, January 31, 2003, 2, 3.

48.   *Ibid.,* 16.

49.   *Health Care Policy Report,* January 10, 2003, 180.

50.   Rebecca Adams, "States Seek More Medicaid Help While GOP Eyes Program Overhaul," *CQ Weekly,* Feb. 2, 2003, 258.

51.   *Health Care Policy Report,* January 20, 2003, 181.

52.   Robert Pear, "Governors Seek Aid from Congress and Decline to Back Medicaid Plan," *New York Times,* February 26, 2003, A-14.

53.   *Health Care Policy Report,* March 3, 2003, 279.

54.   *Ibid.,* June 9, 2003, 752-53.

55.   *Ibid.,* p. 753.

56.   "Medicare Law to Pose Problems for States, NGA, Medicaid Officials Say," *Health Care Policy Report,* May 10, 2004, 624; *Medicine & Health,* March 2, 2004, 7.

57.   *Health Care Policy Report,* p. 624.

58.   Subtitle D, Sec. 231. "MA" is "Medicare Advantage," the new name for "Medicare+Choice."

59.   Not defined, but conditions mentioned were cardiovascular disease, congestive heart failure, osteoarthritis, mental diseases, End State Renal Dialysis (ESRD), and HIV/AIDS.

60.   Cf. "Minnesota Claims that Shift to SNPs May Disrupt Existing Care for Seniors," *Medicare Advantage News,* March 17, 2005, 5; Dealing with additional MCOs, co-pays, and private PBMs unacquainted with Medicaid were additional concerns.

61.   Senate Finance did not require an offset but the House Commerce Committee did. Within Commerce, the Republicans proposed taking the needed offset from targeted case management while the Democrats preferred an increase in the Medicaid drug rebate. *Health Care Policy Report,* June 28, 2004, 872.

62.   *Ibid.,* June 16, 2003, 795. Medicare had already been listed several times.

63.   The drug rebate program was created by OBRA '90 and became effective January 1, 1991. Under this program, drug companies wishing to sell drugs to state Medicaid programs must sign a contract with CMS and submit their "average wholesale price" and "best prices" that CMS uses to calculate the rebate amount, which state programs can then submit for the amount to reimburse the drug companies.

64.   Specifically, the Oversight and Investigations Subcommittee of the Commerce Committee.

65.   *Health Care Policy Report,* February 9, 2004, 175

66.   *Ibid.,* May 3, 2004, 597.

67.   The Medicare/Medicaid and SCHIP Benefits Improvement And Protection Act of 2000 (BIPA; P.L. 105-554).

68.   "Major Management Challenges and Program Risks: Department of Health and Human Services," GAO-03-01.

69. "Medicaid—Improved Federal Oversight of State Financing Schemes is Needed," GAO-04-228, p. 2.

70. The GAO was especially critical of the eight-year transition which seemed unnecessarily long, cost the federal government a large amount of money, and violated CMS's own regulatory criteria for two (Nebraska and Wisconsin) of the eight-year transitions. 5.

71. "CMS Draft Outlines New Process to Enable Pre-Determination of State Medicaid Budgets," *Health Care Policy Report,* February 23, 2004.

72. "Stakeholders Identify Problems with New CMS Budget Proposal," *Ibid.,* March 8, 2004; also Penny Thompson, "Medicaid's Federal-State Partnership: Alternatives for Improving Financial Integrity," (Washington, D.C: Kaiser Family Foundation, 2004).

73. *Medicine & Health,* March 2, 2004, 1.

74. *Health Care Policy Report,* April 5, 2004, 455.

75. "Public Hospitals Question Crackdown by CMS on Intergovernmental Transfers," *Ibid.,* June 14, 2004, 799.

76. *Ibid.,* 799.

77. *CQ Weekly,* January 3, 2005, 10.

78. Joseph J. Schatz and Andrew Taylor, "Bush's Budget: A Thousand Pages of Political Pain," *Congressional Quarterly*, February 14, 2005, 366.

79. *Ibid.,* 366.

80. Messages from Jim Nussle (R., Iowa) and Judd Gregg (R., NH) chairs of the House and Senate budget committees. Cf. *Health Care Policy Report,* February 14, 2005, 205.; also *Medicine & Health, Perspectives*, January 24, 2005, 1.

81. The reductions did not apply to mandatory populations or benefits and was intended to expand coverage by including new groups. Also, the waiver applied only to "primary care networks" and did not include mandatory services or the aged, blind, and disabled. The initiative was troublesome because it could make poorer people worse off in benefiting those better off. Also, the Utah state legislature, applying a bit of incrementalism in reverse, approved benefit reductions and co-pay increments for non-pregnant adult traditional enrollees in 2003; and an approved waiver amendment, "Covered at Work" allowed the state to use Medicaid funds for premium assistance to parents and adults eligible for PCN coverage but with existing employer sponsored insurance. Both of these amendments extended the basic thrust of taking from the poorest to benefit the less poor. Cf., *Utah Sec. 1115 Waiver* (Washington, D.C.: Kaiser Family Foundation, July 2004) 1.

82. offset by $15 billion in new spending.

83. *Health Care Policy Report,* February 7, 2005, p. 166.

84. A repayable advance, not a grant.

85. This from Mitch Daniels, who had been OMB director in President Bush's first term.

86. *CQ Weekly*, April 15, 2005, 1015.

87. *Medicine & Health, Perspectives,* February 4, 2005, 7

88. Statement by Heather Wilson (R., NM) as quoted in *Health Care Policy Report,* April 18, 2005, 497.

89. Even as they were voting, House Republicans complained that the Senate would undermine them. Within less than a month 44 House Republicans sent a letter to Jim Nussle, budget committee chairman, protesting the projected Medicaid cuts. *Health Care Policy Report, Ibid.,* 497.

90. Note in this respect the tradition about Washington's response to Jefferson that House legislation was poured "into the senatorial saucer to cool it." Cf. Donald

C. Bacon, Roger H. Davidson, and Morton Keller, *Encyclopedia of the United States Congress*. New York: Simon and Schuster, 1995. Vol. 4, 1785.

91.   The rate of increase would be cut in half over ten years.

92.   *CQ Weekly,* March 14, 2005, 648-49.

93.   The core group was Smith, Norman Coleman (Minn.), Susan Collins (Me.), and Arlen Specter (Pa.). They were joined on some issues by Olympia Snowe (Me.), Lincoln Chafee (R.I), and Jim Jeffords (Ind., Vt.).

94.   *Health Care Policy Report,* February 14, 2005, 211.

95.   SConRes 18.

96.   Andrew Taylor, "Four Line Up to Blast Budget Plans," *CQ Weekly,* March 24, 2005, 648.

97.   To add to the perceived injustice, Medicare was not tapped for any reductions, and a move to roll back a 5% reduction in physician payments, set to start on December 1st, would have to be offset and require additional savings from Medicaid.

98.   Kate Shriber, "GOP Senators Bolt on Medicaid Cuts." *CQ Weekly,* March 32, 2005, 721.

99.   *CQ Weekly,* April 15, 2005, 1014.

100.   Proposals included (1) a change from AWP to AMP ($4.3 billion savings); (2) extension of the Medicaid rebate program to Medicaid managed care ($1 billion savings); (3) tiered copayments for prescription drugs ($2 billion); (4) increasing the look-back period and penalties for transfer of assets to qualify for Medicaid nursing homes ($1.5 billion); (5) changed treatment of managed care plans under the provider tax regulations ($1.2 billion), "The Medicaid Commission, Report to the Secretary of DHHS and the U.S. Congress," September 1, 2005. The NGA proposal included a number of additional drug savings, flexibility amendments, and premium support options.

101.   *Short-Run Medicaid Reform from the National Governor's Association,"* (Washington, D.C.: National Governors' Association, 2005).

102.   S 1716 was only one of a series of Grassley-Baucus bills dealing with health care that were developed with bipartisan cooperation by the Finance Committee over several years. The Emergency Health Care Relief Act of 2005 was introduced on September 14, 2005, two weeks after Katrina struck, with strong bipartisan support and the endorsement of the NGA. The act would have allowed hurricane survivors relocated to other states and who were below the FPL to establish presumptive eligibility by declaration and would have paid 100% of their Medicaid costs. Pregnant women and children would be covered up to 200% of FPL. Income would be measured on a current basis (i.e., income they had at the time, not their income in their previous location). Disaster Relief Medicaid would last for five months with the possibility of a five-month extension. Other sections of the bill would compensate health care providers with add-on payments for unpaid care; assist Medicaid beneficiaries with prescription drug enrollment; support premiums of persons seeking to preserve their employer based insurance; and provide temporary cash assistance for TANF recipients.

103.   *Medicaid: The Best Safety-Net for Katrina Survivors and States* (Washington, D.C., Center for American Progress, 2005).

104.   Under the secretary's proposal, states were supposedly "compensated in full," but it was not clear by whom or under what authority. They were invited to form uncompensated care insurance pools, but the secretary had no authority to waive the budget-neutral waiver requirement and the proposal left unclear from whence extra funds would come to pay for uncompensated care. Cf. Edwin Park, *Failing to Deliver: Administration's Waiver Policy Excludes Many Katrina Survivors and*

Provides No Guarantee of Full Federal Financing. Washington, D.C.: Center on Budget and Policy Priorities, September 9, 2005, 2,3.

105. *Deficit Reduction Act of 2005: Implications for Medicaid.* Washington, D.C.: Kaiser Commission on Medicaid and the Uninsured, February, 2006), 5.

106. NGA, *Short-Run Medicaid Reform.* The larger agenda, which dealt with Medicaid comprehensively and over the longer term, was the result of months of study and a commissioned report. Cf. Vernon K. Smith and Gregg Moody, *Medicaid in 2005: Principles and Proposals for Reform,* (Chicago, Ill.: Health Management Associates, February, 2005).

107. *Health Care Policy Report,* September 9, 2005, 1194.

108. Kaiser Commission, *Deficit Reduction Act of 2005: Implications for Medicaid,* 1.

109. The House bill also included some specific exemptions, for pregnant women, people in institutional care, and individuals considered "medically frail" or having "special needs" as defined by the secretary. Cf. Victoria Wachino, Leighton Ku, Edwin Park, and Judith Solomon, *Medicaid Provisions of the House Reconciliation Bill: Both Harmful and Unnecessary."* Washington, DC: Center on Budget and Policy Priorities, December, 2005, 9.

110. Smith's Republican allies included Olympia Snowe (Me.) and Susan Collins (Me.), Lincoln Chafee (R.I.), Mike DeWine (Ohio), Arlen Specter (Pa.) and Norm Coleman (Minn.)—with Smith, a total of seven.

111. S. 388, Bipartisan Commission on Medicaid and the Medically Underserved.

112. The Senate would have set lower minimum rebates, used a different price index, and extended rebate requirements to managed care plans.

113. This "stabilization fund," which was part of the Medicare Modernization Act of 2003, was intended as a subsidy for managed care plans reluctant to enter underserved areas. The Senate provision was based squarely on a recommendation by MedPAC that the subsidy was not needed.

114. One Senate initiative that survived was the Family Opportunity Act. The Senate also got some changes in cost sharing and flexibility on benefits. A small but important measure was to allow home and community-based services as an optional benefit rather than requiring a waiver. Under this option, states could also cap the number eligible for such services.

115. On drugs, the House used a less aggressive pricing index and declined to raise the rebate levels or extend them to managed care. Neither the House nor the administration approved of the repeal of the Medicare HMO subsidy. At one point the administration threatened a veto if the subsidy were repealed, though it would seem unlikely from a president that has used signing statements as a substitute for vetoes and, to date, has vetoed only one piece of legislation.

116. In June, 2006, DHHS issued regulations indicating that proofs of citizenship other than passports or birth certificates could be recognized, such as medical certificates or affidavits of parties other than relatives. *New York Times*, June 5, 2006, A-14.

117. The flexibility provisions start with a sweeping disclaimer about "notwithstanding any other provision" of Title XIX, that would seem inconsistent with an EPSDT mandate. The meaning of "wrap-around" in not explained nor is it clear whether wrap-around coverage is mandatory or permissive. The benefit is not accompanied by procedural guarantees or measures to broaden access that were part of earlier legislation dealing with EPSDT, for instance, in 1989. Moreover, nothing is said about the possible impact of enforceable cost-sharing requirements on this benefit. Andy Schneider, e-mail, May 31, 2006. A CMS statement in April, 2006 and a letter from Sen. Grassley and Rep. Barton to Secretary Leavitt stated in terms

that reducing EPSDT benefits were "not an option" and that Congress "intended to make no changes in EPSDT." as quoted by Christie Provost Peters *EPSDT: Medicaid's Critical But Controversial Benefits Program for Children.* Washington, DC: National Health Policy Forum, November 2006. 3.4. How much weight to attribute to these statements is questionable in view of the obvious fact that DRA *did* change the status of EPSDT.

118. Critics have expressed a concern that the DRA flexibility provisions would allow a substitution of EPSDT benefits for existing optional benefits rather than adding to them and that a combination of benchmarking, targeting, co-pays and abandonment of routine screening of children would drastically reduce access to EPSDT. Cf. Peters, *EPSDT* and Sara Rosenbaum, *Defined-Contribution Plans and Limited-Benefit Arrangements: Implications for Medicaid Beneficiaries.* Washington, DC: George Washington University School of Public Health and Health Services, September 2006. 9 ff. The history of EPSDT would seem to indicate that positive measures are needed to reach even a small fraction of those in need and that there are many ways and opportunities to deny access to the program's benefits.

119. *Congressional Quarterly,* December 30, 2005, p. 2.

120. *Congressional Quarterly,* December 22, 2005, p. 2.

121. *Health Care Policy Report,* September 19, 2005, p. 1194.

122. The objections related to the so-called "Byrd Rule," which dealt with reconciliation bills and specified grounds for objection to provisions that were non-germane, did not change revenue or outlays, fell outside the committee reconciliation instructions, would increase the deficit, or change Social Security. The Byrd rule could be waived only by a three-fifths vote of the Senate, so that it was useful not only for assuring appropriate procedures but for delaying a reconciliation bill.

123. Andy Schneider *et al., The Administration's Medicaid Proposals Would Shift Federal Costs to the States.* Washington, D.C.: Center on Budget and Policy Priorities, February 2006, 3-7.

124. *Ibid.,* p. 4.

125. Matthew Salo, telephone interview by Smith, October 20, 2006.

126. *Ibid.,* telephone interview by Smith, December 4, 2006.

127. Tardy and inadequate response to the Katrina hurricane was an important policy failure.

128. However, gains among the young, women, and Latinos may be important and continuing trends.

129. This is a factor that might be important. Richard Nathan has argued that we may be entering a new cycle of federalism in which states are of increasing importance as initiators of change. If that is true, then some of the Medicaid leadership states—an increased number of which are now Democratic—may have a large role in promoting constructive Medicaid reforms. Cf. Richard P. Nathan, *Back to Business With Substantially Changed Political Arithmetic—What Will the Changes Mean?* Albany, NY: Rockefeller Institute. November 16, 2006. 1.

130. Officially the "Bipartisan Commission on Medicaid Reform," but later usually referred to as the "Medicaid Commission" or the "Leavitt Commission.

131. One part of the Commission's charge was to report on specific options that would produce Medicaid savings of $10 billion over five years. This task was successfully completed before the deadline of September 1, 2005. The larger task was to develop and report back to the secretary with recommendations that would ensure the long-term sustainability of the Medicaid program. In November 2006 the Commission adopted its recommendations and issued a final draft report.

132. The Commission had no one generally recognized as an expert on Medicaid policy. The Democratic governor lacked extensive experience with Medicaid. Only ne member was a strong advocate for Medicaid. To many, it seemed more like a task force aimed at articulating views sympathetic to the secretary than a commission seeking what was best for Medicaid.

8

Devolution and Waivers

The Medicaid program may well be unique in its capacity for incremental growth. Created as a weak entitlement[1] and loosely articulated, it has proven to be highly adaptive, capable of vigorous growth, and tenaciously resistant to containment—almost too strong for our federal system. Like the common law, it has developed increment by increment and layer by layer; though unlike the common law, with almost no sustained efforts at reform and no successful ones.[2] In a word, Medicaid tends to grow, by parts, too much or too little, and without adequate means for reform or restructuring.

Over the years, there have been attempts to transform Medicaid radically: by capping or block-granting the program; federal-state "swaps" of responsibilities; or by folding the program into a larger national health insurance proposal. Both the Nixon and the Reagan administrations pushed for 5% caps on federal funding for Medicaid. The Ford and Reagan administrations and the Republican Congress of 1995 sought to block-grant the program. The Nixon administration "federalized" the adult welfare categories and the Clinton administration de-linked Medicaid and welfare. But none of these were considered reforms as such and, except for welfare, never enacted.

One theme common to most of these efforts has been "devolution," the transfer of authority or control from the federal government to the states or a local body. In applying such a notion to Medicaid, it is important to realize that "devolution" can be holistic (a block grant) or incremental (increased waiver flexibility), or somewhere in between. What is devolved is also important: whether it is authority over eligibility and benefits, service delivery and payments, or standards of care.[3] So, too, with the ultimate purpose of devolution: whether to alter the federal-state balance, increase efficiency or shrink the program, encourage de-institutionalization or the privatizing of an activity.

Devolution in Medicaid was only a small part of a broad movement that became important following the Johnson administration and its Great Society programs that left, as part of its legacy, a persuasion that the federal government had grown too large and that "balance" needed to be restored to the federal system. Whatever one may think about the underlying theory of that proposition, an important political fact was that trust in the federal government to redress domestic problems had shifted to a presumption in favor of state and local solutions.[4] The Nixon administration, confronting a strong Democratic Congress, sought mostly to consolidate grants and increase administrative efficiency rather than attack the Great Society programs as such. But for President Reagan, government itself—especially the federal government—was the problem. Accordingly, he aimed not only to devolve but also to shrink federal domestic programs, the largest of which were the entitlements, including Medicaid. Medicaid came in for attention on both these accounts—devolution and disentitlement. It was also a program arguably in need of restructuring because of its institutional bias and traditional claims processing orientation.

For a variety of reasons, seeking to disentitle the Medicaid program has proven to be difficult, unpopular, and divisive. But devolution could be approached incrementally, was perennially urged by the governors, and had bipartisan support in the Congress. The big confrontations over the Medicare and Medicaid entitlements in 1981 and 1995-96 were visible and dramatic, but much of the struggle over Medicaid, especially from 1981 on, has been about "devolution," especially in the form of "flexibility" amendments, managed care and home and community-based waivers, SCHIP, and a new generation of Sec. 1115 waivers. To be sure, disentitlement and devolution often went together, especially with a threat of disentitlement helping to generate concessions that were devolutionist or some mix of both. But most of the "restructuring" of Medicaid—insofar as this has taken place—has been in the form of flexibility amendments, the Sec. 1915(b) and 1915(c) waivers and the Sec. 1115 comprehensive and "superwaivers."

Antecedents

The devolution of Medicaid as a sustained process began in earnest with the Reagan administration and OBRA '81; but some antecedent developments are of interest, both to establish a baseline and to understand why and how devolution occurred.

The original statute is a good place to start. It opens with a statement of purpose following closely one in the earlier Kerr-Mills legislation: "enabling each State as far as practicable under the conditions in such State" to furnish medical assistance and rehabilitative services "on behalf of families with dependent children" and the "aged, blind, or permanently and totally disabled." Unlike Medicare, Title XIX does not employ the language of "entitlement," leaving the concept largely implicit in the text.[5] The entitlement—such as it was—was linked to the traditional welfare categories, with eligibility determination left essentially to state criteria and administration of the means tests. Beyond the five mandated services, benefits were largely up to the states. Subject to a few content-neutral tests—statewideness, comparability, and adequacy in amount, duration, and scope—states could decide which services they wished to provide.[6] There was, of course, Sec. 1903(e), the "comprehensive care" provision, but that was more a vision statement than a mandate and was postponed and later repealed in 1972. Prior to the 1980s, the presumption was that the federal government provided half or more of the money and the states administered the program, subject to a minimum of statutory requirements.[7] This idea of what Medicaid should be—a program run by the states with federal aid and some general standards—fairly well describes the early period, 1966-1983. Even today, many Medicaid directors believe that is the way Medicaid should be—a persuasion that is lasting and powerful.

A brief anecdote illustrates this last point. At a National Health Policy Forum meeting in Washington a few years ago, a number of HCFA administrators were sharing recollections of their experiences.[8] In the "question and answer" that followed, a member of the audience noted that the panelists had spoken almost exclusively about Medicare and asked why more had not been said about Medicaid. The answer by a member of the panel was that their topic had been "administration," and that they had little to do with Medicaid administration since that was a matter for the states. This dictum needs to be set alongside another observation from a HCFA Administrator that one-third to one-half of his time was spent in dealing with waivers and the negotiations and on-going adjustments these involved.

In part, the paradox is a matter of definition: of what is politics and what is administration. Also, waivers have become, over time and especially since the Clinton and Bush administrations, much more powerful instruments of change and of a kind of policymaking, the means and ends of which are not always noticed or well understood. Whether described as "politics" or as "administration," Medicaid issues of federal-state relations and devolution have grown in importance, though not always in visibility or clarity.

The fifteen-year period from 1966 to 1981 could be thought of as "classical," in that Medicaid, during that time, was primarily a claims-paying program of fee-for-service providers delivering health care in the traditional manner. Most of the policy emphasis in both the Johnson and Nixon administrations, as well as in the Democratic Congress, was to establish the program, process and pay legitimate claims and hospital bills, and curb fraud and abuse. A modicum of program planning occurred. Even the Social Security Amendments of 1972, with scores of Medicare and Medicaid provisions, were directed primarily at making the classical model work with greater program integrity and efficiency, not at transforming it.

There were, of course, differences between Democrats and Republicans and between Congress and the administration. Many Democrats, both in the Congress and in the career civil service, identified strongly with the Medicare model and with its priorities—inherited from the Social Security Administration—of program integrity, paying on time, and getting it right.[9] Republicans shared this tradition less and, especially during the Nixon administration, many came to government from the private sector and, in health policy, were more likely to think in terms of private-sector approaches, such as HMOs. Even so, their attention was less on program modification than on ways to increase the economy and efficiency of the Medicaid program as legislated. Democrats and Republicans agreed on the central objectives of implementing and sustaining the original program, although their means varied.

In this initial period, much of the federal emphasis was on "marginal centralization,"[10]—marginal in the sense that it introduced a few limits or procedures rather than changing program structure, content, or mission or directly ordering behavior. Moreover, these limits often came with concessions or adaptations of a devolutionist sort that made them more palatable to the states.

Good examples of this kind of behavior appeared in the Medicaid provisions of the Social Security Amendments of 1967. A number of these were marginally centralizing. They included nursing home standards,[11] the EPSDT mandate, and limiting of the federal Medicaid match for the "medically indigent" to 133% of a state's level of income eligibility. Then or eventually each of these was an important centralizing step—but each was accompanied by or limited by concessions important to the states. Along with the nursing home standards, Congress recognized and defined an "intermediate care facility" (ICF) and made it eligible for Medicaid funding, a measure considerably more important in the short run than the nursing home standards. EPSDT eventually became onerous for the states, but initially implementation was left mostly to good will and did not become a strongly specified and compulsory matter until OBRA '89. The 133% limits on federal matching for the medically indigent were effective[12] in curbing Medicaid expenditures and might seem procrustean in character. But they also left much to the states: for instance, to increase their federal match by raising welfare eligibility and to modify the Medicaid "spend down." Furthermore, the 133% limit was supported by many governors: as a way of sharing the FMAP total amount more fairly, to prod laggard states to raise welfare eligibility, and to protect governors themselves from their own state legislatures.[13]

The approach of the Nixon administration could also be described as "marginal centralization," but with a significant shift in underlying philosophy: toward centralization for the purpose of or combined with operational devolution. This theme was well expressed in the report of the McNerney Task Force on Medicaid. Particularly relevant in the present context was the emphasis there upon management and the use of the state plan to achieve objectives, including a restructuring of the delivery system to align incentives and put insurers, providers, and consumers on the same side in controlling costs.[14] The Task Force supported PSROs and HMOS as entities that could realign incentives more effectively, and with less intrusive intervention, than regulation. In effect, some leadership and strategic intervention would facilitate devolution, eliminate some regulation and, less obviously, reduce the intrusive role of congressional sub-committees.[15]

Two related Medicaid concerns during the Nixon and Ford administrations were fraud and abuse and a Medicaid information system. Like overlapping circles, these initiatives shared common ground but were distinct in part. Recalling earlier history (*supra*, 70), lack of claims data was a major problem in the early implementation of Medicaid. Information systems were needed to pay claims promptly and accurately and to identify and track pervasive fraud and abuse. Such systems along with usable databases, were also important for planning and management, to prioritize activities, and to make the agency case with public authorities.

Fraud and abuse, though, were urgent and had strong political appeal. As a result, the two concerns competed for public attention but were also complementary. Management information systems supported efforts to identify and curb fraud and abuse; and the visibility and appeal of anti-fraud measures supplied some of the political clout needed to fund information systems.

The most significant legislation on this topic was the Medicare and Medicaid Fraud and Abuse Amendments of 1977 (P.L. 95-142). This legislation passed in the first year of the Carter administration by over-whelming majorities in both houses of Congress, the result of a growing concern over fraud and abuse; a desire on the part of both Congress and the administration to clear the way for another try at national health insurance; and a campaign by Sen. Frank Moss and the Senate Special Committee on Aging for protective nursing home legislation. Described broadly, the legislation defined offenses and increased penalties; required various kinds of disclosure by providers; increased the role of PSROs and lengthened their terms; and provided 90% federal funding for three years to help establish and operate separate state offices that would investigate and prosecute suspected Medicaid fraud.

This fraud and abuse legislation was important in itself and provided a template for later legislation. It was a good example of forthright remedial action. But its visibility and appealing righteousness tends to divert attention from the other part of the story: about computers and information systems and alternate approaches to claims processing and program integrity that put more emphasis upon developing capabilities and improving behavior and less upon detecting and punishing evildoers.

The notion of sophisticated management information systems (MMIS) for Medicaid got on the agenda rather early, both nationally and locally. Computers and "automatic data processing" were in vogue. States needed help, to get the millions of claims processed and audited and the federal government wanted and needed data from the states. Some states set about developing their own data processing and information management systems. A few, such as Michigan and Texas, were out in front and provided models. Others contracted with Blue Cross/Blue Shield plans or one of the new data processing consulting firms.[16] The laggards processed what they could, with unpaid claims piling up in filing cabinets and warehouses.[17] State by state, experience differed; but it was widely apparent that management information systems were critical needs.

Early in the implementation of Medicaid, Ellen Winston—the administrator of Public Assistance—proposed a joint initiative that would bring state officials to Washington, D.C. to exchange program data and information about Medicaid best practices and meet with federal officials who would communicate some doctrine and provide technical assistance. One objective was to develop of a model template for a Medicaid MIS. With SRS funds she was able to pay their expenses and scores of state officials did come, even though some were concerned that the information shared might be used against them.[18] Ms. Winston soon departed, but the McNerney task force supported the concept and recommended that a "separate organizational entity," a Division of Management and Payment Systems, be established within Medicaid to pursue this and related aims.[19] One product of these initiatives was a five-volume Medicaid series on MMIS published between 1971 and 1974 that included shared experience and best practices and templates for adding modules to developing state information management systems.

Among major purposes of the MMIS were to combat fraud and abuse and to improve and increase the data flow to federal officials. But MMIS was first and primarily to enable states to administer and strengthen their own programs. It is worth noting, in this context, that the surveillance and utilization review systems (SURS) were late additions, not the central part of the MMIS.

MMIS was devolutionist in its aim to leave much of the monitoring and enforcement to the states. The PSROs were more radically devolutionist since they aimed at turning over much of utilization and quality reviews to local physician committees. These began as an AMA proposal and were touted by Sen. Wallace Bennett, a conservative Utah Republican, as a last chance at physician self-government. They were seized upon by the Senate Finance staff and included as part of the Social Security Amendments of 1972 with emphasis upon case-specific review,[20] but also preserving the educational and quality improvement features.

This noble—or ignoble—experiment failed for a number of reasons: limited jurisdiction,[21] lack of funds and of enthusiasm on the part of physicians, inadequate sanctions, and costs far exceeding the money saved. President Carter sought to eliminate them because they weren't cost-effective and President Reagan because they were "regulative," wasteful, and anti-competitive. One contribution they made, though, was to increase awareness of the conflicts between technical assistance and education versus adversarial investigations and sanctions.[22] This tension was sidestepped for a time rather than resolved. Congress subsidized the development of MMIS but without linking these systems specifically to fraud and abuse; it extended the life of the PSROs for two years and gave the individual states more authority over them; and it provided 90% matching for states to organize separate Fraud and Abuse Control Units (FACUs). Each of these steps were, in part, an additional empowerment of the states.

As the fraud and abuse/MMIS development suggests, much that is important in centralization vs. devolution of activities or authority depends on the amount of collaboration and the spirit with which it is approached—how fair the terms of collaboration are, whether the states are treated as partners or as agents, and how much say they have over what. This first period, from 1966 to 1981, has been described as "marginal centralization," meaning that program administration was largely left to the states. At the time, though, federal officials were struggling to implement the law, get the Medicaid program established, and assure its integrity. Many of the officials were career civil servants, imbued with the Social Security ethos of competence and fidelity to the law. In consequence, some of the centralization, although "marginal," could seem—and sometimes was—both formalistic and oblivious when state perspectives differed or enforcement was involved.

Two important institutions developed from just such circumstances: the National Association of State Medicaid Directors (NASMD) and the Technical Advisory Groups (TAGs). For these, federal actions supplied a stimulus (or two) in the form of penalties for state errors in eligibility determinations.

The Medicaid Eligibility Quality Control (MEQC), begun in 1973 and modified repeatedly, provided for federal review of eligibility determinations, with penalties for error rates above a certain percentage.[23] It had been a continuing irritant, involved significant amounts of money, engendered rancorous disputes, and affected each and every Medicaid program. Moreover, the federal government had gotten more insistent about enforcing it at a time when the Medicaid directors were debating whether and how they should constitute themselves as an independent organization. That decision was made in 1978, in considerable measure because the quality regulations had made these directors increasingly aware that they needed separate representation on matters of national policy. Related to this was a desire to distance and separate themselves from the welfare tradition. They also sought the opportunity to grow as a corporate body and to share more of their best practices—which included not only raising their professional level, but ideas about how to work with or around federal authorities.[24] The National Association of State Medicaid Directors (NASMD) was formed under the umbrella of the American Public Welfare Association in 1978 and is, today, the only national organization representing state Medicaid directors.[25]

The Technical Advisory Groups (TAGs) had a long history. Advisory groups of various kinds were a common practice with HEW (later HHS) programs and a number of informal advisory groups, with specified members from the State Medicaid Directors Association, had been convened over the years in Washington, DC—expenses paid—to consult with federal technical people.[26] In 1981, the new EPSDT penalty regulations were a controversial topic that had both Medicaid and child health advocates aroused. The matter came to a head in a tense Medicaid directors' meeting in Memphis, Tennessee, with a motion for a formally constituted EPSDT technical advisory group. The proposal was readily adopted by HCFA and the EPSDT TAG, though changing over time, lasted for 14 years and set a pattern for other TAGs. It was replaced by the Maternal and Child Health TAG, which continues to this day.

Eventually, the number of TAGS grew to twelve[27] and became an established part of Medicaid policy implementation and administration, dealing with such topics as eligibility, fraud and abuse, managed care, maternal and child health, and quality. As the name implies, they are "technical" and work primarily at a "staff" level where details and technical issues are resolved by federal and state employees working together. They are non-political and do not "make policy," but they are important channels of communication, provide a venue in which federal and state officials can speak frankly, improve implementation and administration, and avoid gaffes and misunderstanding.

Managed Care and Community-Based Services Waivers

The fifteen-year period from 1966 through 1980 was one of "marginal centralization" in which the structure of the Medicaid program remained largely unchanged. In the 1980s, program modifications were vigorously sought: expansion and stronger federal standards by Congressional Democrats, and "flexibility" or devolution by Republican presidents and their allies in Congress. Alternative delivery systems (ADS) and effective methods of cost containment were needed. But divided government, ideology, and increased partisanship prevented comprehensive solutions.

So a natural tendency was to seek Medicaid funding for expanded eligibility and coverage and incremental regulative modifications through the budget reconciliation process on the one side and devolution or added "flexibility" on the other. The original claims-paying Medicaid system needed "fixing;" but it was itself the most available vehicle for change and could be adapted through incremental legislation and waivers. As a result of this historic circumstance, waivers eventually became, almost accidentally, major instruments for structural change.

Sec. 1115 of the Social Security Act, passed in 1962, was the earliest waiver authority for Medicaid.[28] It authorized "experimental, pilot or demonstration" projects, not new program development as such.[29] The 1981 waivers for managed care and home and community-based services[30] were, in contrast, passed specifically to enable states to develop these as program alternatives rather than as research or demonstration projects and are often referred to as "program" waivers.

The history of Sec. 1115 is illuminating. It was a brief, isolated paragraph, part of the Public Welfare Amendments of 1962 (P.L. 81-543 Sec. 1115(a)) which were significant primarily for the addition of social services to welfare cash assistance. The text confers broad authority on the secretary to "waive compliance to any of the requirements" of a number of sections of the Social Security Act for "any experimental, pilot, or demonstration project" which "in the judgment of the secretary is likely to assist in promoting the objectives of title I, IV, X, XIV or XVI in a State or States…"

As written, Sec. 1115(a) invests "the Secretary" with a vast discretion to grant waivers, although for research and demonstration, not for restructuring or the pursuit of various "backdoor" agendas.[31] But if the R&D restriction were lifted or relaxed, then Sec. 1115 could become a powerful instrument for program change, as it was for states seeking welfare reform. In the early years of Medicaid, it was used widely as a substitute for minor state plan amendments. Because of this and similar abuses, the Carter administration tightened the review and approval of the 1115 waivers and largely returned them to their original purpose;[32] but that left the Medicaid program in need of flexibility in addressing such issues as cost containment and service delivery changes.

The legislative history of the Sec. 1915(b) and 1915(c) waiver authority has been recounted (*supra*, 165-168) but in the present context it should be noted that these amendments—though alternatives to the almost complete discretion that governors would have under the House block grant proposals—were still a major devolution of authority to the states to develop service delivery alternatives and that it was based on a bipartisan consensus that they were needed and would be beneficial.

Managed Care—1915(b) Waiver

Medicaid experience with managed care prior to OBRA '81 was mixed and not promising. Early in the history of Medicaid, federal and state officials and policy analysts were keenly interested in "alternative delivery systems," i.e., something other than fee-for-service medicine and especially some form of prospective payment, including hospital budgets, capitation, and HMOs.[33] The Social Security Amendments of 1967 authorized state Medicaid programs to contract with HMOs and other organizations that paid on the basis of capitation or prospective budgets.[34] Under the authority of Sec. 1110, the federal government funded a series of ADS demonstrations, conducted between 1971-1973. These were followed by more series of demonstrations in the mid-to-late 1970s that, according to a comprehensive evaluation, helped to move the states from "buyers of HMO services to designers of alternate delivery systems."[35] The demonstrations were markedly less successful, though, in stimulating managed care. In general, urban poverty agencies did much better by starting local managed care plans for welfare recipients. As of June 1980, only 17 state Medicaid agencies had managed care contracts, only one state had more than one contract, and slightly more than 1% of all Medicaid beneficiaries were enrolled in these plans.[36]

The one state with multiple contracts was, of course, California with its "Prepaid Health Plans," that almost permanently blighted Medicaid managed care. The PHPs were part of the Medi-Cal Reform Act, passed in August 1971 in an effort to curb dramatically rising Medicaid costs. Under Part II of the Act, PHPs could contract with the state to provide comprehensive care to Medi-Cal enrollees for a negotiated per patient fee. No capitation rate could exceed the Medi-Cal fee-for-service rates or payments; and 10% in global savings were required. The Department of Health had to approve the contracts, but other requirements were minimal—especially with respect to plan structure, marketing procedures, financial reserves or tangible assets, standards of access or quality, or rights of enrollees.

To this day, the California experience is remembered as a cautionary example of the evils of inadequate regulation, illustrating almost every imaginable abuse,[37] and involving industrial espionage, terroristic threats, and organized crime. There were other, less lurid examples, most notably New York City and Chicago, but California was exceptional. It was also a particular embarrassment to the Nixon administration that responded with a go-slow policy on Medicaid HMOs and with Project PHRED,[38] aimed specifically at improving Medicaid managed care and preventing a recurrence of the kind of abuses that occurred with the California PHPs.

OBRA '81, with its 1915(b) authorization of waivers opened a new phase in the development of Medicaid managed care. In addition to the waiver, OBRA '81 repealed the requirement that Medicaid HMOs had to be federally qualified, allowing states to qualify the plans so long as they could demonstrate capacity and solvency. The 50% limit on Medicaid enrollees was replaced with a less stringent (and more realistic) 75/25 rule. Sec. 1915(b) provided several options including selective contracting, acting as a central broker, and even requiring Medicaid beneficiaries to enroll in a primary care case-management plan (PCCM) or choose as between several HMOs, PHPs, or a fee-for-service PCCM.[39] The scheme was both imaginative and adaptable: providing strong encouragement but allowing for minimalist versions of managed care, such as fee-for-service PCCMs. As noted previously (*supra*, 166) both Democrats and Republicans supported the waiver for its cost saving potential though, beyond that. Democrats saw managed care more as a way to increase access and Republicans to promote better management.

Evaluating the experience with these waivers is much like deciding whether the glass is half empty or half full. During this period, the rate of increase in Medicaid managed care enrollees lagged far behind that in private sector plans.[40] In 1989, Medicaid enrollments in all forms of managed care stood at two million, about 10% of total number in Medicaid.[41] As of 1991, only 28 states had applied for or implemented Medicaid 1915(b) projects.[42] Also, many of the plans were fee-for-service PCCMs or left provider relations much as they found them, so that cost savings were small or non-existent. In the early '90s, Medicaid managed care took off dramatically, though largely for reasons that had little relation to the Sec. 1915(b) waivers as such.

On the positive side, by encouraging PCCMs, the 1915(b) waiver helped establish the concept of a "medical home." Although little in-depth case management occurred and the "case manager" tended to become largely a managed care "gatekeeper," the idea of case management and of a medical home represented an important step in exchanging a rather empty "freedom of choice" for a commitment to provide the Medicaid enrollee access to care and some management. As reported in a voluminous program evaluation, the waiver was also a learning experience—about the difficulties of organizing managed care, the necessary preliminary steps and expertise required, and what worked and what did not.[43]

In the early 1990s, Medicaid managed care enrollments began increasing sharply, from about half the rate of growth for commercial managed care to two times that rate.[44] That rate of growth continued throughout the decade and could be considered something of a "revolution." Over ten years the number of Medicaid beneficiaries enrolled in managed care plans grew from 2.7 million (9.5%) in 1991 to 18.8 million (56%) in 2000.[45] Some of the factors involved in this growth are of interest, because they had little to do with Sec. 1915(b) waivers or, for that matter, with the evolution of the Medicaid program as such.

One important development was the re-establishment of the Medicaid Bureau in 1990. The Medicaid program had been merged with (or submerged under) Medicare by the Califano reorganization and remained in limbo from 1977 to 1990. Midway through the Bush administration, Gail Wilensky was appointed as the HCFA administrator. She was struck both by the inefficiency of the merged arrangement and by the frustrations of state officials and politicians seeking to get action on waivers, state plan amendments, and other concerns.[46] One of her first actions was to re-establish the Medicaid Bureau. She appointed Christine (Tina) Nye, a Medicaid state director, to be head of the newly reconstituted bureau. Nye brought with her an understanding of and sympathy for state perspectives as well as openness to new approaches and a presumption in favor of waivers, including some of the new Sec. 1115 "super-waivers."[47] These attitudes were also supported by the Clinton administration and by Nye's successor, Sally Richardson, who had also been a state employee.

The growth and comparative success of commercial managed care plans was important for showing the way, providing examples of what worked, and demonstrating the impressive cost-savings that were possible. Commercial HMOs expanded into the Medicare and Medicaid markets, especially during that phase in their development when they sought primarily to increase or consolidate market share rather than maximize profits. Eventually, the commercial HMOs pulled back, but their leadership was important in accelerating developments in the 1990s.

Rising state Medicaid expenditures during the early 1990s was another factor. The whole issue of why and how such expenditures were increasing is complex,[48] but the main elements can be identified. Health care costs were increasing generally and affected Medicaid along with other programs and health plans. Enrollments were up, especially among the costly elderly and disabled. The recession of 1991-92 added to Medicaid rolls and reduced state resources. Then, there were the "unfunded" mandates: not only the Waxman children and pregnant women but the dual eligibles,[49] EPSDT, and the nursing home standards.[50] AIDS was another expense. And so forth. Governors and state legislatures sought relief: protesting the mandates, resorting to provider taxes and DSH schemes, and turning to managed care.

The failure of health care reform in 1993-94 was a stimulus for managed care waivers in part because its demise freed the health policy agenda and because President Clinton and some governors—mostly Democrats—resolved to expand Medicaid as a way of moving incrementally toward national health insurance.[51] These additions to Medicaid were largely achieved not with Sec. 1915(b) waivers, but with Sec. 1115 "super-waivers" and the imaginative use of Sec. 1902(r)(2).[52]

Although much of the action recently has been with the Sec. 1115 waivers, the 1915(b) waivers were, and are, important. They helped establish the concept of a "medical home" for Medicaid beneficiaries. They were useful in facilitating a lengthy learning process at the state level. Also, states have been creative with this authority in devising carve-outs or step-by-step restructuring of their own systems. Even the PCCM option remains important, especially for areas not populated with HMOs or Medicaid programs preferring a more limited version of managed care.

The time elapsed—a decade—from the creation of the 1915(b) waiver authority until Medicaid managed care developed momentum and volume significantly affected both how the waiver was used and the results achieved. By then, the emphasis had shifted more toward cost-saving and away from other managed care objectives such as preventive health, increased access, case management, or quality of care. Ironically, this shift of emphasis was taking place even as a lengthy HCFA sponsored evaluation of managed care was concluding that "the cost-effectiveness of alternative delivery systems for Medicaid has yet to be determined."[53]

One reason to be skeptical about the cost-saving potential of Medicaid managed care was apparent early on—that Medicaid providers were already underpaid, so that trying to get large savings was likely either to drive them out of the Medicaid market or deteriorate the quality of service, or both. When squeezed, the commercial plans "tended to withdraw with the result that Medicaid managed care organizations became increasingly Medicaid only," making them even less attractive to risk-bearing commercial HMOs.[54] Many of these withdrew or reduced their offerings so that Medicaid managed care is today dominated by "Medicaid focused" or Medicaid dominant plans, many of them sponsored by safety-net providers.[55]

Another important issue that should have been apparent is the basic conflict between insurance (or risk) and the Medicaid entitlement.[56] HMOs seek to control risk while Medicaid guarantees access. There is an inherent tension, which would have been evident if managed care had been extended, early on, to more of the frail elderly and persons with disabilities.[57] Medicaid not only covers "uninsurable" populations but provides a much larger array of services than offered by standard commercial plans—or by Medicaid itself for most of its beneficiaries. As a consequence, Medicaid programs have to be "customized" with additional offerings, carve-outs, risk-adjusters, or other adaptations. One effect of this tendency is that Medicaid agencies often negotiate with one or a few providers for a list of services for a set population—the opposite of competition in a health care marketplace.

Over time, Medicaid managed care has diverged widely from the HMO model contemplated early in the 1980s: dominantly Medicaid in membership rather than mainstream; and subsisting on negotiated prices rather than risk adjusted rates. Yet the Medicaid plans provide a medical home, assure access, and manage care for their members within contract limits. States have gained sophistication in operating with them; and the plans accept their special role and are content with modest prospects. It remains to be seen how well they can be adapted to the needs of the frail elderly, the chronically ill, and persons with disabilities. Yet they seem to be achieving some of the objectives contemplated by the Sec. 1915(b) waiver and the early demonstrations.[58]

Home and Community-Based Services Waivers—Sec. 1915(c)

The home and community-based waiver is another initiative that achieved less than expected of its intended objectives and more than expected of some unintended ones. It diverted fewer from nursing homes and saved less money and had minimal impact upon placement of the chronically mentally ill, but was enormously successful in promoting home and community-based services for the mentally retarded. Behind this brief summary there are some stories and a context.

One source of support for this type of waiver was a broadly based movement in the 1970s toward services in communities as an alternative to institutional care. A 1977 initiative backed by Rep. Claude Pepper (D., Fla.) and the House Special Committee on Aging sought to extend and liberalize home care for the elderly. In 1980, the Medicaid Community Care Act (HR 6194), introduced by Rep. Henry Waxman (D., Calif.), renewed support for this objective, broadening it to include mental retardation and mental illness. Another unifying concern for these proposals was the cost and disproportionate share of nursing home care: 40% of total Medicaid expenditures for 6% of the Medicaid enrollees.[59]

The presumption underlying the Sec. 1915(c) legislation was that large, remote institutions were likely to give inadequate care and that better care for the same money or less could be provided in smaller institutions, residential settings, and community-based services. In large measure, this waiver authority built upon the de-institutionalization movement, though not uncritically. Close attention was given to level of care, cost-shifting opportunities, and assuring that the HCBS option did not become an open invitation to add all sorts of new services under the rubric of "medical assistance."

Sec. 2176 of OBRA '81, which followed the House Commerce Committee bill in broad outline, authorized home and community-based services waivers for individuals who, without such services, would require "the level of care provided in a Skilled Nursing Facility or an Intermediate Care Facility the cost of which could be reimbursed under the State Plan" (Sec. 2176(2)). No mention was made of other institutions, such as HMOs or ICF/MRs, or of other developmental disabilities. But the committee print included ICF/MRs, though not IMDs; and Sec. 123 of TEFRA (1982) allowed states to include children with disabilities living at home who would be eligible for Supplemental Security Income if institutionalized.[60]

Quality of care was a matter for concern, especially given the past history of ICF/MRs and of de-institutionalization; and the Commerce Committee made much of the need for early and individual assessment, comprehensive treatment plans, and standards of care. On the other hand, a major purpose of the HCBS waiver was to give states greater flexibility, especially important with the local variation and mushroom-like growth of community-based services.[61] The latter view prevailed in the legislation, which relied primarily on state plans, though it did require individual assessments, written plans of care, "assurances" (satisfactory to the secretary) about "safeguards" to protect health and safety, and reporting on type and amount of "medical assistance" provided and its effects on the "health and welfare" of the recipients.[62]

Measures to contain costs were especially important for this particular waiver because of the number and variety of services that might well be added: such as case management; home health and homemaker services; physical, speech, and other therapies; adult day care, habilitation; respite care, and such "other services requested by the State as the secretary may approve." Not only was experience with these services limited, some of them—like "habilitation" for instance—seemed almost an invitation to invent and spend. Another concern was the so-called "woodwork" effect, i.e., the needy persons, deficiencies, and afflictions that would be revealed (crawl out of the woodwork) when some condition was treated.[63] In a word, what seemed like a money-saving venture could wind up costing a lot of money.

The statute addressed the issue of costs in two ways. One was a budget-neutral (or cost-neutral)[64] requirement—supplied by the House bill—that the average per capita expenditures for recipients under the waiver could not exceed the amount that the state "reasonably estimates" would have been made in that fiscal year if there were no waiver. The presumption was that the waiver would produce some savings, but a common objection to the requirement as phrased was that it did not allow start-up costs to be spread over the life (three years) of the waiver nor total expenditures to be off-set by savings from other parts of the state Medicaid budget.[65] The other element, which came from the Senate, stipulated that services provided had to be for persons who "but for" those services would require the level of care in a SNF or ICF "the cost of which could be reimbursed under the State Plan." This was the foundation for what came to be known as the "bed capacity" or "cold bed" test, to wit, that there had to be an institutional bed freed up by such services or that would not have to be built in their absence.

Medicaid agencies that were experienced and well placed in their own state administrations had little trouble with the HCBS waiver as such, but for others it occasioned difficulty and anguish. At the time, most states had little experience with waivers, and for some of the less sophisticated ones, the HCBS waiver involved major tasks of trying to understand HCFA requirements, assemble the data, and write the applications.[66] A complicating factor was that this waiver involved a multi-disciplinary effort—coordination between Medicaid and other departments at the state level and collecting data and program schema from a number of agencies, which were both clueless and resentful where HCFA was involved. Moreover, some of the justifications and supporting data—for instance, those relating to calculations of per capita costs, bed occupancy, and cost-neutrality—were made yet more difficult because of inexperience and having to work with an assortment of agencies at different levels of commitment and experience.

The situation within HCFA made the waiver process even more onerous. With the formation of HCFA, the merger of Medicare and Medicaid, and the move to Baltimore in 1977-78, a large number of the Medicaid staff resigned, diminishing Medicaid representation within HCFA and leaving Medicare officials in control of most important decisions and, specifically in point, oversight of rulemaking and review of activities relating to this waiver. A consequence was that state Medicaid officials, interested in their waiver, often had difficulty navigating the Bureau of Program Policy (later, Bureau of Eligibility, Reimbursement, and Coverage) or getting a fair and responsive hearing from Medicare officials little interested in Medicaid affairs.[67] These officials, with a background in Medicare or the earlier SSA Bureau of Health Insurance, brought with them an ethos of "getting it right" and an approach of taking a topic firmly in hand, looking to the statute, declaring the rule (or program memorandum) and enforcing it—an attitude at which the remaining Medicaid veterans would "roll their eyes" and wait for their Medicare counterparts "to learn why they call them 'sovereign states.'"[68] These BPP/BERC officials spent hours on the telephone, teleconferencing and negotiating with state agency representatives, often walking applicants through the process step-by-step. But they would also challenge definitions of services and inclusions of particular items,[69] discrepancies in numbers,[70] the qualifications and payments for specialists, and methods used for calculating expenditures and savings. A former official said, in retrospect, that they imported Medicare methods into Medicaid, and that may have been a mistake.[71]

The bed capacity test, aka the "cold-bed" test, was a blunt, powerful instrument used by HCFA,[72] to assure cost-neutrality and that the HCB services covered in the waiver represented a genuine substitution for institutional care and not another add-on. Under the statute, cost-neutrality is required. Therefore, the costs of care under the waiver should not exceed the cost of care without the waiver: in other words, care under the waiver should be offset by actual reductions in institutional care or not "building beds" that would need to be added without the waiver. But just saying that was not enough, as early state behavior soon demonstrated. California, for instance, simply declared that it was putting 6100 Medicaid enrollees under waiver with the matter of bed reduction left for surmise. Other states would secure certificate-of-need (CoN) authority for new beds then rescind the authority and claim a reduction of beds. The HCFA response was the "bed capacity" test: that, for waiver purposes, beds were limited to their total of certified beds plus a turnover allowance.[73] This bed capacity limit was not inflexible, since nursing homes often did need to add capacity. But for that, more than a mere CoN was needed: the institution would have to show that beds had been built or would be built, and would be certified without the waiver.[74] Sometimes, allowances were also made for surplus beds that would be permanently retired.[75]

The "cold bed" language was pejorative and imprecise, but it made good sense as applied to the ICF/MR. Few long-term residents of nursing homes return to the community, so that states seeking HCBS waivers had to rely primarily on beds not built, turnover, or diversion rather than deinstitutionalization. At that time, though, there were over 300,000 mentally retarded or developmentally disabled living in large, often remote "asylum" type institutions, even though therapists much preferred smaller, community-based settings. There was also deinstitutionalization of an undesirable type: to the "bed and care" rooming houses in which the mentally ill or retarded could vegetate while their "hosts" lived off the SSI checks of their "guests."[76] As long as the "cold-bed" rule was in effect, it restrained waivers for developmentally disabled HCB services, though not as stringently as for nursing homes. Still, many supported it since it retired beds in larger, older facilities, encouraged smaller residential and community settings, and kept Medicaid funds out of the hands of unqualified and sometimes unethical providers.[77]

Another source of vexation for the states and for HCFA was the Reagan OMB that regarded waivers with suspicion and reviewed them zealously to see if they were consistent with the president's priorities. This wariness about waivers did not begin with the Reagan administration. In the Carter administration, especially during Patricia Harris's tenure as DHHS secretary, OMB had objected to the extravagant use of Sec. 1115 waivers to provide subsidies for inner-city hospitals and long-term care demonstrations which it saw as "back door" agenda building. As to that, one holdover from the Carter administration was a batch of waivers subsidizing over 60 Medicare HMOs—not only a questionable expense but at odds with TEFRA and the Reagan administration's emphasis upon "competition." In 1982, the deficit was being taken seriously so that the new administration was concerned about covert agendas and about the budgetary impact of the "social pork barrel," the "woodwork" effect, and programs that turned into add-ons rather than instead-ofs. Also important was David Stockman's experiment with "top-down" policy making,[78] which cast OMB as the premier staff agency and defender of the faith in domestic policy issues. Practically, that meant that key program areas within OMB, such as Human Resources, Veterans, and Labor and, under that, Health and Income Maintenance, should be headed by political appointees and civil servants who shared the administration's goals and who would be proactive, assiduous, and loyal in protecting White House priorities.[79]

Particularly important with waivers was to be proactive, to deny or modify costly waivers or ones that moved programs in undesirable directions or were likely to become a political embarrassment. These were prime administration objectives, though not directly related to the substantive merits of the waivers as perceived by the states or by HCFA. Also, they were not grounds for refusal that the administration wanted voiced or noised about. As a result, waivers were often delayed or returned, sometimes with repeated demands for more data, improved methodologies, or a reduction in the size and scope of the request, when these objections may have been and certainly seemed "pretextual" (not the real reason) and possibly related to an entirely different HHS activity or a larger struggle over control of the executive branch.[80] Whatever the ultimate reason(s), these interventions caused delays, frustrated health care officials, and angered state administrators and governors. HCFA officials were not allowed to blame OMB, so they were put in the embarrassing and untenable position of having to explain delays and seemingly arbitrary decisions without mentioning the key determinant.[81] Under these circumstances, governors began to intervene more frequently. Also, the existing waiver procedures lost credibility and HCFA gained some important enemies, among them William Jefferson Clinton, then governor of Arkansas.

Such impediments helped reduce the number and size of HCBS waivers so that, as late as 1990, only 40,000 of the MR/DD population and 135,000 of the frail elderly were under HCB waivers. Only one state, Vermont, was operating a 1915(c) waiver specifically targeted on the mentally ill.[82] By then, federal and state expenditures under this waiver were over $1.5 billion, but that sum represented only 4.7% of long-term care expenditures and 1.9% of total Medicaid expenditures.[83]

Between 1987 and 1990, various measures eased the waiver require-ments for nursing homes and for the mentally retarded and developmen-tally disabled. OBRA '87 added a new 1915(d) waiver for the elderly that eliminated the budget-neutral and bed capacity tests and substituted an annual cap on federal spending that would be determined by updating from a base year.[84] Although this option met with little response,[85] the bed capacity test was gradually relaxed and finally repealed in 1994.[86] An important modification for the mentally retarded and developmentally disabled was to allow states to meet the cost-neutrality test for residents of nursing homes who required an ICF/MR level of care by counting those costs rather than those for a nursing facility.[87] In OBRA '90, Congress added a new optional Medicaid benefit for the elderly with functional disabilities that had a cap on annual expenditures, but required only a state plan amendment rather than a waiver.[88]

Numbers served under 1915(c) waivers grew throughout the 1990s at roughly two times the rate before 1990s[89] because of many factors, including the demise of the cold-bed test, state caps on nursing home construction, the continuing movement toward deinstitutionalization, and more favorable attitudes toward waivers under the first Bush and the Clinton administrations. But the main growth was not that intended.

Initially intended primarily to provide a community-based alterna-tive for nursing homes, the HCBS waiver was much more successful with respect to the MR/DD population. In large measure, that was because the waiver worked better for a situation in which extensive de-institutionalization was either in process or in prospect. For nurs-ing homes, beds could not be built or potential residents could be diverted, but few long-term elderly residents were good prospects for de-institutionalization. Home and community-based services for the elderly grew rapidly over the decade, but more as an add-on than as a displacement of nursing home beds. HCBS waivers were "sold" as cost-savers, but often increased total costs because of the woodwork effects and expected savings from diversion that did not materialize.[90] By 2002, more than half of the expenditures for home and commu-nity-based services were under the mandatory Medicaid home health benefit and the optional state plan personal care, not for beneficiaries under 1915(c) waivers.[91]

With the mentally retarded and developmentally disabled, the situation was quite different. As a result of earlier efforts in a number of states, (*supra*, 103-104) Congress had created the ICF/MR which helped fund the building of a large number of facilities, some huge and remote, but others small and community-based. Advocacy groups were well organized and vocal at national, state, and local levels and pressed hard for normalization and community-based facilities and services.[92] There was a natural fit. Parents supplied energy and intensity. States had surplus beds, money for additional services, and could often adapt smaller residential facilities for HCB waivers. With the relaxing and eventual demise of the bed capacity limit, 1915(c) waivers for MR/DD took off: in 1990, 40,000 of this population were under waivers; in 2002, 358,000 were.[93] In 1977, 54,000 developmentally disabled persons were in large state institutions. In 1998, 3000 were.[94]

As for the severely and chronically mentally ill, the story was different. Mental health advocacy groups were not as united or mobilized; and both advocates and providers had been historically divided between the state and local institutional facilities and the community mental health centers. In addition, the IMD exclusion (*supra*, 49) effectively barred use of the 1915(c) waiver by excluding use of federal funds for these institutions. This exclusion applied not only to long-term care mental hospitals but also to nursing homes and other long-term facilities primarily serving persons with mental illness. It also worked indirectly to discourage 1915(c) waivers, since savings from deinstitutionalizing long-term facilities could not be counted toward cost-neutrality,[95] nor could they be used as a comparison group.[96]

Actions by Congress and by HCFA between 1987 and 1992 modified the IMD exclusion, greatly reducing its importance. One step was the addition of a subsection[97] that required treatment and services for mentally ill or mentally retarded nursing home residents and the inclusion of "mental and psychosocial well-being" as a specified objective applicable to all residents. A related measure was included in the Medicare Catastrophic Coverage Act of 1988, defining IMDs largely by excluding facilities of 16 beds or less.[98] HCFA regulations, based on this legislation, pushed states to upgrade care for the mentally ill or mentally retarded in nursing facilities and/or provide treatment for the more serious cases in smaller, personalized facilities. The IMD exclusion would still apply to large, warehouse-type facilities that provided little or no therapy and would continue to be bar them from Medicaid funding.

Had the change in the IMD exclusion been made earlier, it might have had a significant impact upon 1915(c) waiver activity. But state agencies from the mid-1980s on were finding different ways to draw upon Medicaid funds, especially under new standards for SSDI and SSI established by the Social Security Disability Benefits Reform Act of 1984 (P.L. 98-466).[99] This development made it easier for states to pay for a whole array of services in a community setting and collect federal matching funds for services that had previously been paid for by state-supported public institutions. This combination of flexibility and incentives was critical in enabling state Medicaid programs to respond to the challenge and the promise of a new generation of psychotropic drugs. At the same time, the need for both coordination of care and cost containment provided a great stimulus to behavioral health managed care "carve-outs" which could offer access to many but had an incentive to select against the sickest or most disabled and, unlike the safety-net providers, might be of little or no help to the uninsured. It is worth noting, in passing, that one of the important uses for DSH funds in some states has been to subsidize state mental health institutions.[100]

These developments may well have been, on balance, better outcomes than would have been achieved if the 1915(c) waiver had been more appropriately designed for mental health program needs from the beginning or more effectively modified along the way. Be that as it may, the example of mental health adds to the concerns about waivers as instruments of program development. Waivers, by definition, suspend or relax controls on Medicaid, itself a weakly institutionalized program, subject to many exogenous influences. Program waivers are sought to deal with present predicaments or objectives, but they are developed and implemented over time, in a changing and imperfectly understood environment with a dynamic of its own. Experience with these two program waivers—1915(b) and 1915(c)—suggests that they are good ways to give states more say but as instruments of programmatic changes they are likely to achieve both less and more than contemplated in their original design—less of their prime objectives and more of some others, with unintended consequences that may be of great importance.

The State Children's Health Insurance Program (SCHIP)

It may seem inappropriate to consider the State Children's Health Insurance Program (SCHIP) in a discussion about devolution and waivers, but it is both a significant precedent and an interesting example of

devolution. In 1997, there was strong, bipartisan concern about an estimated 10.5 million uninsured children and an additional number who,
though insured, were receiving inadequate care. Also important were
the numbers of unemployed and the working poor without insurance,
concerns that gained added salience as employers cut back on insurance
and men, women, and children lost insurance because of changes in the
welfare program in 1996, which severed the automatic link between
receipt of welfare and Medicaid eligibility.

None of these developments had any necessary connection with Medicaid. Early on, some version of a child health block grant and tax credits
for the working poor seemed likely. Medicaid entered as an option in
April 1997 with a proposal from Sen. Chafee and Sen. Rockefeller to
extend Medicaid coverage to children in families up to 150% of poverty.
Within the House, some budget funds had been earmarked for a health
benefit, but Ways and Means preferred tax credits to purchase insurance,
while Commerce supported a child health grant to the states. When Ways
and Means eventually receded, the way was open for the Commerce
Committee to develop a block grant proposal, resembling the block
grant proposal of 1995, but adapted for child health. The final legislation combined the two approaches, allowing states to opt for SCHIP or
for Medicaid expansion or combine the two.

The resulting legislation may seem fortuitous, taking the form and
direction it did largely because it could be done in the course of a budget reconciliation, while competing alternatives, such as a child health
block grant or tax credits, would have been unlikely to pass as stand-
alone bills. In the context of the present discussion, SCHIP was also a
significant devolution of programmatic control with important and unforeseen consequences: an add-on to Medicaid that would pay the states
handsomely—if they chose this option—to cover children in families
up to 200% of poverty and with much greater flexibility with respect
to benefits, cost-sharing, and service delivery. The statute included a
small opening for family coverage,[101] and states were encouraged, in the
conference report, "to consider such innovative means as vouchers and
tax credits." In sum, legislation that seemed on its face a straightforward
effort to cover children also opened up possibilities for covering families
and childless adults and for experimenting with additional devolution
and even privatization.

The combination of a popular cause (children's health), an enhanced
match, and program flexibility was appealing and states were vigorous

and inventive in their outreach, enrollment, and retention efforts, adopting methods encouraged over the years by federal Medicaid officials and developing approaches of their own.[102] Outreach was of special importance. Many in the target population were hard to enroll because of lack of previous experience with insurance, transience, linguistic and cultural barriers, and fear of officials (especially INS agents). These activities were of interest not only because effective in increasing enrollments, but also for reducing the stigma traditionally attaching to Medicaid and because they led states, in some instances, to extend them their Medicaid programs as well.[103]

With respect to the main objective, enrolling uninsured children, SCHIP has worked well. According to a recent estimate, 4 million children are currently enrolled or 6 million, if enrollees for a full year are counted, and over 600,000 adults. All fifty states, the District of Columbia, and the territories participate and 41 states have opted for coverage up to 200% of poverty. To be sure, the program started slow, had its ups and downs and some losses, but has come close—by a generous interpretation —to the original target of five million.[104] At the same time, the legislation, written as it was, influenced events in some unexpected ways, largely because of the combination of flexibility and incentives and the temptations these offered, especially when combined with the unique politics of Sec. 1115 waivers. In a way, the statute did too much and too little, especially in the light of political dynamics since its passage.

One element was the SCHIP model itself: the combination of an enhanced match with increased flexibility and a non-entitlement status. The basic scheme derived from the Commerce Committee's Republican proposal of 1995, one which Republican governors had welcomed at the time, even with reduced fiscal support, and which soon got a renewed endorsement as a model to "modernize" Medicaid for the new century.

An important part of the political dynamic was a concern for the uninsured and the working poor. Both Democrats and Republicans wanted these groups covered. The Democrats saw SCHIP as another step on the way toward national health insurance, while Republicans hoped for more emphasis upon the working poor as such and moving away from Medicaid toward tax credits or premium support. As noted, the statute made a small gesture in the direction of "family" coverage, though none at all toward single persons without children or disabilities. Furthermore, the family coverage option was introduced with language so restrictive that it was difficult to tell whether it was intended as a new opening or a closing off.

At the same time, SCHIP waivers were specifically authorized and they were an attractive route because they were encouraged by the Clinton administration, the cost-neutral (technically, "allotment-neutral") requirement was relatively easy to meet,[105] and the coverage provisions were much less onerous than those for Medicaid.

As for coverage, the legislation combined a modicum of prescription with a large amount of flexibility (*supra*, 263-265). The House bill was minimal, requiring only basic services and wellness care for babies and children, including immunizations. The Senate bill added the concept of benchmark plans including actuarial equivalence; and the conference contributed the notion of health care "generally available to state employees," as well as "any other benefits plan" that the secretary determines "upon application by a State" provides "appropriate coverage for the targeted population." As for the scope of services offered—how many days or visits and what would be included, such as dental, vision, or hearing or mental illness—that also depended upon benchmark plans, actuarial equivalence, or what the secretary would approve. Critically important, though, is that the referent for actuarial equivalence is "privately insured children,"[106] with no mention, for instance, of special needs children or of EPSDT with its array of preventive and wrap-around services and its distinctive concept of "medical necessity" as it applies to children.[107]

SCHIP was not, to be sure, intended to be like Medicaid. And it is hard to quarrel with an objective of extending health care for needy children up to 200% of poverty. Almost immediately, though, this new initiative added to the tension between flexibility and protectiveness and to the distributive issue of how much to devote to the neediest as opposed to the needy. The inclusion of a Sec. 1115 waiver authority as part of SCHIP increased the likelihood that such distributive issues would be devolved—settled at the state level. And observing the synergy of Sec. 1115 waivers, SCHIP, and Medicaid helps to make two points: (1) that exercises in devolution or privatization need to be considered not by themselves but cumulatively and in their historic and political context; and (2) designed not just with regard to their beneficial use but also with an eye to how they could be misused and put to different objectives by a another administration.

Section 1115 Waivers for Medicaid and SCHIP

Although beginning with the Public Welfare Amendments of 1962 (*supra*, 332) and intended primarily to authorize a variety of social service demonstrations, the Sec. 1115 waiver authority has become, over the years, quite possibly "the most powerful health policy tool" possessed by the executive branch for restructuring Medicaid and SCHIP.[108] In principle, this does not mean that the executive branch can legislate or defy statutes, though how far it can go remains to be seen. Without doubt, this waiver authority is a powerful instrument, especially with a Congress sympathetic to executive branch objectives or not disposed or able, as a practical matter, to object to the use of this authority. In recent years, it has been and continues to be a major tool for incrementally restructuring the Medicaid and SCHIP programs, raising serious doubts about the future of these programs, the entitlement status of Medicaid, and some constitutional issues about the role of the executive branch in determining Medicaid policy, up to and including restructuring of the program as a whole.

Sec. 1115 waivers were, for Medicaid, relatively insignificant until the Clinton administration. Although intended for demonstrations, little attention was paid to their design or subsequent evaluation and they were casually sought—usually to avoid a regulation or modify some minor provision in a local program—and so easily granted that, until the late 1970s, they were often seen as an easier way to make changes in the program than to seek a state plan amendment.[109] One persistent tendency, though, was programmatic use with consequences that were sometimes unwelcome or even embarrassing. In the late 1970s, the Carter administration sought to restore these waivers to their original purpose of research and demonstration. The Reagan administration was suspicious and even hostile to waivers because they often cost money or led to follow-on expenses and because they could thwart administrative priorities or be used for "back-door" agenda building. One expression of this concern was the distinction made in OBRA '81 between R&D waivers and "program" waivers, i.e., the Sec. 1915(b) and Sec. 1915(c) waivers, which narrowly limited the provisions that could be waived. Waivers were subjected to rigorous budget reviews and in 1983 an agreement between DHHS and OMB formalized the budget-neutral policy.[110] The harshness of these OMB examinations is legendary (*supra*, 341-342) and are credited with reducing the scope and number of Medicare and

Medicaid waivers, although this effect was partially offset by an increase in congressionally mandated projects.[111]

An important development in the first President Bush's administration was the widespread use of Sec. 1115 waivers by states that were seeking a measure of welfare reform in the absence of a federal initiative. These waivers were used for food stamps and to extend Medicaid eligibility and benefits beyond the existing 12-month period for welfare recipients returning to work.[112] They were used both for demonstrations and for programmatic changes. The federal government also permitted replication across state lines—another move away from research and demonstration as such. TANF and the welfare legislation of 1996 owed much to this earlier experience.

This renewal of Sec. 1115 activity gave only a hint of the enormous potential of such waivers, especially for a program like Medicaid that was complex and highly regulated, but much in need of change. For an item, Sec. 1115 waivers are not bound by requirements of statewideness, comparability, or choice of provider, but can be used to modify Medicaid program structure selectively as well as comprehensively. The secretary's discretion is largely unfettered, allowing almost any demonstration that "in the judgment of the Secretary is likely to promote the objectives" of the various grants under the Social Security Act (42 USC 1315).[113] The secretary has authority to match state expenditures not otherwise matched under the Medicaid statute. And Sec. 1115 waivers can be statewide or multi-state, are typically approved for a five-year period and can be re-approved. So far, none have been terminated except at the request of the state.

Although these provisions put enormous power in the hands of the secretary—or those that influence the secretary—they have never been codified through rulemaking or effectively challenged in the courts.[114] One might wonder what Congress thought it was doing in authorizing such discretion. Part of the answer lies in the fact that the original statute, passed before Medicare or Medicaid, and taken in context seemed aimed at small, relatively inconsequential demonstrations in connection with local welfare experiments and, possibly, child health programs, with no thought of how they might be substituted for legislation as an instrument of large-scale programmatic change. Be that as it may, Sec. 1115 waivers later became an important part of overall Medicaid policy, first in the Clinton and then in the second Bush administrations.

The Clinton administration favored waivers, especially those used to extend eligibility. Governor Clinton had chafed at HCFA and had been an active chairman of the NGA and sympathetic to the demands of fellow governors for more flexibility both with respect to welfare and Medicaid. In the beginning of his administration, more lenient and expeditious treatment of Medicaid waivers was made a priority. After the defeat of health care reform, additional reasons for supporting Medicaid waivers, especially Sec. 1115 ones, were to extend coverage to the uninsured and working poor as well as to advance the administration's goal of moving incrementally toward national health insurance.[115] In time, another incentive was the amount of savings from some of the "super-waivers" that helped substantially in lowering the Medicaid baseline.[116]

Early in 1993, the incoming Clinton administration made a commitment to the National Governors' Association to "streamline" the waiver process and make it more responsive to state needs. It actively promoted use of Sec. 1115 demonstrations, encouraging proposals that would "preserve and enhance beneficiary access to quality service."[117] The administration quickly approved five major waivers: Oregon, Hawaii, Rhode Island, Tennessee, and Kentucky. Subsequent to these approvals, and after negotiation with the NGA, the administration published a "guidance" in the Federal Register[118] setting forth options and procedures formally and publicly. This notice gave explicit recognition to statewide and multi-state waivers, indicated that waivers would be approved for five years or more, and suggested that states might use funds from various sources to finance their projects, such as payments redirected from DSH hospitals and savings from managed care.

The speed and informality with which the early waivers were granted was disturbing to some, especially advocates for the poor, who complained about the inadequacy of public notice and comment, the secrecy of the negotiations between state and federal officials, and the lack of legislative accountability.[119] Protection of the Medicaid recipients was also an issue, since all of the waivers utilized managed care and generally sought to achieve budget neutrality through managed care savings, reallocating DSH funds, and reducing utilization of FHQCs.[120] Taking a negative view, which some did, these new super-waivers could be seen as a design to herd the poor into HMOs and deny them access to their accustomed Medicaid sources, especially the safety-net providers.[121]

By 1997, HCFA had approved 14 statewide Medicaid waivers, all of them with mandatory managed care, with a cumulative enrollment of eight million recipients accounting for 20% of all Medicaid expenditures.[122] SCHIP was passed in 1997 and immediately created a surge of interest for waivers under this program as well. At the time, HCFA did not wish to prejudice future developments and declined to grant waivers until general policies had been set forth in July of 2000. Meanwhile, SCHIP expenditures lagged and Clinton administration faced the unpleasant options of reallocating SCHIP funds or allowing them to revert to the U.S. Treasury.

In this dilemma, HCFA further liberalized waiver requirements. One step was to consider waivers that included parents of SCHIP children and pregnant women if the state was already covering children up to 19 with family incomes up to 200% of poverty.[123] A related approach, described as "buying out the base," allowed states that had expanded coverage to higher levels to refinance this coverage under SCHIP, with its higher match.[124] Still another concession to the states was to use "allotment neutrality" rather than budget-neutrality, which was especially helpful since it enabled states to get the higher SCHIP match and count the allotted amount rather than historic or actual expenditures.[125]

Only a few SCHIP waivers were granted under the Clinton administration. New Jersey covered parents as well as pregnant women and children up to 200% of poverty. Wisconsin covered parents under its BadgerCare demonstration. A Minnesota waiver application begun under the Clinton administration was approved in the first year of the Bush administration. It may seem a paradox that the main beneficiary of increased flexibility with respect to Sec. 1115 waivers was the Bush and not the Clinton administration, but that is a reprise on the familiar theme that waivers are shaped by those who use them, often in ways widely different from those intended by those who authorized them.

Much of the background for the new Health Insurance Flexibility and Accountability Demonstration Initiative (HIFA) has been discussed (*supra*, 281-284) so a few summary comments should suffice. This effort failed as legislation after which the main effort shifted to administrative action with the announcement of the HIFA and the Pharmacy Plus[126] waivers in the summer of 2001. At the time, HCFA/CMS said that it would expedite these waivers and that states could use their excess SCHIP funds to help pay for eligibility expansions. Under the new waiver—and contrary to policy under the Clinton administration—states were permitted to reduce benefits and increase cost sharing by existing beneficiaries in order to cover the uninsured. States were also encouraged to redesign their programs and experiment with private sector initiatives, such as premium assistance.[127]

Inasmuch as states were already in fiscal difficulty by 2001 and considering various kinds of reductions in their Medicaid programs, the HIFA waiver could be seen as an invitation to reorder priorities as between existing Medicaid beneficiaries and the uninsured. This might be praiseworthy, but was also contrary to long-settled Medicaid policy and had never been authorized by Congress—or so thought the GAO.

In a June 2002 report to the Senate Finance Committee—one of a series dealing with SCHIP—the GAO called attention to several deficiencies with the HIFA and Pharmacy Plus waivers.[128] The GAO expressed concern that the expedited procedures might leave inadequate opportunity for beneficiaries and others to learn about and comment on the waiver and that some of the savings claimed, though imaginative, were not allowable. The most serious complaint dealt with use of unspent SCHIP funds to cover single adults, a practice that the GAO deemed to be unlawful and, at the least, a misinterpretation of the Sec. 1115 authority.[129] It requested that Congress consider legislation specifically prohibiting the use of unspent SCHIP funds for uninsured childless adults and require the secretary to improve the public notice and participation requirements, assure "valid methods" for demonstrating budget-neutrality, and make clear which should prevail: the SCHIP statute or the secretary's interpretation of his authority under Sec. 1115.[130] The Secretary responded with an argument that Sec. 1115 authorizes expenditure under any title of the Social Security Act. The GAO thought this argument historically incorrect and contrary to the plain language of the statute.[131] For several years Sen. Grassley, the Finance Committee chairman, and Max Baucus, the ranking member, sought to address this matter without success. Finally, the Deficit Reduction Act of 2005 stated in terms that unspent SCHIP funds could not be spent for new or additional coverage for childless adults. That may not end the matter, but the episode is a good illustration of the classic tension between law and administration and of the conflict in health policy over coverage of the neediest vs. coverage for a larger number of needy.

In any event, HIFA waivers were not much sought—largely because they provided no additional resources.[132] Over a four year period, from 2001 to 2005, Sec. 1115 waivers accounted for only 2% of the growth in Medicaid and HIFA waivers for less than 1%. Moreover, two-thirds of the coverage gains were in New York under a waiver that predated

HIFA.[133] Even these modest gains were offset by states that reduced benefits and added cost sharing with no gains in enrollment, and by enrollment declines in Oregon and Tennessee.[134] Meanwhile, the number of uninsured in America continued to rise to an all-time high in 2004, of 46 million or 15.7% of the population.

In January, 2003, President Bush put forward a new proposal for restructuring Medicaid. States could receive additional federal payments—that would be budget-neutral over ten years—if they would accept spending caps, and restructure their programs along lines similar to SCHIP (*supra*, 293). Mandatory populations would be protected, but states would have increased freedom to impose enrollment caps and cost-sharing and to cut back on optional categories and services—which at that time amounted to about two-thirds of Medicaid expenditures and included additional services for many of the sickest and most severely disabled. Several Republican governors endorsed this plan, but the National Governors' Association rejected it as a block-grant in disguise. Congress added its own $10 billion relief plan[135] to a $350 billion tax reduction bill, which the president signed in May of 2003. There the matter rested until after the election of 2004.

The second term of the Bush presidency brought renewed attempts at Medicaid reforms as well as a new approach to Sec. 1115 waivers. That approach was signaled by President Bush's endorsement of the Utah waiver and the nomination of Michael Leavitt to be the new secretary of DHHS. The administration would use Sec. 1115 waivers strategically in promoting the administration's restructuring priorities in addition to or instead of efforts by Congress. Several of these waivers give a good sense for the direction of this new path, though not what its terminus might be.

The Utah Sec. 1115 "Primary Care Network" waiver of 2002 is a good example of the use of one set of techniques. Under this waiver, Utah increased cost-sharing and reduced benefits for 17,600 parents with incomes below 150% of poverty,[136] and used the savings to expand eligibility for other poor and near-poor adults without dependent children. This second group was capped at 19,000 and its members had to pay an enrollment fee. Benefits were limited to primary care, with no coverage for mental health, other specialists, or inpatient hospital care other than emergency care. These enrollees were also subject to significant cost-sharing obligations. When the 19,000 limit was reached, enrollment was closed although over 50,000 additional applications had been received. In August 2003, the waiver was amended to provide for premium supplements ($50 for individuals and $100 for families) for those who had access to employer-sponsored insurance. The obvious merits of this waiver is that it provides some basic coverage to (small) cohorts of parents, childless adults, and working poor though at the expense primarily of a welfare population.

TennCare was another interesting example since it involved a daring experiment by a Democratic administration to cover the entire uninsured population in the state under a Sec. 1115 waiver. After a rocky start, the program seemed to work well and was widely acclaimed. Under increasing fiscal pressures, though, the original waiver was modified in 2002 to restrict eligibility and benefits for both children and adults. Then, in November 2004, Governor Phil Bredesen announced that he would seek to terminate TennCare and revert to Medicaid and SCHIP coverage. At the time, he estimated that 430,000 low-income enrollees would lose coverage—about one-third of those currently enrolled—the largest single reduction in the history of Medicaid. A concurrent study by McKinsey and Company, consultants, indicated that the savings would be less than projected and, moreover, that with a matching rate of 65%, Tennessee would lose two federal dollars for every dollar it saved and that the loss of TennCare coverage would lead to an increased demand for uncompensated care. The McKinsey report concluded that Tennessee would "have to contribute additional money from state funds largely offsetting the savings from reduced enrollment."[137]

Mississippi provides an illustration of how a waiver could be used to disentitle the dual eligibles. The basic proposal came from Governor Haley Barbour, formerly the chairman of the Republican National Committee. As a first step, the Mississippi legislature passed HB 2434, which terminated Medicaid coverage for 65,000 Poverty-Level Aged and Disabled (PLAD) beneficiaries and directed the governor to apply for a waiver. This waiver, capped at 17,000, would continue limited Medicaid benefits to those dual eligibles who would retain their Medicare coverage, but not the more comprehensive benefits of Medicaid. Exceptions were made for some dual eligibles, such as cancer patients receiving chemotherapy or radiation, kidney patients on dialysis, organ transplant patients on anti-rejection drugs, and mental patients on anti-psychotic medication.[138] For those without Medicare whose Medicaid benefits were also being terminated, a schedule of reduced benefits would be provided, up to a limit of 5000 persons. With the waiver capped at 17,000, though, almost 50,000 of the PLAD beneficiaries would lose all Medicaid coverage. Moreover, the coverage for those under the waiver would be less than current Medicaid coverage and last only for the term of the waiver. The services lost would be especially those important for dual eligibles, such as long-term care, vision and dental, and services helpful for maintaining patients in a community setting. Progress of this waiver was briefly delayed by a court order staying the legislative exclusion of the PLAD beneficiaries, but the waiver was eventually implemented for five years, beginning in 2004.

Florida's "Medicaid Reform" waiver—submitted on October 3, 2005 and approved sixteen days later—has attracted broad interest as a possible template for national Medicaid reform. The key notion is the use of risk-adjusted premiums (or vouchers) that could be used for Medicaid managed care coverage or, outside of Medicaid, to subsidize the purchase of employer-supported insurance or for individual coverage. To promote competition, the plans could vary optional benefits so long as the package was "actuarily equivalent" to the current Medicaid program, covered pregnant women and children (including the EPSDT benefit), and was broadly representative of the needs of the majority of the population. Beyond the per capita limit, individuals would be responsible for their care, except that those participating in state-defined healthy activities could receive credits usable for additional coverage or to purchase private insurance. The waiver is being implemented as a pilot program in Duval and Broward counties and will cover 2.2 million children, parents, disabled and elderly beneficiaries, with full state implementation to follow in 2007.[139]

This initiative could be of great importance. In one large demonstration it would test many of the ideas that Republicans and some economic theorists have championed for years: a defined contribution, competition and consumerism, a large measure of privatization and individual self-direction. As with the "super-waivers" generally, this effort could be primarily a covert attempt to transform the federal Medicaid program by increments. Yet it also seems aimed at a serious testing of a number of important new options. There are obvious problems: such as how to develop an adequate risk adjuster and control risk selection by health plans and how and how much to support the safety-net providers and the Medicaid infrastructure. But the waiver is touted as a template for reform of Medicaid nationally and, should it work well, would be an important coup for Governor Jeb Bush.

These examples are not representative of much of the Sec, 1115 waiver activity over the last few years. Most of the 1115 waivers since January 2001 have expanded coverage and used redirected DSH or SCHIP funds rather than benefit reductions or cost-sharing to meet the added costs. The most popular change was to cover parents or childless adults. A few states imposed co-pays or reallocated optional benefits; but aside from the examples cited (and Texas and South Carolina) they have not sought major structural changes. Instead they tried to husband resources, find additional revenues, and keep their programs intact. Whether the more radical waivers are just that or are portents of a growing national trend remains to be seen; but there are reasons for doubting the latter possibility.

So far, only a few states have shown strong interest in use of "super-waivers" to recast Medicaid in a major way. Those that did were southern or traditionally conservative and had Republican governors.[140] In three of the states, moreover, there were strong political ties or ideological sympathy with the Bush administration.[141] The trend—if there is one—would seem worrisome not because it is national but because it would amend Medicaid regionally, without national sanction, might further divide "Red" and "Blue" states, and widen racial disparities in Medicaid coverage and access to care.

Other concerns have centered on the activities and intensions of CMS in the administration of waiver policy, especially that CMS has played favorites and pushed ideological priorities of the Bush administration in negotiating caps on spending and setting the "special terms and conditions"[142] for individual waivers. There was a larger question about the role of CMS in what appeared to be an administration strategy of incrementally deconstructing Medicaid in much the same way the Democrats had incrementally built up the program.

There were CMS activities that gave rise to such concerns, but how objectionable they were and what to make of the suspicions about motives is debatable. One example was approving waivers in which unspent SCHIP funds were used to cover single adults—which, according to the GAO, was contrary to the intent of the statute (*supra*, 353). CMS would also negotiate over "budget neutrality" and required global caps for the Pharmacy Plus waivers and for the Vermont and Florida "super-waivers—all of which seemed reasonable, given the nature of the programs. Another occasion for such negotiations has been the tying of Sec. 1115 waiver approvals to the modification or phasing out of existing UPL and

IGT methods for generating matching funds in favor of certified public expenditures (CPEs) and the creation of dedicated Uncompensated Care Pools (UCPs).[143] Desirable or not, this policy had a precedent in similar efforts by the Clinton administration and some legal foundation in BIPA 2000. Finally, CMS has been faulted for a laxity in the determinations of budget neutrality that amounted to favoritism toward waivers it liked—an abuse of administrative discretion, but hardly new with the Bush administration.

When sorted out and explained, these CMS activities do not seem especially alarming as such. For the most part, there were precedents from the Clinton administration and some foundation in earlier legislation. One interpretation or rationale for the present activities is that they are drying up or transforming objectionable Medicaid maximizing schemes and seeking to shift these funds from provider payments (to DSH hospitals and other safety-net institutions) to insurance products (HMOs and HSAs) that would increase coverage for the working poor and advance administration objectives such as competition and private initiative.[144] That might be seen as a praiseworthy aim. Moreover, even if these activities were part of a covert strategy to use waivers to deconstruct Medicaid and make it more and more like SCHIP, that effort doesn't seem much different, in principle, from earlier Democratic efforts to enlist Medicaid in a march toward national health insurance.

Several observations are in order. One is that waiver negotiations that hold the DSH funds hostage seem coercive to the states.[145] Many within the Medicaid community are disturbed by what they perceive as an ideological bent in these initiatives and fear that allegedly legal activities may conceal or be used to promote covert and illegitimate purposes.[146] They seem to be one more effort to pursue administratively an objective that Congress has refused to ratify legislatively. CMS's commitment to apparently ideological purposes and willingness to proceed with dubious legal authority or test the limits of the law, though not confirmative, are consistent with such an attribution. Meanwhile, CMS has done little to dispel this kind of distrust and has resolutely resisted a simple remedy, which would be a notice and comment procedure for Sec. 1115 waivers at the national level, as already required for the states. Sunlight may not be enough; but reducing the opacity that has characterized CMS waiver proceedings would help. Little is known about what ulterior purposes may or may not be at work and that is a large part of the problem.

The Sec. 1115 waiver initiative was, of course, not the only thrust in the campaign to devolve and disentitle Medicaid. The DRA contained a whole array of provisions increasing flexibility with respect to cost-sharing, benefits, and making changes without waivers easier to make. Several states have already chosen this route rather than a Sec 1115 waiver to restructure benefits.[147] Moreover, Medicaid provisions in the president's budget for FY 2007 (*infra*, 409) that would reduce federal matching percentages and administratively eliminate payments for various Medicaid benefits and halve allowable hospital taxes would in effect push states to take greater advantage of their newly bestowed flexibility.

Some of the bad news is that efforts to devolve or disentitle Medicaid are well into their third decade. The good news is that the program continues to survive and find unexpected sources of political support, and that moderate political shifts either within individual states or the Congress may be enough to slow or deflect efforts to deconstruct the program and open the way for needed and moderate reforms.

Notes

1. Timothy Stolzfus Jost, *Disentitlement? The Threat Facing Our Public Health Care Programs and a Rights Based Response*, New York: Oxford University Press, 2003, 3.
2. The McNerney Report of 1970 (*supra*, 97 ff.) was an exception, though it was not implemented. The staff work that preceded the Social Security Amendments of 1972 contained specific Medicaid recommendations, but not for comprehensive reform. Under the Reagan administration, HCFA undertook an array of program evaluations and sent a list of recommendations to the Administrator which were passed on to the White House, but no action was taken.
3. A useful discussion is Thompson and DiIulio, *Medicaid and Devolution,* 16 ff.
4. John D. Donohue, *Divided States.* New York: Basic Books, 1997, esp. ch. 1.
5. Especially in the state plan requirements and the mandated services.
6. Although matching was restricted to services listed in Sec. 1905(a).
7. Cf. Paul Offner, *Medicaid and the States.* New York: Century Foundation Press, 1999, 6; Frank Thompson aptly describes this period as one of "marginal centralization," Thompson and DiIulio, *Medicaid and Devolution,* 18. Both Offner and Thompson date this period as 1966-1983, the latter date being the year in which a long series of congressional legislative mandates began.
8. The Forum was entitled "Reflections on HCFA: Former Administrators Speak Their Minds." It met on February 23, 2001 and included four former HCFA administrators: Nancy-Ann Min DeParle, William Roper, Bruce Vladeck, and Gail Wilensky.
9. Fidelity to the law, program integrity, and administrative competence were ideals that inspired many Social Security civil servants from the inception of the program through the 1970s with a solidarity and purposiveness characteristic of the public health service, the forest service, the foreign service, graduates of the military academies, or other elite career services.

10. This apt term is borrowed from Thompson and DiIulio, *Medicaid and Devolution,* 18-19.
11. Based on the Moss Amendments.
12. Savings were projected to rise to 45% in four years. On the effects of this amendment, see Stevens and Stevens, *Welfare Medicine in America,* 156-166.
13. Another concession along with the 133% limit was to liberalize the benefit requirements for the medically indigent, stipulating that any five of the allowable services would suffice—and early instance of offsetting limits on Medicaid expenditures with added flexibility.
14. *Report of the Task Force on Medicaid,* 2, 26, 27.
15. A popular doctrine at the time was "Grodzins' paradox," that centralization often had to precede decentralization for the latter to operate appropriately. Cf. Morton Grodzins, *The American System: A New View of Government in the United States.* Chicago: Rand McNally, 1966, 384 ff.
16. One problem with contracting out was that most of these agents were paid by the number of claims processed and had little or no interest in whether the claims were repetitive, excessive, or fraudulent. Also, the data collected was often proprietary and the agents were reluctant to share, so that states could not use such data for planning or even to counter fraud and abuse.
17. In a few instances it was literally true that boxes of unpaid claims piled up in warehouses. Late payment led some providers to withdraw from the Medicaid program and others to resort to "factoring," *i.e.,* discounting their claims to a factor who would seek to get them paid—a practice that led to conspiracy and fraud and was soon outlawed.
18. J. Patrick McCarthy, telephone interview by Smith, July 14, 2004.
19. *Report of the Task Force on Medicaid,* 122. Lawrence Lewin, interview by Moore and Smith, November 7, 2002.
20. Case-specific review would facilitate identification and censoring or penalizing individual physicians, as opposed to aggregate surveys, good for educational or hortatory exercises.
21. Initially, PSROs covered only inpatient facilities and did not include either ambulatory care or physician services.
22. Many seasoned administrators were skeptical about the value of enforcement proceedings and, for that matter, about the importance attributed to fraud and/or abuse. Keith Weickel, who was the Medicaid Commissioner from 1974 to 1977, strongly supported an educative approach and once said "we have known for a long time that the best treatment for fraud and abuse is preventive and the best prevention is efficient management." He believed that the first and primary emphasis should be upon getting the MMISs up and running, an endeavor requiring cooperation with the states. Cf. Martin Judge, "Progress in the War on Medicaid Fraud," *Health Care Financing Administrative Record,* Vol. 2, 1977, 24-27, at p. 26. Rozanne Abato, who began her career in Medicaid in 1976 as a temporary hire recalls conducting fraud and abuse reviews by examining records in physicians' offices, laboratories, nursing homes and hospitals and the shock and animosity these invasions engendered. This mode continued for eighteen months, when it was abandoned and a different emphasis pursued by the new Office of Program Integrity in Baltimore. Telephone interview by Moore and Smith, September 17, 2003.
23. The MEQC began in 1973 as an adaptation of a similar penalty procedure applied to public welfare eligibility determinations. States were required to set up their own MEQC or "Quality Control" systems for review of eligibility determinations,

from which "the Secretary" would select and review a sample, with penalties to be assessed for error rates above a percentage limit. For example, a 3.5% error rate, with a 3% limit would mean a fine of 0.5% of the federal payment for the category affected.

From the start, MEQC had a troubled history. Aside from the penalty itself—often sizable and disruptive—the states complained about mistakes, the statistical methods, and the ways in which the penalty was determined and waivers granted. The MEQC gave rise to lawsuits, GAO investigations, and congressional intervention over the years. At present, the program appears to be in administrative limbo, but it was an important source of discontent and controversy during the early years of NASMD. For some background, cf. *Maryland v. Mathews*, 415 F.Supp. 1206 (C.C.C., 1976) and HHS Departmental Appeals Board, Decision no. 1332, May 26, 1992. With special thanks to David P. Smith, OGC, DHHS and Larry Bartlett of Health Systems Research.

24. Larry Bartlett, interview by Moore and Smith, March 14, 2003.
25. Although independent, NASMD is an affiliate of the American Public Human Services Association, which is a successor to the APWA.
26. Vernon Smith, telephone interview by Smith, November 23, 2005.
27. Ten is the current number; and the role of TAGs has been considerably reduced under the Bush administration.
28. Medicare has a number of waiver authorities, including Secs. 1110 and 1115 of the Social Security Act, Sec. 402 of the Social Security Amendments of 1967, and Sec. 222 (a) and (b) of the Social Security Amendments of 1972.
29. Cynthia Shirk, *Shaping Public Programs through Medicare, Medicaid and SCHIP Waivers: the Fundamentals.* Washington, D.C.: National Health Policy Forum, 2003, 3, 4.
30. The Sec. 1915(b) waivers are sometimes referred to as Sec. 2175 (their designation in OBRA '81) and as "freedom of choice" waivers since they allowed waiver of the Medicaid recipient's right to free choice of providers. The Sec 1915(c) HCBS waivers were Sec 2176 in OBRA '81.
31. Jay Greenberg, Walter Leutz, Bruce Spits, and Stanley Wallack, "A Historical Note on Medicare and Medicaid Waivers." Waltham, MA: Health Policy Consortium, 1983, 3. This essay was part of a multi-year evaluation of Medicare and Medicaid waivered experiments that was mandated by OBRA '81 and conducted by HCFA between 1983 and 1985. It provided a wealth of information on waivers, helped to launch numerous articles and research careers, and was expanded into a general survey of the Medicaid program—which was forwarded to the administrator, William Roper, and then to the White House, where it was ignored. The authors are much indebted to Gerald Adler, HCFA/CMS, for sharing with us a number of the reports from these projects.
32. *Ibid.,* 3.
33. Cf. Falkson, *HMOs and the Politics of Health System Reform,* Ch. 2, esp. 14 ff.
34. Jerry Cromwell and Sylvia Hurdle, *Impact of Demonstration Projects on Medicaid and General Health Policy.* Waltham, MA: Health Policy Research Consortium, 1987, E-9.
35. Jerry Cromwell, Sylvia Hurdle, Janice Singer, and Margaret Macadam, *Impact of Demonstration Projects on Medicaid and General Health Care Policy.* Waltham, MA: Health Policy Research Center-Cooperative Research Center, 1987, 4-3.
36. *Ibid.,* 4-2.
37. High pressure and fraudulent marketing; inadequate and/or incomplete staffing; selective enrollment and disenrollment; minimal services and hours; phantom

facilities; dishonest consultants and contractors; forgery and falsificiation of documents; kickbacks and self-dealing. One contractor realized a 4000% profit on his investment. One of the most telling statistics was that less than half of the PHP premiums went for patient care. Cf. *Prepaid Health Plans,* Hearings, Permanent Subcommittee on Investigations of the Committee on Governmental Affairs, United States Senate, 94th Congress, 1st Session (Washington, D.C.: Government Printing Office, 1975), especially testimony of David Vienna, 5 ff. Also, interview of David Vienna by Moore and Smith, April 2, 2003.

38.   Prepaid Health Research, Evaluation, and Demonstration Project—a number of demonstrations developed in collaboration with California but with strong leadership and supervision by the federal government.

39.   *Medicaid Source Book,* 376. The mandatory enrollment feature was repealed by TEFRA in 1982, but selectively reinstated by BBA '97.

40.   Robert E. Hurley, "Medicaid Confronts a Changing Managed Care Marketplace," *Health Care Financing Review,* Vol. 14(1) 1992, 11-25, at 12.

41.   *Medicaid Source Book,* 1025.

42.   *Ibid.,* 1025.

43.   John Holahan, James Bell, and Gerald A. Adler. eds., *Medicaid Program Evaluation, Final Report.* Baltimore, MD: Health Care Financing Administration, 1987, 4-43-44.

44.   Hurley, "Medicaid Confronts a Changing Managed Care Marketplace," 12.

45.   "Medicaid Managed Care," *Fact Sheet.* Washington, D.C.: Kaiser Commission on Medicaid and the Uninsured, December, 2001, 1.

46.   Gail Wilensky, telephone interview by Smith, November 17, 2005.

47.   Christine Nye, interview by Moore, August 8, 2005.

48.   Cf., Rowland *et al., Medicaid Financing Crisis,* 1993.

49.   Added by the Medicare Catastrophic Coverage Act in 1988 and retained as a Medicaid responsibility when the major part of MCCA was repealed in 1989.

50.   EPSDT and the nursing home standards both became much more expensive as a result of amendments.

51.   Even before the failure of health care reform, governors were interested in expanding Medicaid to cover uninsured workers.

52.   John Holahan, Teresa Coughlin, Leighton Ku, Debra J. Lipson, and Shruti Rajan, "Insuring the Poor Through Medicaid 1115 Waivers," *Health Affairs*, Vol. 14(1) 1995, 200-216. Sec. 1902(r)(2), first passed in 1988, permitted expansion of coverage to pregnant women, children under 19 years if age and QMBs, largely without regard to income.

53.   Jerry Cromwell, Sylvia Hurdle, Janice Singer and Margaret Macadam, *Impact of Demonstration Projects on Medicaid and General Health Policy,* 4-49.

54.   BBA '97 eliminated the 75/25 rule, substituting quality improvement regulations.

55.   Debra A. Draper, Robert E. Hurley, and Ashley C. Short, "Medicaid Managed Care: The Last Bastion of the HMO?' *Health Affairs*, Vol. 23(2) 2004, 155-167 at 160-61.

56.   Cf. Sara Rosenbaum, "Negotiating the New Health System—a Nationwide Analysis of Medicaid Managed Care Contracts," in Stephen M. Davidson and Stephen A. Somers, *Remaking Medicaid—Man-aged Care for the Public Good.* San Francisco: Jossey-Bass Publ., 1998, 197-218; also Sara Rosenbaum and associates, *Negotiating the New Health System: A Nationwide Study of Medicaid Managed Care Contracts.* Washington, D.C.: George Washington University, Center for Health Policy Research, 1977, and successive reports under this title.

57. According to Robert Hurley there was little initial awareness of this problem. He cites Robert Masters in Boston as one of the first to become serious about taing on this challenge. Interview by Moore and Smith, June 10, 2003; also Masters, "Medicaid Managed Care and Disabled Populations," in Davidson and Somers, *Remaking Medicaid.* 100-117.

58. Draper *et al.,* "Medicaid Managed Care: The Last Bastion of the HMO?," 155-167.

59. Omnibus Budget Reconciliation Act of 1981, United States Congress, House of Representatives, Report 97-158, Vol. 2, 316.

60. A regularization of the "Katie Beckett" model waiver. Cf. Carol O'Shaughnessy and Richard Price, *Medicaid "2176" Waivers for Home and Community-Based Care* (Washington, D.C., Congressional Research Service, 1985),16-17.

61. Robert Gettings, telephone interview, Smith, January 12, 2006.

62. Sec. 2176(2).

63. At the time, HCFA was sponsoring a National Long-Term Care Channeling Demonstration which showed, *inter alia,* that alternative community based systems were often more expensive than institutional care, because of the "woodwork" effect and other factors such as transportation, overhead expense, and loss of economies of scale. Other important issues were how to count the time and effort of unpaid caretakers (mostly spouses or relatives) and how much of this effort would be displaced by paid-for home and community based services.

64. In this context, "cost-neutral," though "budget neutral" was the more generic and commonly used term. Later regulations clarified that what was meant was total per capita expenditures (including physician services, acute hospital care, dental and pharmaceutical services, and not just HCB services).

65. Later "flexibility" proposals have urged that offsets be allowed from any part of the Medicaid budget or from any health services supported by the Social Security Act, or under any title of the Act.

66. Lu Zavistovich, interview by Moore and Smith, August 3, 2004. HCFA provided a review guide that went through the application process step-by-step and HCFA staff would often, over the telephone, walk applicants through the steps. Nevertheless, inability to understand what HCFA required and lack of a template or "model" waiver was a frequent complaint. Cf. O'Shaughnessy and Price, *Medicaid "2176" Waivers,* 25-26.

67. Lu Zavistovich, *ibid.*

68. Robert Wardwell, interview by Moore and Smith, April 13, 2003.

69. Does "habilitation" include job counseling? Does it include paying for patients' TVs and VCRs?

70. For instance, different amounts claimed for Medicaid payments and as expenditures in a waiver renewal application.

71. Hoyer, telephone interview by Smith, December 8, 2005.

72. Credited to Robert E. Wren, then Director of Provider Services and Coverage.

73. A simplified example: a nursing home has 100 beds which, on average, turn over once every two years. The turnover allowance would be 50 beds/year, so that the nursing home's total bed capacity for waiver purposes would be 150.

74. Some states did not have CoN authorities. At this time, moreover, health planning and local CoN agencies were being phased out. Without a CoN—which by then would probably have been rather easy to acquire—the state would have to provide convincing evidence that construction would actually take place along with other pertinent data about occupancy rates, waiting lists, and so forth. O'Shaughnessy and Price, *Medicaid "2176" Waivers,* 25-26.

75. Wardwell, telephone interview by Smith, January 17, 2006.
76. Wayne Smith, telephone interview by Smith, January 13, 2006. There were exceptions—residential facilities run by gentle, caring, and dedicated "house parents," but most such residences were abominations.
77. *Ibid.,* January 23, 2006.
78. Cf. Smith, *Entitlement Politics,* 150 ff.; also Peter M. Benda and Charles H. Levine, "Reagan and the Bureaucracy: The Bequest, the Promise, and the Legacy," in Charles O. Jones (ed.) *The Reagan Legacy: Promise and Performance* (Chatham, NJ: Chatham House Publishers, 1988).
79. Key figures at OMB were John Cogan, program associate director for human resources, veterans, and labor; David Kleinberg, the deputy associate director and head of health and income maintenance; and Steven Lieberman, health and income maintenance. Cogan was a political appointee; Kleinberg and Lieberman were civil servants.
80. Reviews were described as "irrationally stringent," with irrelevant questions and frequent demands for more and more documentation. One anecdote involved a young budget examiner who was told to "go back, ask more questions, and find a way to deny it [the waiver]." Wardwell, telephone interview by Smith, April 3, 2003.
81. Wardwell, who was in charge of 1915(c) waivers in HCFA during this period, once complained of a waiver being held up by OMB. John Cogan, the program associate director (PAD), telephoned him asking why he was "lying about OMB" and misleading people. He intimated that he might have to complain to the secretary about a civil servant who couldn't do his job properly. *Ibid.*
82. *Medicaid Source Book,* 390, 960.
83. *Ibid.,* p. 406.
84. *Ibid.,* p. 408.
85. During the first years, only Oregon applied for this waiver. States were wary because of the cap. Also, under this waiver, they could not use the more liberal standards for eligibility, such as the 300% of poverty for nursing homes and more liberal asset tests and spousal impoverishment provisions. *Ibid.,* 409.
86. Gettings, telephone interview by Smith, January 12, 2006.
87. *Medicaid Source Book,* 388.
88. *Ibid.,* 409. This option was extended by the DRA of 2005 to include all HCB services.
89. "The 1915(c) Home and Community-Based Services Program: Data Update," (Washington, D.C.: Kaiser Commission on Medicaid and the Uninsured, July 2005), 1.
90. Joshua M. Wiener and David G. Stevenson, "State Policy on Long-Term Care for the Elderly," *Health Affairs,* Vol. 17(3), 1998, 81-100, at 90-91. This article is especially good for illustrating some of the complexities of nursing home policy.
91. Some important discussion of this trend can be found in John Holahan, James Bell, and Gerald S. Adler (eds.) *Medicaid Program Evaluation: Final Report, op. cit.,* Ch. 8, 20-21.
92. Including advocacy, lawsuits, and political mobilization. Care for the mentally retarded and mentally disabled is a long-term and expensive responsibility, so that parents are well motivated to organize and seek aid for their charges.
93. Cynthia Shirk, *Rebalancing Long-Term Care: The Role of the Medicaid HCBS Waiver Program,* (Washington, D.C.: National Health Policy Forum, March 2006), 4.

94. Bruce C. Vladeck, "Where the Action Really Is: Medicaid and the Disabled," *Health Affairs,* Vol. 22(1) 2003, pp. 90-100, at 94.

95. Richard G. Frank, Howard H. Goldman, and Michael Hogan, "Medicaid and Mental Health: Be Careful What You Wish For," *Health Affairs*, Vol. 22(1), 101-113, at 105.

96. Allen J. Leblanc and M. Christine Tonner, "Medicaid 1915(c) Home and Community-Based Services Waivers Across the States," *Health Care Financing Review,* Vol. 22(1) 2000, 159-174 at 163.

97. 1919(b)(A)(vii) developed at the staff level by Thomas Hoyer (HCFA) and Andy Schneider (of the House Commerce staff). Hoyer, telephone interview by Smith, January 23, 2006.

98. Amending Sec. 1905(i). "The term 'institution for mental diseases' means a hospital, nursing facility, or other institution of more than 16 beds, that is primarily engaged in providing diagnoses, treatment, or care of persons with mental diseases, including medical attention, nursing care, and related services." P.L. 100-360 (1988).

99. This particular legislation was the culmination of a two-year bipartisan effort within Congress to curb the Reagan administration's purging of the SSDI rolls of allegedly ineligible recipients. Ineligible recipients had been a continuing issue, addressed earlier in the Carter administration by periodic reviews of the rolls; but disability advocates claimed that the Reagan administration pushed the reviews with excessive zeal, intending to shrink the program itself as part of an overall objective of reducing the size of the government. This act passed Congress by a unanimous vote and within weeks the United States Supreme Court directed Secretary Heckler to reconsider terminations in thousands of cases from California and other western states. Most of the fight had been about SSDI, not SSI, but the same standard for disability applied to both. As for mental health, the important part of the act was to bar termination of disability benefits only if there was substantial evidence that the recipient's medical condition had improved and that he or she was able to work—a standard that was of decisive importance for the severely and chronically mentally ill and that has not been subsequently challenged. This episode was another instance in which the Medicaid program was protected by and benefited from the political strength of another constituency. Cf. Katherine P. Collins and Anna Enfer, "Social Security Disability Reform Act of 1984: Legislative Histories and Summary of Provisions," *Social Security Bulletin* Vol. 48(4) 1985, 5-32; also *Congressional Quarterly Weekly,* September 22, 1984, 2332, and December 15, 1984, 3119.

100. Cf. Frank, "Medicaid and Mental Health: Be Careful What You Wish For," also, Michael Perry and Nell Robertson, *Individuals with Disabilities and Their Experiences With Medicaid Managed Care—Results From Focus Group Research*, (Washington, DC: Kaiser Commission on Medicaid and the Uninsured, 1999) and Sharon K. Ling, Teresa A. Coughlin, and Stephanie Kendall, "Access to Care Among Disabled Adults on Medicaid," *Health Care Financing Review*, Vol. 23(4) 2002, 159-173.

101. The "families" being covered had to include "targeted low income children" and satisfy the secretary that the purchase was "cost effective" when compared with existing coverage and would not substitute for existing health insurance coverage. "Cost effective" meant that the family coverage could cost no more than coverage for the child or children.

102. States took steps to simplify and facilitate enrollment, remove demeaning and stigmatizing procedures such as asset tests, encourage mail applications, and

minimize verification requirements. Some adopted presumptive eligibility and 12 month continuous eligibility and simplified renewal procedures—measures that increased enrollment and reduced the need for personal visits and onerous paperwork.

103. *Living Without Health Insurance*, Hearings, Unites States Senate, Committee on Finance, 107th Congress, First Session, 2001 (Washington, D.C.: Government Printing Office, 2001), Prepared statement by Donna Cohen Ross, pp. 187-194 at 188-189.

104. Statements of this kind are hazardous. The initial start up was slow. In addition, early estimates of SCHIP enrollments were inflated, but SCHIP performed well by more realistic CBO estimates. The BBA '97 deficit reduction schedule required a three year 20% reduction in SCHIP allotments from 2002 to 2004 which caused a three-year lag in enrollments, often referred to as the "CHIP-dip." Recession and a relatively stagnant or non-existent recovery led to unemployment and cutbacks in employer-sponsored insurance, increasing the number of uninsured. And single men (unless disabled) and many immigrants were ineligible so that reductions in the number of uninsured were less impressive. Still, SCHIP grew and preserved gains though it might not have done so without cutbacks in eligibility, cost-sharing, and benefit reductions. Also, the number of enrollees actually declined in 2003-2004. But managing to grow most of the time, retain enrollment, and reduce the number of uninsured children by over a million in a recession, with large numbers of unemployed and states in severe fiscal distress would seem like a qualified success.

105. Especially in the first years, since a number of states had unspent funds carried over from previous years or reallocated from states that had not met their allot-ments. Cf. Jeanne Lambrew, *Section 1115 Waivers in Medicaid and the State Children's Health Program: An Overview*. Washington, DC: Kaiser Commission on Medicaid and the Uninsured, 2001, 17.

106. Sec. 2103(b)(4)(D).

107. Cindy Mann and Elizabeth Kenny, *Differences that Make a Difference: Compar-ing Medicaid and the State Children's Health Program Federal Benefit Standards.* Washington, DC: Georgetown University Health Policy Institute, 2005. Under EPSDT, "medical necessity" covers medical services necessary "to correct or ameliorate defects and physical and mental health conditions," which has been in-terpreted to include—in addition to treatment and cure of illness or injury—chronic illness and disability and preventive and ameliorative services.

108. Lambrew, *Sec. 1115 Waivers,* 1.

109. Jay Greenberg, Walter Leutz, Bruce Spitz, and Stanley Wallach, *A Historical Note on Medicare and Medicaid Waivers,* Waltham, MA: Brandeis University, Health Policy Center, 1983), 11.

110. Cynthia Shirk, *Shaping Public Programs Through Medicare, Medicaid, and SCHIP Waivers: The Fundamentals*. Washington, D.C.: National Health Policy Forum, 2003, 5.

111. *Ibid.,* also, Allan Dobson, Donald Moran, and Gary Young, "The Role of Waivers in the Health Policy Process," *Health Affairs*, Vol. 11(4)1992, 72-96 at 85-86.

112. Shirk, *Shaping Public Programs,* 12-13.

113. Some provisions of the Medicaid statute cannot be modified by waiver: the statu-tory matching rate, quality assurance requirements, statutory limits on cost-shar-ing, and some provisions relating to dual eligibles. Cf. Lambrew, *Section 1115 Waivers,* n4, 15.

114. There have been a few court cases and some occasional minor limitations imposed by Congress, for the most part to insist on a procedure or curb an activity with respect to a specific situation, not limit the power or discretion of the secretary as such. *Ibid.,* n3, 4.
115. Richard Hegner, *Section 1115 Medicaid Waivers: Demonstrations or Strategy for Incremental Reform?* Washington, D.C.: National Health Policy Forum, 1995, 5.
116. Christopher Jennings, interview by Moore and Smith, June 23, 2004.
117. Lambrew, *Sec. 1115 Waivers a* 4.
118. "Medicaid Program: Demonstration Proposals Pursuant to Section 1115(a) of the Social Security Act: Policies and Procedures," *Federal Register* Vol. 59. no. 186, September 17, 2004, p. 49249.
119. Hegner, *Section 1115 Medicaid Waivers,* 3.
120. Cynthia Shirk, *op. cit.,* pp. 13-14. A 1994 lawsuit challenged the first five waivers as violating the Administrative Procedure Act and Medicaid statutory and regulative requirements, especially with regard to patient protections. The suit was brought by the National Association of Community Health Centers.
121. All of the new waivers utilized managed care and, under a Sec. 1115 waiver, could make managed care enrollment mandatory. BBA '97 limited the need for a managed care waiver, requiring only a state plan amendment in most instances. It should also be noted that the Oregon waiver, which had been turned down by the Bush administration, made use of a prioritizing of benefits that was often denounced as "rationing." Initial enrollment under the Tennessee waiver approached the chaotic. And earlier managed care waivers in Philadelphia had been denounced as "genocidal" because of their impact on racial minorities.
122. Cynthia Shirk, *op cit.,* p. 14.
123. Jennifer Ryan, *1115 Ways to Write Medicaid and SCHIP Rules.* Washington D.C., National Health Policy Forum, 2002, p. 8. Another important reason was that the statutory requirement for "family coverage" was difficult to meet—a showing that family coverage would be cost-effective in comparison to coverage for children alone.
124. *Ibid.*
125. Cynthia Shirk, *op. cit.,* p. 15.
126. The Pharmacy Plus waiver allowed states to expand prescription drug coverage to low-income seniors not eligible for Medicaid.
127. Cynthia Shirk, *op cit.,* p. 27.
128. *Medicaid and SCHIP—Recent HHS Approvals of Demonstration Waiver Projects Raise Concerns,* GAO-92-817. Washington, D.C.: Government Printing Office, 2002. Commenting on four approved waivers (of 13 submitted) three of which—Arizona, California, and Utah—sought to reduce the number of uninsured and one—Illinois—extended drug coverage to low-income seniors.
129. *Ibid.,* 16-17. In the larger scheme of things an appropriate resolution of this matter is not obvious. The SCHIP statute required that unspent SCHIP funds be reallocated (to states that had spent their allocations—which makes sense if the obligation to spend that money on children is all that is at stake. But what about spending the money on other programs for children, or enrolling parents especially if that gets more children enrolled? The Clinton administration also had a role in stretching the waiver. Under the SCHIP statute, the requirement for family coverage was that it be "cost-effective" which meant costing no more than coverage for the child or children alone. As of April 1999 only two states had qualified under this test. HCFA announced on July 31, 2000 that it would

consider Sec. 1115 waivers that used unspent SCHIP funds to cover parents of SCHIP or Medicaid eligible children and was silent on the cost-effectiveness test. In other words, the Clinton administration was also ignoring or stretching the law, although it did not encourage reduced coverage or increased use of cost-sharing as a way to cover more uninsured. *Ibid.,* 19. Another issue raised by the GAO report was which should take precedence—the absence of such authority under the SCHIP legislation or the broad authority conferred by the Social Security Act in authorizing the Sec. 1115 waiver.

130. *Ibid.,* p. 31.
131. *Ibid.,* p. 17.
132. Samantha Artiga and Cindy Mann, *New Directions for Medicaid Section 1115 Waivers: Policy Implications of Recent Waiver Activity.* Washington, D.C.: Kaiser Commission on Medicaid and the Uninsured, 2005, 2.
133. Samantha Artiga and Cindy Mann, *Coverage Gains Under Recent; Section 1115 Waivers: A Data Update.* Washington, D.C.: Kaiser Commission on Medicaid and the Uninsured, 2005, 5.
134. *Ibid.,* 1.
135. The Medicaid relief took the form of an 18-month 3% increase in the FMAP. *Health Care Policy Report,* June 2, 2003, 713.
136. Primarily current or recent TANF cash benefit recipients or Medicaid recipients qualifying by spend-down. *Overview of the Utah Section 1115 Waiver.* Washington, D.C.: Kaiser Commission on Medicaid and the Uninsured, July 2004, 4.
137. As quoted in Leighton Ku and Vikki Wachino, *The Potential Impact of Eliminating TennCare and Reverting to Medicaid: A Preliminary Analysis.* Washington, D.C.: Center on Budget and Policy Priorities, November, 2004, 3.
138. *Ibid.,* 3.
139. The "Medicaid Reform" plan covers infants under 200% of poverty; ages 1-6 at 133% of poverty; and 6-20 at 100% of poverty. Non-institutionalized disabled and elderly SSI recipients are covered but not those receiving Medicare. Parents and pregnant women are covered only up to 23% of poverty or about $300 for a family of three. This latter figure for parents and pregnant women may seem gratuitously stingy, but it makes sense if a major purpose is to have a general test of the concepts.
140. Vermont might be regarded as an exception to this generalization; but it is traditionally conservative and had a Republican governor.
141. Florida (Jeb Bush), Mississippi (Haley Barbour) and South Carolina (Mark Sanford).
142. Sec. 1115 waivers all include a number of "special terms and conditions" which set forth the CMS conditions for waiver approval. These often involve lengthy negotiations and can be both complicated and "political" in some of their requirements. Jennifer Ryan, *Medicaid in 2006: A Trip Down the Yellow Brick Road?* Washington, D.C.: National Health Policy Forum, March 2006, 15 and n29.
143. *Ibid.,* 16-18.
144. Charles Milligan, interview by Moore and Smith, October 26, 2006.
145. One Medicaid official, as reported by Milligan, called it "financial plea bargaining."
146. *Ibid.,* p. 15.
147. Kentucky and West Virginia. Also, South Carolina withdrew its Sec. 1115 waiver and is, for now, proceeding under this new authority. *New York Times,* May 24, 2006, p. A-24; Ryan, telephone interview by Smith, June 16, 2006.

9

Past and Future

What of value about Medicaid policy for the future can be learned from a history of Medicaid politics and policy? A philosopher has said that those who ignore history are condemned to repeat it; and some historians that history teaches no lessons.[1] Not much is to be gained by attempting to resolve this difference or decide where a historical account of Medicaid falls between the extremes. Some of the program's historic behavior seems fairly predictable and some not. Combining a generous federal match with program flexibility, Medicaid has grown and adapted consistently to become the largest health insurer in the United States and the "workhorse" of the American health care system. Yet the program—decentralized and polycentric and much affected by external influences—is cyclical, quirky, and even perverse in its responses, like an eccentric associate one has known for years who remains full of surprises.

The metaphor of character or personality helps frame a central question addressed in this chapter: what do we know about the persistent behavior or 'character" of Medicaid politics and policy that can help improve the current program, make it work better, or enable it to respond successfully to the challenges of a changing political and fiscal environment?

Any formulation of "persistent" properties or "characteristic" behavior may be well-grounded in history and endorsed by authorities, but will also be subjective, contextual, and broadly thematic rather than sharp in detail so that, at best, it can support a small number of general policy recommendations rather than a large number of specific ones.

Before proceeding, a few of the premises on which this discussion is based should be made clear. In our view (*supra,* ix-x), a single-payer or strongly integrated national health insurance (NHI) proposal is not likely to become law in the near future. Any version that might succeed would likely be an "aggregative" model,[2] combining various mandates and preserving Medicare and Medicaid along with other nationally funded programs, such as the Veterans Administration and CHAMPUS, or even SCHIP. Another assumption is that the historic, long-term commitment to providing health insurance and/or health care for the poor, pregnant women and children, and the elderly and disabled will remain so that, with or without NHI, there will be a question of what to do about Medicaid.

As stated in the preface, our preference would not be to end the Medicaid entitlement, but to save it and make it "work"[3] a statement that can have widely different significance depending on what is meant by "it" or "entitlement." As for the first—which raises the issue of the multiple roles of Medicaid in providing insurance or paying for health care—Medicaid is described, at times, as a program for the poor, as providing coverage for the uninsurable and uninsured, or as a way-station on the road to NHI. Historically, Medicaid has moved some distance in each of these directions, but our view is that such extensions, though appropriate as pioneering or joint ventures, can threaten Medicaid's more established and legitimate obligations, the program's institutional integrity, and even its long-term political survival. Another view, also stated in the preface, is that Medicaid has flourished as a relatively weak entitlement—compared, for instance, to Medicare or Social Security—and should continue as such, although with some carefully designed and mostly incremental changes to restore and strengthen the entitlement in some ways as well as limit and contain its expansive potential in others.

Medicaid So Far

The Medicaid program's capacity for steady growth and adaptation has been its most striking feature. Estimated in its first year to cost half a billion dollars in combined federal and state expenditures, that year's growth doubled the estimate and thereafter the program[4] grew at rates typically between 15% and 20% a year.[54] Today, with an estimated enrollment of 55 million and combined federal and state expenditures of $300 billion, it is, by far, the largest health insurance program in the United States and one of the largest in the world.

The combination of flexible funding and a generous federal match has facilitated, over the years, a transformation of Medicaid from a narrowly based welfare-linked system of categorical eligibility into a program that often takes on a broad mission of comprehensive care for the poor. In addition to growing vigorously, the program has been extensively adapted to address unmet needs, encourage service delivery changes, and sustain an infrastructure on which health care delivery for the poor depends. It has been aptly described as a "workhorse" of the U.S. health care system, because of its capacity to address difficult tasks that others avoid.[6] It is also useful to think of the Medicaid program as a kit-bag of tools, some of them old and clumsy, but field-tested and familiar.

Some of the *additional* benefits and program activities that have developed over time that were *not* contemplated in the original statute include:

- Comprehensive benefits for pregnant women and children (to age 18) with minimal or no co-payments even though not receiving or eligible for welfare.
- Wrap around coverage of low-income Medicare beneficiaries, including drugs, medical devices, and many optional benefits.
- Comprehensive and community based services for persons with disabilities.
- Extending coverage to persons with mental illnesses and HIV/AIDS.
- Coverage for persons transitioning from welfare to work, for working persons with disabilities, and emergency and childbirth services for undocumented aliens.
- Support for safety-net providers and the healthcare infrastructure, including safety-net hospitals, community and migrant health centers, mental health services,[7] and school health programs.
- Statewide waivers restructured many state programs comprehensively and in ways differing radically from the original Title XIX.

Aside from growing, the Medicaid program has undergone three major systemic changes and is currently moving toward a fourth. The program began as a payment mechanism for categorically linked vendor payments to traditional fee-for-service health care providers. It has changed into one increasingly based on contracts negotiated with managed care organizations, especially for mothers and children. Initially, the program took service delivery for acute care and institutional placements as a given. Today, the emphasis is increasingly upon shaping benefits and service delivery to enable Medicaid beneficiaries to live and function effectively and independently in the community.[8] A major transformation was initiated by SCHIP, which offered a version of "Medicaid Lite" that encouraged growth in a new direction, especially reaching more of the uninsured children and parents among the working poor with easier enrollment procedures and coverage options similar to those offered in the commercial insurance market.[9]

Another development of great potential significance has been the venturing by a number of states into premium assistance,[10] paid for by SCHIP funds, Sec. 1115 waivers, or HIPP[11] programs. This approach would come much closer, in principle, to covering the uninsured as such and would also involve the Medicaid program in the evaluation of private insurance products and policies toward private industries.

While it is unclear how far any of these tendencies will or should go and supporters of the Medicaid program differ in their appreciation of them, the point remains that they show a capacity for systemic adaptation even within the presently existing legislative and regulative framework.

Medicaid is also a thrifty purchaser of health care. The big drivers of Medicaid costs have been increased enrollment, often occasioned by recession and unemployment; high levels of health care inflation including prescription drugs; and governmental mandates.[12] When allowance for such factors is made, Medicaid regularly outperforms the private sector or Medicare, especially in expense per enrollee. Moreover, these cost constraints are reliably effective, since they come largely from Medicaid's advantages as a single payer, the large market share occupied by Medicaid MCOs, and the infrastructure of providers accustomed to surviving on lean diets.

Inventory: Things to Do or Change

The sustained change and protean adaptability of the Medicaid program over four decades can be attributed in large measure to a generously matched entitlement with latitude for incremental development along a variety of paths and to the skill and determination in taking advantage of these program characteristics at both the federal and state levels. Much of this growth and adaptation was opportunistic and politically responsive with little effort or capacity to do much about uneven or excessive growth. So there is a downside to this pattern of growth: patches of neglect and excess, and a lack of systemic reform.

Despite the robust growth, Medicaid remains an uneven, 50-state program, not available for many it could reach, with eligibility, income and asset limits, cumbersome enrollment procedures, great variations in benefit levels, and "disparities" in access to and quality of services as between rich and poor, urban and rural, and racial and ethnic groups.

For an item, the statute itself—even as amended over 40 years—is much less inclusive and equitable than generally supposed. Children, the blind and disabled, and low-income elderly are automatically eligible for

Medicaid if they qualify for SSI, but the SSI income limit is only 74% of the FPL[13] and eleven "Sec. 209b" states have even lower income limits. Over the years, eligibility levels for pregnant women and children have been raised dramatically and mandated at levels above the FPL. But childless adults are ineligible, no matter how poor they are, and only about one-third of parents, including non-pregnant mothers are covered. Those that are covered, primarily under TANF, are subject to state income limits, which average about 40% of the FPL.[14] Many of the elderly poor qualify only for partial Medicaid benefits. Undocumented immigrants are eligible only for emergency and pregnancy-related services and legal immigrants must have entered the United States on or after August 12, 1996 or have resided in this country for five years.

Although less important today, several omissions or exclusions from coverage have shaped the development of the Medicaid program. One of the most important of these was the IMD exclusion. Another was coverage for disability arising from alcoholism or drug abuse. Coverage for disabilities generally was delayed by a restrictive definition of disability. Omission until recently of coverage of HCB services except under a waiver delayed development in this area. And a failure to include HIV and AIDS-related conditions held back coverage for these maladies. These omissions increased the overall "swiss-cheese" nature of the program and helped perpetuate its institutional bias. Eventually, coverage was extended one way or another to most of these areas, which testifies to the flexibility of the program; but many in need of care went without coverage for years until these changes were made.

Fifty states add to this diversity with their own determinations of eligibility and coverage. Income eligibility for adult populations in Alabama is 13% of the FPL, and the average for all states, not counting children, is only 41% of poverty.[15] Moreover, it is up to the states to decide how far they will go in extending eligibility to optional populations or what optional benefits they will cover. Here, the variations are enormous, with some states covering less than 15% of the poor and others as high as 36% and with expenditures for Medicaid recipients varying between different states by a factor of four if federal matching is included and by 12 to 14 if state expenditures alone are considered.[16]

These interstate variations are accompanied by "disparities" between and within states in health care treatment and outcomes,[17] some of them attributable to racial and ethnic discrimination, either deliberate or by letting local "folkways" and institutions prevail largely unchanged. As for Medicaid, these disparities have resulted mostly from "institutional" racism, rather than intentional discrimination, yet it is disquieting to realize how pervasive the problem is,[18] the lack of attention to it, and how little has been done about it, even though the issue has been prominently on the federal agenda since 1985.[19] True, the Medicaid program has little effective leverage with respect to this problem, but racial and ethnic disparities are especially troubling for a program that rests much of its moral authority upon a claim of supporting health care for the neediest.

As Medicaid has opportunistically grown beyond its original categorical and welfare-linked coverage, one broad and persistent issue has been whom Medicaid should insure and why? Should it, for instance, include an unemployed father with the eligible child?; the working poor who have no insurance or inadequate insurance?; the poor and near-poor who are uninsurable?; the unemployed transitioning between welfare and work?; middle-class persons with disabilities who would otherwise be impoverished? And so forth. These are all questions that have been historically controversial, with some still at issue today, especially over how best to cover more of the poor and the near-poor who are uninsured.

Medicaid's "institutional bias" is a historic legacy that has been reduced but is still present in modified forms. Waivers, managed care "carve-outs," and HCBS waivers have reduced the imbalance and helped change the locus of care and treatment. But we still wrestle with the question of how best to organize the delivery of services at the community level and what the role of Medicaid—a financing mechanism—should be. A former HCFA administrator, Bruce Vladeck, notes that the "de-institutionalization" struggle has largely been won. The challenge for "the next decades is how to build an adequate supply of high-quality community-based service systems"[20] for those with disabilities.

What to do about the "dual eligibles" more generally is a troublesome issue with deep historic roots. Both Kerr-Mills and the Medicaid statute included a category of "medically indigent," which provided one way that coverage could be extended to the poor not otherwise categorically eligible. The Medicaid statute also allowed states to "buy into" Medicare Part B or pay the Part A and Part B deductibles and co-pays for Medicare beneficiaries who met Medicaid income eligibility standards.[21] The establishment, by the Social Security Amendments of 1972, of Supplemental Security Income increased Medicaid eligibility and with it the numbers of those dually eligible. Sixteen years later, the Medicare Catastrophic Coverage Act (MCCA) mandated Medicaid coverage for Medicaid beneficiaries with incomes below the FPL. At the time, this burden was to have been shared by the establishment of a Medicare prescription drug benefit; but the repeal of the MCCA left the dual-eligible mandate in place without the fiscal relief originally part of the MCCA. Other federal requirements coming about the same time—costly federal nursing home standards, EPSDT penalties, and expanded coverage for pregnant women and children—helped make the dual-eligibles along with other "unfunded mandates" a touchy federal-state issue that has persisted for years. Today, it is hard to say whether the establishment of a Medicare prescription drug benefit with its "clawback" feature has soothed the troubled waters or only roiled them more, but the distribution of federal-state responsibilities for the dual eligibles continues to be in dispute.[22]

Another category—that overlaps with the dual eligibles—is beneficiaries with severe and chronic conditions that typically require multi-disciplinary protocols of treatment and are hugely expensive over time. Some of the most important are cancer, diabetes, emphysema, cardiovascular disease, strokes, arthritis, asthma, Alzheimer's disease, HIV/AIDS, back problems, depression and anxiety. Medicaid provides varying amounts of coverage for most of these conditions, often more generous than either Medicare or private insurance. These conditions, important for their aggregate cost, are also an area where significant enhancements in quality as well as cost savings might be realized by the reorganization of care and the adoption of disease management protocols and information technology.[23]

Cost containment is a major issue that has been dealt with more reactively and piece-meal than thoughtfully or systematically. At first, little attention was given to the topic, in part because Medicaid was likened to Kerr-Mills and the state response was expected to be modest and restricted by the matching requirement. With costs growing at an alarming rate, the federal government responded with various *ad hoc* and partial measures: the 133% limit on medical indigency; utilization review and PSROs; and percentage cuts or global caps on federal matching. Because of public assistance, states would tend to keep payments low but, attracted by the generous federal match, would respond to health care needs with little concern about aggregate costs until there was a fiscal crunch, at which point they would devise *ad hoc* remedies such as reducing payments to providers and cutting back on optional benefits or eligibility.

Meanwhile, Medicaid has grown so vigorously over the years—at twice or more than the rate of health care price inflation—that aggregate expenditures have become a serious matter and one of the major reasons adduced for scrapping the Medicaid entitlement outright. At the federal level, much of the concern is about the size of the non-discretionary budget, of which Medicaid, along with other entitlements, is a large part. At the state level, it is the growing share of Medicaid in state budgets and its encroachment upon other priorities such as education, highways, and prisons. The fiscal perversity of the Medicaid entitlement is important: often burgeoning when times are good but cut back with a recession when most needed and states   constrained by other needs and lower tax revenues. Some refer to it as a "boom and bust" cycle—of which more later—but, for now, the point is that the aggregate amount, the rate of growth, and the relation of Medicaid ups-and-downs to the business cycle are continuing issues.

Medicaid managed care in its various manifestations is a powerful and constructive way to increase access, coordinate service delivery, strengthen accountability, and save money. Yet there are limits and downside risks or side effects. For an item, cost saving is likely to be less than hoped because Medicaid service providers have already been squeezed repeatedly and thoroughly. Also, managed care is about managing risk, so that there is a persistent danger of risk selection to avoid high cost enrollees, such as those with severe disabilities or chronic diseases. Moreover, MCOs are geographically selective and not always available in the inner city or sparsely populated or medically underserved areas, which raises a further question of the role of the more traditional safety-net providers, such as the public hospitals and community health centers, what their role should be, and how they will be sustained and compensated for the no-pay or high-cost patients the MCOs don't take.

This mention of managed care and the safety-net providers leads toward a complex of unresolved issues and technical problems that can be summarized under the heading of developing, sustaining, and monitoring programs for the acute and long-term care of the frail elderly and persons with disabilities. Both managed care and the safety-net institutions (which include many of the great medical centers and teaching hospitals as well as public hospitals and clinics) will have major roles in developing the organizational entities, protocols, and working relationships for these tasks; but devising service delivery models that could be successfully brought to scale within individual states, deliver quality and contain costs, and be held accountable could be the challenge of a decade or more.

Changes of this sort, which draw heavily upon collaboration, shared aspirations, and inventiveness, highlight another issue of the appropriate roles of rulemaking and enforcement versus other methods of assuring program integrity, quality in performance, and effective access. To be sure, legalistic rules and enforcement will not disappear. But revising modes of service delivery will bring opportunities to reassess this balance as well as experience in implementing approaches that could be less burdensome and work more efficiently in preventing fraud and abuse or assuring continuity and quality of care. This approach might be a more productive way of "modernizing" Medicaid than most or all of the proposals usually found under this heading.

An urgent and politically charged topic is Medicaid waivers, which have grown, under the Clinton and Bush administrations, from modest dispensations to a method for remaking whole state Medicaid programs and "restructuring" the federal program state-by-state following state or administrative priorities without authorization by the Congress. This is a development that has progressed quite far without, as yet, any systematic review to determine what federal interests need to be protected and what the role of waivers should be, for instance, in testing new models of service delivery in contrast to adopting them as a fiscal bailout or way to dismantle existing Medicaid programs.

Federal-state relations in Medicaid have mostly been a kind of "antagonistic cooperation," the balance shifting over time toward one pole or the other with periods in which mutual trust and collaboration between federal and state officials prevailed and others characterized by lack of communication or candor, imputing of bad faith or perversity, even denunciations and defiance. Sometimes the federal authorities would be the offenders—for instance, OMB under the Reagan administration or Congress and the "unfunded" mandates. Other times, it would be the states, with fraud and abuse, or various schemes of "Medicaid maximization." Waivers have been a fruitful source of discord. To be sure, a balance of cooperation and antagonism can be useful, much as they would be in contractual negotiations or collective bargaining; but the contemporary level of antagonism and distrust needs to be reduced, especially when seeking to create new entities that combine increased discretion with an accountability that is both effective and rests lightly.

The politicizing of Medicaid both nationally and locally trended sharply upward in the mid-1990s and remains a serious issue. Among the factors in this development have been the increased visibility of the

Medicaid program, its dramatic growth and impact on both the federal and state budgets, and the controversies over mandates, regulation, and Medicaid maximizing. The election of 1994 heightened attention to a number of domestic programs, including entitlements such as Medicare and Medicaid. It was also interpreted as a mandate by conservative and ideological Republicans to complete the unfinished "Reagan revolution," and led to a highly mobilized and ideological party politics that continues to this day.

This politicizing, especially with a strong ideological thrust, works against moderate and carefully articulated improvements. Focusing conservative effort on an ultimate goal of "restructuring" Medicaid or ending its entitlement status may be good for solidifying the party's "base" and the ideologues, but it also mobilizes opponents and stymies even mutually beneficial compromises because they might diminish a strategic or tactical advantage in the larger struggle. The *immobilisme* or "gridlock" produced by this kind of politics discourages those who work at developing moderate and actionable policy options so that there is less to discuss or negotiate and more that reduces to energizing the faithful and counting the votes.

The Medicaid Entitlement

One of the most contested items in the history of Medicaid has been its entitlement status: both its nature and whether it should exist at all. It is perennial and has come up in a number of different ways: in federal-state "swaps;" attempts to "block-grant" the Medicaid program or cap aggregate expenditures, in federal-state antagonisms over flexibility vs. mandates, in budgets and deficit reduction, and in fundamental ideological disputes about the role of the state and its moral obligations toward the less fortunate. The entitlement struggle is also holistic—involving Congress, the administration, the courts and federal-state relations—so that almost any major change in Medicaid policy will bear upon this conflict either directly or indirectly. As with warfare, it often helps to clarify what the fighting is about.

In considering the Medicaid entitlement, an initial identification of several elements of that entitlement may be useful. Narrowly, the entitlement requires the federal government by law to pay states a formula-determined percentage of covered and medically necessary expenses incurred by its enrolled (or prospectively enrolled) beneficiaries. The federal government has a duty to the beneficiaries to see that the statutory requirements are met. The states, in turn, are obligated both to the federal government and to the beneficiaries to spend the funds for lawful and agreed-upon purposes. Providers have a right to lawful payments. These are all "hard" obligations, implied by the law itself, but there are budgetary, political, and moral aspects that help convey some of the larger significance of "entitlement."

From a budgetary perspective, the Medicaid entitlement obligates the federal government to make payments for all eligible recipients, typically authorizing "such funds as may be necessary" for that purpose. Entitlement authorizations can be annual or for several years, but for Medicaid, it is permanent, which is important since it does away with the need for periodic reauthorizations and creates an ongoing, unlimited (uncapped) commitment to match expenditures for the specified purposes. This is the aspect of the Medicare and Medicaid entitlements especially at issue in the budget reconciliations and that gets much of the publicity. Medicaid would cease to be an "entitlement" without this feature; but it is not always the most consequential in shaping the program.[24]

The Medicaid entitlement from a legal perspective is a claim to health care goods and services that can be legally enforced.[25] This definition presupposes the American legal system, the Medicaid program with its federal and state rules and regulations, and the health care industry and Medicaid beneficiaries and health care providers with their claims to services or payments and their means of legal redress. It also hints at some important truths: that lawsuits and courts have been important in establishing beneficiary and provider claims and for enforcement of other instruments of accountability, such as the state plan or regulations. From another perspective, the role of the courts underlines the relative weakness of other means of assuring programmatic compliance.

The political dimension of the Medicaid entitlement is important. In this respect, it is a commitment or pledge to a clientele and those who serve them. That pledge is institutionalized to some extent in the continuing, open authorization. But for many Medicaid supporters it is a deep obligation, taking on a cause that transcends ordinary politics or elections. For politicians that have to win elections, though, a political defense of Medicaid can be difficult: it is not an "earned" entitlement like veterans' pensions or "paid for" like Social Security or Medicare and its constituency is poorly organized and lacks resources. Of course, Medicaid advocates work with politicians and are an important resource. But the Medicaid cause is often a "hard sell," which is a major reason for describing it as a "weak entitlement."

There is a distributive issue of practical morality that is different from and in addition to the political and legal considerations: who is the Medicaid entitlement for? As noted, the entitlement runs to the recipients and to the states and, derivatively, to the providers.[26] Read as a whole, the statute would seem to imply that the neediest came first, but it doesn't say so, and that leaves open issues of practical morality that arise in the distribution of benefits as between the neediest and the needy; shifting the risk from the insurer to the insured; and sharing the burdens of cost containment. That is not to say that such issues can be ultimately resolved, only that they come up and that it helps to recognize them and understand some of the implications.

The Medicaid entitlement is weak in political support and in provisions for assuring program integrity and administrative implementation, especially at the state level. But it should be noted that it is strong in another way: in its mandate for generous and redistributive matching payments to the states. Practically, this combination of weakness and strength led to some fraud and abuse, but it also allowed for local flexibility and encouraged states to expand their programs—a boon to some and a bane to others.

For the Entitlement

These statements in support of the entitlement have both theoretical merit and popular appeal but are not, therefore, either right or conclusive. At the same time, they do support the entitlement as such and a view that it should be retained and not abandoned for some other approach, such as health care grants to the states, vouchers, or health savings accounts.

Support for the entitlement can be found in the fact that it has been repeatedly ratified. Over the years, various attempts to substitute a block grant or a capped entitlement have been rejected, largely because they lacked ensured protections for the core Medicaid populations. Put somewhat differently, a major argument for the Medicaid entitlement is not just that it has been around for a time, but that it has protected and improved the condition of pregnant women and children, persons with disabilities, and the elderly and has been formally approved because it does so. There is both an historic and a present commitment to these populations and, so far, none of the alternatives to the Medicaid entitlement seem to provide assurances of adequate protection for them or that the commitment will continue.

The entitlement is important to sustain the infrastructure of Medicaid and safety-net providers that make possible the delivery of a variety of health care and services of tolerable quality at a low cost. The argument is that the experience and long-term commitment needed to make Medicaid work as well as it does are possible because many who are part of this infrastructure are willing to accept a tradeoff of lower income for long-term stability: they will, in a sense, make a career of Medicaid if they can make a living.[27] If the support—whether political or fiscal—is too small or uncertain, they will have to go elsewhere. In effect, political and fiscal stability nurture some other-regarding and non-pecuniary motivation and support an infrastructure that helps give it practical effect.

Another reason for preserving the Medicaid entitlement is that it often allows our better angels to prevail. It institutionalizes a legislative politics that is both generous and protective. Incrementalism and a continuing authorization facilitates extensions of eligibility and improvements in coverage while the ethos (and pathos) of taking away entitlements for the poor and afflicted make it difficult to rescind them. For a country distinguished for its stinginess and punitive attitudes toward the poor and still without a system of national health insurance, this tilt toward generosity and protectiveness is a desirable change from our typical behavior.

Against the Entitlement

One of the arguments against the Medicaid entitlement is that it has encouraged too much growth—that it has been too seductive or successful. At first, attacks upon Medicaid were a reaction to the Great Society programs and a part of efforts to reduce the size of the federal government and restructure American federalism. As the program developed, its rate of growth was a perennial concern. Late in the 1980s a dominant theme was that Medicaid, along with other entitlements and mandatory spending, was eating up too much of the federal budget and, at the state level, that Medicaid was largely driving budget growth and crowding out other vital priorities, such as education, highways, and prisons.

Without doubt, the Medicaid rate of growth—averaging 10-15% or more per year—was and is a matter of general concern. It should be noted, though, that these high growth rates are largely attributable to such factors as high unemployment, rising medical and prescription drug prices, and extensive "Medicaidization" of programs already supported by state budgets. Furthermore, increases in Medicare costs *per patient* have been low and compare favorably with private insurance, even while providing more services. But the rates of increase are perceived to be high—by many, unsustainably so--and in politics appearances are often more important than reality.

The entitlement is thought by some, especially governors, to be a bad trade: bringing with it mandates, over-protectiveness, and regulations that stand in the way of local initiatives and Medicaid adaptations that could save money and still enhance service delivery. Of course, waivers are one kind of remedy, but a partial and often exasperating one that raises issues of its own. The appeal of "super-waivers" and the SCHIP model are evidence that there is a genuine problem. The entitlement, with its strong political support, defends the Medicaid program against radical change; but it also preserves the layered complexity of the Medicaid program and its incremental pace of change, which are good as a conservative defense, but give rise to demands for drastic change.[28]

Critics of the entitlement have opposed it because it inhibits change; and most of them have in mind a direction and an agenda to follow. Often proposed amendments have been described as ways to "restructure" or "modernize" Medicaid, though their intent might more accurately be termed "deconstruction." Agenda items have included block-granting, capping the entitlement, making Medicaid like SCHIP, and a number of specifics aimed at devolution, shifting incentives or risks and adopting "market-like" devices, easing or dispensing with waivers, encouraging managed care, and generally shifting more "responsibility" to consumers by adding co-pays and sharing premium costs. Among the objectives of this approach would be to "empower" and "incentivize" the beneficiary to plan and manage their own care; stimulate competition among providers; and increase efficiency and reduce costs.

There is enough merit to either point of view to suggest that framing the issue as entitlement versus non-entitlement is not good policy and that a major victory for either side would likely produce widespread discontent and future entitlement wars. Meanwhile, the partisan mobilization, alarmist prophecies, and obscurantist ideology that characterize much of our current scene work against bipartisan compromise and crowd out reasonable and supportable reforms that might help to defuse some of the controversy over this and other Medicaid issues.

A Modest List of Proposals

The recommendations that follow are described as a "modest list" for two reasons. They are proposals that are familiar, have been around for a time, are moderate in content, and might generate substantial bipartisan support. The list is also modest because it is not extensive. Many possible improvements in the Medicaid program are not included because this historical account provides little or no foundation for their discussion. For the recommendations made, we have tried to stay close to themes or conclusions that, in our view, the record of events supports. For much the same reason, these proposals are set forth broadly, without working out the details.

Underlying these recommendations is a view that Medicaid should be kept, at least until something better comes along. For more than a decade, though, partisan warfare over Medicaid has threatened its existence and hindered moderate, broadly acceptable reforms. With this history in mind, the recommendations have two major purposes. One is to achieve something like a truce or peace settlement that would reduce partisanship and federal-state tensions. The other is, to pursue the peace-making metaphor a step further, to improve or "modernize" the program in ways that would prolong a period of peaceful development and additional negotiation.

Much of the battle has been over flexibility versus protectiveness—especially the balance between the two and particulars relating to each—without reaching an ultimate agreement or compromise. Some sense of what the fighting has been about and the outcome of some of the contests can provide useful perspective. Almost from the beginning of the Medicaid program, most Republicans have sought for greater flexibility and less federal intrusion, both to set priorities and to manage the state programs more effectively. The opposition—Democrats, and some Republicans—have been primarily concerned about protectiveness for pregnant women and children, the frail elderly and chronically ill, and persons with disabilities.

This distinction or dichotomy figured critically in three budget reconciliation acts that dealt comprehensively with Medicaid. The "Medicaid Transformation Act," which was part of the vetoed Balanced Budget Act of 1995, featured a capped entitlement with percentage set-asides for protected categories of Medicaid beneficiaries to which the Senate added a list of specific protections for these groups. The Balanced Budget Act of 1997 allowed greater flexibility, especially with respect to managed care, but held the vulnerable Medicaid beneficiaries harmless and mandated quality improvement programs for managed care. It also added SCHIP, which enrolled uninsured children as well as providing a vehicle for

extending eligibility to some of the working poor. The Deficit Reduction Act of 2005 continued this distinction: an SCHIP-like program for
most of the adult program, but with exemptions for pregnant women and
children, the blind and disabled, and those in long-term care.

At the heart of this controversy over flexibility versus protectiveness
is a familiar question of distributive justice about how much of limited
resources should go to help the neediest as opposed to benefiting a larger
number of less needy. This was an issue recognized in the original statute[29] by prohibiting discrimination against the welfare population in favor
of other categories; and it was largely for this reason that the original
requirements of statewideness and comparability were included. In its
modern form, it is a question of how protective to be of the sickest, most
vulnerable, and often "uninsurable," as opposed to an added flexibility to
cover more of uninsured, working poor, parents and children.

One trouble with this conundrum is that it lacks a satisfactory answer.
How does a politician—or a philosopher—choose between the neediest
and most expensive beneficiaries who are also the least likely to make
future contributions to the society, as opposed to the pregnant women
and children, the uninsured, and the working poor (who may be taxpay-
ers and voters)?[30] This is a tough choice with no rationally compelling
solution[31] that begets passionate advocacy on both sides and that persists
despite numerous political engagements and electoral cycles. It would
seem to be an impasse appropriate for compromise and some kind
of "treaty" or informal, even implicit, agreement that accommodated
strong differences, reduced tension, and promoted less bellicose modes
of dispute settlement.

The Deficit Reduction Act of 2005 may have done little to remedy
Medicaid's underlying defects or omissions, but it could be an important
contribution to framing the public debate and leading it into constructive paths. On the one hand, it increased "flexibility" substantially by
importing the SCHIP model with its "benchmark equivalent" plans and
encouraging more cost-sharing in the form of tiered co-payments and
Medicaid premiums for those above the FPL. But the DRA also acknowledged the importance of safeguarding the traditionally protected
categories, especially pregnant women and children and those with disabilities. In this respect, the Act reaffirmed the differential needs of these
categories and the importance of meeting them. In two different ways,
this informal truce could be a significant natural experiment: seeing
whether the tenuous settlement will hold and prove useful and how well

the protected and the non-exempt populations fare with this combination of increased flexibility and specific safeguards.

It should be noted that the DRA kept the Medicaid entitlement: the FMAP and the open and continuing authorization are still there. True, the practical benefit of the entitlement is limited and hollowed out; and a next installment could reduce it further. But deficit reduction and budget reconciliation are perennial exercises and the Medicaid chapters are loaded with exemptions, add-ons, and formula changes. What has been done can also be undone, almost with the stroke of a pen, and with little structural displacement.

An area where there may be scope for extensive cooperation between Republicans and Democrats and between state and federal governments is increased coverage for the uninsured working poor, many of whom are not enrolled in Medicaid because of categorical exclusions and the vagaries and indignities associated with establishing Medicaid eligibility. The SCHIP and HIFA waiver initiatives address this issue, but in ways that at times seem like robbing Peter to pay Paul: helping the uninsured at the expense of the needy and already entitled. States have experimented with premium assistance, Medicaid buy-ins, and super-waivers, though with meager results.

One way to cover many of the uninsured that has received recent attention would be to combine tax credits with Medicaid coverage. Tax credits for the working poor has been a long-term favorite of conservative Republicans because of its apparent simplicity and its private sector approach, but unacceptable to Democrats largely because it was seen as another "voucher" scheme that would undermine both traditional employer-sponsored insurance and Medicaid. But tax credits have gained support in recent years because of proposals to use the Earned Income Tax Credit (EITC) to purchase health insurance, creation of a health insurance voucher for workers displaced by the Trade Act,[32] and the steady erosion of employer-sponsored insurance. Even with this acceptance, the tax credits in most proposals are too low to buy adequate health insurance. But a tax credit combined with Medicaid and additional state support could provide a reasonable amount of coverage. Tax credits could also be combined with employer-sponsored insurance to produce a robust insurance package.[33]

The gains from such an approach could be important and lasting. It has wide appeal and might promote bipartisan collaboration and a partial settlement of a long-disputed issue. It could divert some of the pressure from Medicaid and SCHIP, save money for Medicaid and ease the distress of service-net providers. Successfully combined with premium assistance, it might help stabilize employer-supported insurance.[34] It could also be designed to bypass traditional categorical eligibility and further erode this relic from the past and create political pressure to abandon it entirely.[35]

The greatest challenge confronting Medicaid in the near future may well be, as Bruce Vladeck has argued, devising, implementing, and paying for a next generation of programs and service delivery options for those with disabilities and severe, chronic diseases. At present, this challenge lacks detailed specification and reaches far beyond the capabilities or jurisdiction of the Medicaid program, but past experience may provide some guidance in confronting an uncertain future.

A threshold question is that of the proper extent of Medicaid's responsibility for those with disabilities. Initially, the disabled was a small category, inherited from the Social Security Act of 1935, and not expensive. Much of the growth in these categories has been a result of the failure of private insurance, states unloading expenses by "Medicaidization" of care for these populations, or federal expansions of eligibility.[36] As these expenses have grown, they have put increased strains upon state budgets, with governors asking for relief, including a complete takeover of the dual eligibles.[37]

Takeover of state Medicaid responsibilities is not in favor lately, nor is it likely that the federal government would either repeal or assume the dual eligible mandates that were part of the MCCA. One modest proposal, though, would be for the federal government to reduce the "clawback" and give the states more of the benefit they had expected from the Medicare pharmaceutical drug provision. Another would be to include an allowance in the FMAP or even a separate match for the numbers of those with disabilities served. Such steps would ease the financial pinch for the states and help restore a sense of fairness. Some portion of this added money might also be earmarked for program development, especially administrative expenses and enhancements.

A more diffuse topic is what, beyond measures in effect, should be done to save money and promote quality in programs for those with disabilities and the chronically and severely ill. One answer is that Medicaid already does a good job of containing costs on a per case basis and could probably do better with its managed care and carve-outs, negotiated contracts, drug rebates, use of less costly home- and community-based alternatives, and monitoring of provider payments. There is also a kit bag of tools, such as electronic medical records, HEDIS, quality assurance and improvement, and performance based competition and purchasing that have been or could be adapted to specific programs and a Medicaid setting.[38]

Much recent thought about program development for persons with disabilities has converged on the notion of combining recent advances in care or treatment with services that would enable them to live in a community setting and have "a job, a home, and a date on Saturday night." A number of waivers and demonstrations have shown the feasibility of such a concept for individual cases or small numbers, raising a question of how this approach might be 'brought to scale," *i.e.,* designed in such a form that it will work in "real time," could be widely adapted, and wouldn't break the budget. With this goes a second question of the role of Medicaid as a program and an administrative agency. These are not, as yet, questions that have answers; but past history may help decide how to approach such problems—or how not to.

Such a grand design transcends the reach of the Medicaid program, both nationally and locally, since it would require coordinating services, such as education, affordable housing, socialization, counseling and direction, job opportunities and training, and administrative remedies and civil rights enforcement. It is hard to imagine Medicaid as the lead agency riding herd on such an effort, either nationally or locally.

An instructive example from the past was the Bush administration's response to the Olmstead decision (*supra*, 285 ff). This decision was interpreted as a mandate for "community-based alternatives" for those with disabilities and helped point to the New Freedom initiatives. It also led to a national commission on mental health and a task force draft from six different departments and agencies charged with "removing barriers to independent community living" and "working cooperatively" to provide services to persons with disabilities in "the most integrated setting." So far, some barriers have been removed but few services added, no follow-up on the mental health commission's report, and only two small programs begun, aimed primarily at promoting "independence" in navigating the health care system.

Another possible approach would be to center efforts on the MiCASSA[39] approach. This initiative, not yet law, would create a new Title XIX benefit for home and community-based services with a short-term enhanced match to pay for new services and provide financial assistance for "real system change" that moved toward home and community-based services for those with handicaps. MiCASSA has strong support within the Senate Finance Committee and a national advocacy group dedicated to this effort. In practical terms, it would support an "umbrella" organization at the state level, open a path for more comprehensive funding, and put Medicaid in a leadership position. But it lacks support from the "big categories" such as mental health, mental retardation, or the aged, and has failed to get significant support at the sub-committee level in either house of Congress, after a decade of effort.

These examples of MiCASSA and the Bush administration's post-Olmstead response suggest that efforts of "going to scale" are likely to center on the big categories: mental health, mental retardation, physical disabilities, the chronically ill and frail elderly, HIV/AIDS, and alcohol and drug abuse. Each of these big categories has its own care-giving traditions and theories. They also supply the energy and political clout at the national and local levels to push for legislation and funding and to ward off political attacks.

One reason for seeking service delivery models or templates that can be brought to scale is that—like education or manufacturing—a prescribed curriculum or mass-produced product may provide good or desired outcomes for the largest number of people. But the energies devoted to this kind of quest suggest some less obvious considerations: that these efforts focus the aspirations of professionals, mobilize advocates, facilitate leadership and federal-state cooperation, and provide a template or "paradigm" that can be evaluated and reformed over time. In brief, it is a way to organize service delivery, but also to create a political process with a continuing push toward expansion and improvement.

Waivers could be valuable in this process, though recent experience suggests that they have been mostly used for devolution of policy, de-institutionalization, and diffusion of managed care rather than as learning opportunities or the development of significant innovations in health care service delivery.[40] Innovations such as "money-follow-the-person" or "cash and counseling" (*supra,* 289) that are useful across categories of disability could be elements of a new service delivery template. But these are elements or tools, not a new template or paradigm. And they involved years of R&D effort within HCFA, numerous demonstrations, and collaboration with outside entities. They resembled old-fashioned R&D projects more than waivers.

About such elements or tools, one observation is that devices like the Prepaid Health Plans (PHPs), the ICF/MRs, Managed Behavioral Health Care (MBHC). the SNF Resource Utilization Groups (RUGs) and, more recently, "cash and counseling" and "Independence Plus" have been, or could be, important contributions in the programmatic development of Medicaid. But they are tools that can be misused or overworked and have unexpected consequences: for instance, the introduction of the ICF/MR or the use of the RUG-based PPS for SNFs.[41] Looking ahead to the future and the expense and complexity of programs for those with various categories of disability, it would seem even more important to test in advance, with well-designed projects, real-time experience, and careful evaluation. This is not to argue that Sec. 1115 waivers should be used only for their original purpose, rather that there is a serious need for a variant or category of the Sec. 1115 waiver that would be rededicated to the traditional R&D mission and used—with in-house expertise and strong outside involvement—for the testing and evaluation of such options.

As for the Sec. 1115 "superwaivers," most of them have dealt with the adult and SCHIP populations, not the dual eligibles or disabled. Only one, the Mississippi PLAD initiative, has sought specifically to cut back on the dual eligibles. And some states, most notably, Florida and Massachusetts, have used Sec. 1115 waivers to develop experiments of great national interest. Yet these superwaivers have also been used by both the Clinton and Bush administrations in ways that seem legislative in nature and amount to a restructuring of Medicaid, state by state, without benefit of public debate or legislative authorization.

Congress has done little with respect to these superwaivers in part because of uncertainty about the nature and gravity of the problem and lack of a suitable procedure for intervention.[42] One way of increasing both the transparency and the visibility of the waiver process that has been advocated and should have strong bipartisan support would to require a notice and comment procedure at the national level as it already is for the states. Another would be for Congress to establish a specific oversight responsibility combined with reporting requirements.[43] To be sure, such procedures will further complicate the waiver process. In considerable measure, though, that is what procedures are for—they complicate a process in order to provide assurances that it is legal, constitutional, and trustworthy.

The need for monitoring leads to a recommendation for a Medicaid advisory commission similar to the existing Medicare Payment Advisory

Commission (MedPAC),[44] that could oversee developments within the federal and state Medicaid programs and provide ongoing summaries, data, and policy options for action by the Congress.[45] It would be essential that such a commission have credibility with both Democrats and Republicans. Such a commission must have the capability to discern trends within the Medicaid program and to formulate policy options for the Congress. Such a body could, for instance, track the impact and state responses to a recession or rising prescription drug costs; the effects of managed care on the status of the safety-net providers or clientele;[46] or "crowd-out" occasioned by premium assistance plans. It could review and comment upon controversial waivers and/or proposals for restructuring benefits as well as technical payment mechanisms such as performance based purchasing. If its work is well done, it would help bridge the partisan gulf within Congress and provide the House and Senate with alternatives to the administration's versions of reality.

One area where some neutral competence might be helpful is in revising the FMAP formula, a project that is vital and not without difficulty. It is essential because of the mounting pressure upon state budgets and state Medicaid programs, especially in times of economic recession. And it is difficult because of politics and because it has parts that move at varying rates and affect fifty different states plus the territories.

One major element should be a counter-cyclical adjuster big enough and responsive in a way that moderates the so-called Medicaid "boom and bust" cycle.[47] The other part of the problem is the variables to be considered in calculating the FMAP—other than the inverse of per capita income—such as a medical CPI, rising drug costs, numbers of unemployed or uninsured, dual eligibles, undocumented immigrants, and so forth. These are matters that Congress will ultimately have to decide, but when the time comes, such a commission could be vitally important in collecting and evaluating the data, framing the alternatives, and monitoring and updating the formula.

A Medicaid commission could also be helpful in dealing with the long-festering problems of DSH, UPLs, and other forms of "Medicaid maximization." Measures that increase Medicaid enrollment and coverage or reduce the numbers of uninsured will reduce the need for such subsidies; but recalling their origins, and the continuing gaps in coverage and numbers of the uninsured and no-pay patients, it is doubtful that the need for subsidies and safety-net providers will disappear, at least not immediately. And a Medicaid commission could assess that need specifically and help target funds more accurately.

Two long-standing historical trends should receive consideration in planning for the future. One is the steady move away from categorical eligibility; and the other, the continuing shift toward community-based and "consumer" oriented modalities of care. Each presents important opportunities along with matters for concern.

There has already been important progress toward a non-categorical eligibility: covering children, non-pregnant mothers and other family members, SSI recipients and persons transitioning from TANF, to mention the most numerous groups. Today, many advocacy groups propose the adoption of the federal poverty level as a non-categorical eligibility based upon economic need. Such a step would especially cover in families and single adults, the most numerous of those presently excluded. It would also greatly simplify Medicaid application, remove some of the stigma and indignity, and reduce class and racial disparities.

This step would be a large one for many states,[48] and a source of discord between them and the federal government if it took the form of an immediate mandate. A reasonable compromise, recommended by a NASHP workshop would be a requirement—phased in over four years—that states fully cover all individuals with incomes up to 100% of the FPL, but allow the states to use their own methods of counting income.[49] A variant would be a proposal by the National Governors' Association that individual states have the option of adopting the FPL as a standard, with encouragement to do so. Either way, an important point is that such a standard would become a goal to be sought nationally.

Much has already been said about waivers, devolution, de-institutionalization, community-based services, and consumer initiatives. It is also important to be aware that Medicaid has been substantially transformed by such developments and in ways not likely to be reversed. Some "marginal centralization" may be needed; but our semi-sovereign states are hard to coerce; and community-based health care has to succeed most of all at the local level. Therefore, these devolutionist and privatizing tendencies should not be seen as a call to "take back the night," but as an opportunity to move federal-state relations in a new direction: one that puts less emphasis upon mandates and regulations and more or less intrusive influences or incentives, such as data collection and publication, quality assessment and improvement, changing reimbursement formulas, prudent purchasing, and federal-state and public-private collaboration in adapting techniques and developing and implementing service delivery models.

This approach to federal-state relations has antecedents that suggest it might have wide appeal. A major objective of the vetoed Medicaid Transformation Act of 1995—which later became the model for SCHIP—was to shift the emphasis from federal mandates and regulations to more internalized influences such as quality improvement programs and growing competence and professionalism within state programs. It would also facilitate or, at least, not get in the way of adapting and implementing various techniques for cost containment and quality improvement such as redesigning the process of treatment or care, collection and use of outcome evaluation data and "buy right" or prudent purchasing techniques especially useful, for example, in complex and costly cases involving long-term care for the chronically ill and disabled.[50] Viewed this way, long-term and extensive devolution opens opportunities to move in this direction. It also makes creative adaptation essential.

Racial disparities as an issue can be used to provide illustrations of how a more traditional approach of mandates and standards might be combined with a new emphasis upon quality improvement and the communication of information. It illustrates ways in which different approaches can supplement each other to meliorate a potentially intractable and politically explosive issue with a minimum of direct regulation or intrusiveness.

One part, involving a bit of marginal centralization would be some culturally sensitive amendments to the enrollment procedures and access standards that remove barriers but do not affect medical practice directly. These could be supplemented by collection and dissemination of data on racial disparities as part of auditing the quality of care as well as working collaboratively with private plans to devise methods for reducing such disparities. A next step might be to release performance standards, share data and experience, and encourage states to consider such information in their purchasing activities.[51] There are formidable obstacles confronting this approach, not the least of which would be generating and standardizing the data, but it would be minimally regulative, rest lightly upon the states, and could hardly be less effective than the existing approaches.

The Deficit Reduction Act of 2005 (chapter 6) included authorizations for a number of demonstration grants that are especially important as a bipartisan acknowledgment of the need for a concerted and monitored R&D effort. They also lay some important foundations upon which to build. Most of these proposals came from the Senate bill and passed largely intact, including two major demonstration projects: one for the development of community-based alternatives to psychiatric residential treatment for children (Sec. 6063) and the other a "Money Follows the Person Rebalancing Act" (Sec. 6071) to test the value of the MFP approach for increasing the use of home and community-based services as an alternative to long-term institutional care.

These two demonstration projects had strong evaluation components with state-by-state comparisons mandated for the MFP demonstrations and funding for the costs of evaluation and report preparation The MFP project would also pay for oversight and technical assistance to upgrade quality, disseminate information about promising practices, provide guidance on design or trouble-shoot projects in process (Sec. 6071(f)). Apart from the substantive merits of these initiatives, they are significant because they may indicate increased involvement by the Congress in the design and development of home and community-based service delivery as well as a disposition to cover additional administrative costs.

These efforts are far from a comprehensive design that would, for example, provide a template for one of the "big categories" such as mental health or the physically disabled. They deal more with the parts or elements of such a design. And the partial nature of these efforts makes a strong case for a Medicaid commission that could provide independent monitoring and keep Congress informed about related and systemic developments and alert to impending trouble. But these particular initiatives seem well planned and crafted to provide a basis for future program development.

In moving toward designs that could be brought to scale, a next step might be to extend the Sec. 6063 demonstration beyond children to programs for adults with mental or developmental disabilities who—at their age—have deep needs for "a job, a home, and a date on Saturday night." Grants could be combined with waivers and awarded competitively,[52] with an emphasis upon such criteria as quality improvement, cost-effectiveness, and wide applicability. This approach would squarely address a difficult problem and could be valuable in learning what works and what does not at a local level and in real time. For this reason, the implementation and evaluation of such projects would be especially important along with resources for adequate reporting and, as needed, technical assistance and concurrent involvement of federal officials.

Nursing homes remain a huge, unresolved mare's nest of problems. The issue is unresolved because of the absence of a successor to an ailing institution, misaligned financial incentives, and lack of alternative placements and community infrastructure. The problem is huge in terms of aggregate expenditures: $115 billion in 2004, 45% of which was contributed by Medicaid, representing 22% of the total federal-state Medicaid budget.[53] Beyond that, the population as a whole is aging, "baby boomers" are retiring in increasing numbers, and the percentage increase of those over 85 years of age—the "old old"—is more than any other age cohort.

Much in the way of resources or statutory authority needed to address the nursing home issues lies beyond the normal reach of the Medicaid program or even of the DHHS. But past experience may be useful in suggesting some principles and specific, largely incremental, modifications that may have promise as a beginning or as pointers.

Following a theme already developed, nursing homes for the aging is another area where Medicaid beneficiaries might like to have alternatives such as a home, a job (or meaningful activity) and even a "date" (or socializing) on Saturday night. Because often frail and missing some ADLs, nursing home occupants are not usually regarded as good candidates for deinstitutionalization, but diversion from nursing home placement is an important option. Furthermore, many nursing home placements are short-term, especially if there is a workable—preferably attractive—alternative at home or in the local community. Therefore, it would seem reasonable to set, or reaffirm, a goal of restricting nursing home placements to the frailest and upgrading the quality of the remaining nursing home beds[54] and HCB services, enabling most aged Medicaid recipients to live in a community setting for as long as they can and chose to do.[55]

A major obstacle to such an agenda is the historic burden of the past: a persistent encouragement of nursing homes by federal fiscal policies and a failure to develop cost-effective alternatives or an infrastructure that would support living at home. Several measures might substantially improve this situation both for the elderly beneficiary and for the Medicaid program itself.

A good place to begin would be incremental changes that eliminate some of the provisions or dispensations that encourage over-utilization of nursing facilities as compared with home and community-based alternatives: for instance, tightening eligibility for nursing home admissions and making it easier for states to manage HCB services or systems.[56] A related measure would be to offer an enhanced match, similar to that for SCHIP for innovations that would systematically improve HCB programs and relate them effectively to institutional care.[57] An initiative of this sort might provide, as well, an opportunity to coordinate care and control the well-documented tendency of HCB services, in the aggregate, to cost more than nursing home placements.

Long-term care insurance, especially of the sort that includes coverage for community-based services, would not only reduce public expenditures but could enable more people to continue living in their own homes or local communities. To turn this option into a robust prospect would require actuarial computations, program design, and tax legislation; but a minor Medicaid change that made appropriate insurance policies eligible for tax credits and Medicaid premium support would most likely have substantial bipartisan support.

The importance of supportive programs and infrastructure has been recognized in a small way by such initiatives as the National Family Caregiver Program of the Administration on Aging and the System Change Grants for Community Living administered by CMS. It remains to be seen how effective such grants will be. Meanwhile, the Medicaid program already has a large role in this effort through its access to and support of the safety-net providers, who are likely to be yet more essential in a system of care without walls. That reflection prompts a further observation that the need for federal-state collaboration, leadership, and strong incentives in developing infrastructure and coordinating efforts strengthens the case for a Medicaid agency with increased resources and presence.

With all of this said, nursing homes are a case in which a new model or successor institution would be desirable but a residual need for nursing homes is likely to remain and we do not yet know how well alternative placements or community-based services will serve. It is worth noting, furthermore, that various modifications, such as the ICF, SNFs, and assisted living did not work out as expected. Therefore, this would seem to be an area for moving incrementally and feeling the ground ahead as we proceed.

A different set of problems is presented by those with severe and chronic illnesses and conditions, other than mental illness or mental retardation. Among these diseases, some of the most prevalent and/or costly are Alzheimer's, asthma, cancer, diabetes, emphysema, heart disease, HIV/AIDS, spinal cord injury, and stroke. Unlike mental illness or retardation, or the frail elderly, the concern is not so much maintenance in the community or an alternate placement, but the high cost of treatment, especially over time.

Most of these diseases or conditions share characteristics that help in devising a strategy for coping with them. They are chronic or persistent which typically implies that they require frequent professional intervention to palliate or prevent them from getting worse. They are often accompanied by secondary complications, such as bedsores or pneumonia, that call for preventive measures or early intervention to avoid deterioration of the patient or a medical crisis.[58] Treatment of such diseases or conditions is costly, so that strategies that are effective in changing the behavior either of the patient or the provider can save large sums of money and justify extensive reorganization of care or investment in sophisticated technology such as electronic medical records, continuous quality improvement, and disease management. The hope or promise of such an approach is that it could be a win-win situation: that improving communication, educating the patient and the health care provider, reducing errors, early intervention and preventive care, choosing the best sites of care, clinical paths, and medically appropriate procedures and medication would both improve medical care and save money.

Disease management is useful as a concept to sharpen the limitations of some of the approaches currently popular. For example, most managed care plans do little to change medical practice. Rather, they "impose a management overlay on top of the existing service system,"[59] mostly intended to cut back on services not produce better care. Even those managed care plans that purport to be part of the next generation of managed care—replacing utilization management with case management and disease management—have relied mostly on changing patient behavior rather than that of the providers.[60]

Possibly, disease management or movement in that direction could become the service delivery model of choice for those in priority categories of chronic diseases and conditions. One lesson from Medicaid experience, though, is that service delivery models seldom work in broader application the way they do in demonstrations or as developed by talented and dedicated pioneers. For instance, one study of efforts to integrate managed care and disease management revealed that disease management was often outsourced by HMOs and done episodically by contract, with financial control, data, and most of the care remaining with the parent HMO, so that much of what passed for disease management was largely soft-ware gadgetry rather than service delivery modification or even effective management.[61]

Another lesson from Medicaid history is that we are always where we are—that is, dealing with existing institutions, relationships, and vested interests. And as the chief medical officer of a managed care network pointed out, disease management rightly done would involve an enormous amount of change and displacement of professional personnel. In his opinion, his network, Health Partners, could save more money and improve care in the short-run by doing a better job with the management tools they already had.[62]

At this juncture, ways of melding both approaches are needed. Disease management can be important for moving beyond the traditional Medicaid managed care model. But managed care is here, now, and is important for integrating care, saving money, providing a medical home (of sorts), and an organizational framework that enables Medicaid officials to plan for the future and enforce a broad accountability. In this area of chronic illness and physical disabilities there is also a need for system design that can be brought to scale. Some multiple grants, combined with waivers, might be a good place to start. Steps toward building an infrastructure are already being taken, such as experimentation with quality improvement data, electronic medical records, and performance based purchasing. In several states, experiments with melding disease management and managed care are pursuing a variety of different approaches and accumulating experience. It is a large assignment that cannot be done overnight.

Assuming that the Medicaid program survives the present fiscal and political crisis, the major challenges confronting the Medicaid program will be to help provide some effective leadership in the development of service delivery options for the disabled and chronically ill; broaden coverage for the working poor in ways that are fair, workable, and politically acceptable; improve quality of care and reduce disparities; maintain fiscal integrity; and devise and implement methods of cost containment consistent with high quality and more than minimally tolerable for providers as well as beneficiaries.

This agenda will require sizeable long-term commitments of resources and effort. It requires thinking about old problems in new ways, so that both innovation and adaptability are important: developing new tools and methods and suiting them to existing, local Medicaid programs. This agenda will also need a fair hearing in Washington and increased collaboration between the federal, state, and local governments.

The DRA of 2005 was a significant precedent because of the importance assigned to Medicaid R&D and for the authorization of funds to pay for added administrative responsibilities, such as program evaluation and technical assistance for agency leadership and to strengthen federal-state collaboration. A related development worth noting was the Senate version of the fraud and abuse provisions (ch. 3, esp. Sec. 6034) which put special emphasis upon information and education, more effective oversight, comprehensive planning and review, and the establishment of a "Medicaid Integrity Program," with "significant" increases in full-time equivalent staff dedicated to this activity.

A similar kind of approach might be adopted for quality improvement and R&D, not necessarily to separate Medicaid from Medicare in these endeavors but to recognize the importance of Medicaid activities, to given them greater visibility, and the kind of staffing and administrative presence needed to collaborate more effectively with the states in their development efforts and to represent Medicaid's interests effectively in working with other agencies, before the Congress, and with the advocacy community.

One of the greatest obstacles to improving the Medicaid program is political partisanship that, especially since 1994, has led to a partisan mobilization and grid-lock that has made sensible compromise or needed modifications difficult if not impossible. Some of the proposals already mentioned—such as a Medicaid commission or combining Medicaid and premium support—are initiatives that need bipartisan support and could, in turn, help moderate partisan conflict over a longer term. The pursuit of quality improvement as a common goal would tend to put a damper on partisanship as would the activities of a Medicaid commission. Congress could aid immensely in this effort, by its response to such a commission, by creating or supporting opportunities for bipartisan legislation, collaborating on oversight or investigations, and by promoting staff cooperation at the committee and sub-committee levels.

Historically, Medicaid has often been protected from partisan assaults because of its layered complexity, which baffled and impeded those who would tamper with the program but also made needed change difficult. A new kind of infrastructure, with less emphasis upon regulations and mandates and more upon steady quality improvement, new and imaginative methods of cost containment, and developing win-win situations would not only be a source of pride, both for the individual states and the nation, but could generate a strong interest in preserving this infrastructure and utilizing it with competence and awareness.

In thinking about such a future, one available resource is the varied and large community of those who make a life work or vocation of Medicaid: the Medicaid directors, public officials at the national and state levels, policy and legal experts, legislative staffs, advocates and providers. These Medicaid "lifers" are repositories of institutional memory, strengthen policy considerations, and add some elements of a career service, with a long-term commitment to the best interests of the Medicaid program and those it serves. Our book is dedicated, with respect and affection, to this worthy company.

Notes

1.   The philosopher was George Santayana (1863-1952). Among the many historians who have expressed that thought are John Toland, Sir George Trevelyan, and Gordon Wood. Also, Winston Churchill and G. F. W. Hegel. With thanks to Prof. Timothy J. Burke.

2.   Illustrations would be The National Health Insurance Partnership (NHIP) proposed by the Nixon administration or Sen. John Kerry's presidential campaign proposal of 2004.

3.   Cf. *Making Medicaid Work for the 21st Century*, Report prepared for the National Academy for State Health Policy by Vernon Smith, Neva Kaye, Debbie Chang, Jennie Bonney, Charles Mulligan, Dann Milne, Robert Mollica, and Cynthia Shirk, December, 2004.

4.   The average was high, but there were peaks and valleys with years under 10% or over 30%, for instances, during the early years of the Reagan and Clinton administrations. One of the lowest growth rates was between 1995 and 1999, in part because of SCHIP but also a response to a high level of prosperity. Another historic low was the period from 2003 to the present, largely because of recession and fiscal stringency. Cf. Alan Weil, "There's Something About Medicaid," *Health Affairs,* Vol. 22(1) 2003, 13-30 at 14. And Leighton Ku, *The Slowdown in Medicaid Expenditure Growth*, Washington, D.C.: Center on Budget and Policy Priorities, Mar. 16, 2006, 1.

5.   Vernon Smith *et al., Making Medicaid Work,* 15.

6.   The original statute pointedly excluded mental institutions for adults, with the exception of beneficiaries 65 years of age or older. The Social Security Amendments of 1972 allowed optional coverage for persons 21 years of age and below in psychiatric hospitals. The mentally ill could also be treated in institutions not specializing in mental health care, such as nursing homes. SSI recipients, who were eligible for Medicaid, could receive psychiatric services in acute care hospitals. And a number of states used their DSH funds to support long-term care in mental hospitals. Over time, and despite the initial "freeze out," Medicaid became the largest source of public funding for mental health services: an example of the program's adaptability. HIV/AIDS would be another striking example. *Ibid.,* 22; also *Medicaid Source Book,* 915 ff.

7.   Cf. Bruce Vladeck, "Where the Action Really Is: Medicaid and the Disabled," *Health Affairs,* Vol. 22(1) 2003, 90-100.

8.   Jeanne Lambrew, *The State Children's Health Insurance Program: Past, Present, and Future,* Washington, D.C.: National Health Policy Forum, July, 2006, 3, 4.

9.   According to one study, at least 15 states have premium assistance programs, about 25 states are considering expanding coverage through employer mandates, and 13 are pondering some form of universal health insurance coverage. Cynthia Shirk and Jennifer Ryan, *Premium Assistance in Medicaid and SCHIP: Ace in the Hole or House of Cards?* Washington, D.C., National Health Policy Forum, July 2006, 2.

10.   Health Insurance Premium Programs, first authorized in OBRA 1990, with amendments in BBA 1997.

11.   John Holahan, Teresa Coughlin, Leighton Ku, David Heslam, and Colin Winterbottom, "Understanding the Recent Growth in Medicaid Spending," in Rowland, Judith Feder, and Alina Salganicoff (eds.) *Medicaid Financing Crisis,* 28-34.

12.   74% for singles; 82% for couples. Schneider, *The Medicaid Resource Book*, 30-31.

13.   *Ibid.,* p. 10.

14.   Children and the disabled (with higher levels mandated) bring the average up to 67%. But only 17 states cover adult populations up to the FPL. Cf. Donna Cohen Ross and Laura Cox, *In a Time of Growing Need: State Choices Influence Health Coverage Access for Children and Families,* Washington, D.C.: Kaiser Family Foundation, Oct. 2005, 17.

15.   John Holahan, "Variation in Health Insurance Coverage and Medical Expenditures: How much is Too Much," in John Holahan, Alan Weil, and Joshua M. Wiener, *Federalism and Health Policy.* Washington, D.C.: Urban Institute Press, 2003, 111-143 at 129, 132-133.

16.   The distinction between treatment and outcomes is important. The 1999 report of the U.S. Commission on Civil Rights, for instance, emphasizes health *outcomes*, i.e., what measurable effects disparities have on health, while the Institute of Medicine Report of 2002 emphasizes health care *treatment* such as differences in access or care given. The first tends to trail off into abstruse issues of measuring effects, while the latter gets into specific barriers to access and discrimination in treatment. Cf., U. S. Commission on Civil Rights, *The Health Care Challenge: Acknowledging Disparities, Confronting Discrimination, and Ensuring Equality.* Washington, D.C.: Commission on Civil Rights, 1999, and Brian D. Smedley, Adrienne Y. Stith, and Alan R. Nelson (eds.) *Unequal Treatment: Confronting Racial and Ethnic Disparities in Health Care.* Washington, DC: National Academies Press, 2003; also, Deborah Stone, "Reframing the Racial Disparities Issue for State Governments," *Journal of Health Politics, Policy, and Law*, 127-152.

17.   Affecting not just refusal to admit to health care institutions, but discrimination in enrollment, geographical and linguistic barriers to access, discrimination in treatment prescribed and in clinical encounters, lack of referral options, ineffective appeals procedures, and so forth.

18.   Cf. *Report of the Secretary's Task Force on Black and Minority Health.* Washington, D.C.: Government Printing Office, 1985. Discussion of the relation between social class and racial or ethnic disparities and health status goes back much farther. One author cites Friedrich Engels, *The Condition of the Working Class in England* (1845); another W.E.B. DuBois, *The Health and Physique of the Negro American* (1906). Some also cite the famous "Black Report" of the British Department of Health and Social Services of 1980. (*Inequality in Health: Report of a Research Working Group*) These citations remind that the topic is broad and historic, but American public engagement with the issue of health disparities has been limited and mostly related to the civil rights struggles.

19.   Bruce Vladeck, "Where the Action Really Is: Medicaid and the Disabled," *Health Affairs, loc. cit.,* at p. 99.

20.   Sec. 1902(a)(10)(B)(15).

21.   For a succinct discussion of the background, see Richard Hegner, *Dual Eligibility for Medicaid and Medicare: Options for Creating a Continuum of Care.* Washington, D.C.: National Health Policy Forum, May 1997.

22.   Cf. *Crossing the Quality Chasm* (Washington, D.C.: National Academy Press, 2001); and Douglas Waller, "How VA Hospitals Became the Best," *Time,* September 4, 2006, 36-37.

23.   For details, see Allen Schick, *The Federal Budget: Politics, Policy, and Process,* Rev. Ed. Washington, D.C.: Brookings Institution, 2000, 291 ff. The authors are also indebted to Andy Schneider for clarification of some aspects. Smith, telephone interview, October 15, 2002.

24.   Jost, *Disentitlement?,* 23.

25.   Cf. this definition of an entitlement: "A program that imposes a legal obligation on the federal government to any person, business, or unit of government that meets the criteria set in law." Schneider, *The Medicaid Resource Book,* 167.

26.   We are indebted to Andy Schneider for this argument. Examples that illustrate this thesis would be health care providers working in safety-net institutions, not-for-profit MCOs, and many of the "lifers" who make a career of Medicaid administration or advocacy.

27.   Thomas Hoyer, an experienced and thoughtful HCFA regulator (now retired), dismayed at the complexity and dubious merit of much of the Medicaid regulative corpus, expressed the heretical view that a block grant might be desirable if it did little more than clear out the accumulated jumble and make possible some fresh starts. Telephone interview by Smith, July 12, 2006.

28.   Sec. 1902(a)(10)(A)(i).

29.   One might compare "quality adjusted life years" (QALYs), but this approach imports a utilitarian bias and tends to assume what was to be proven, so that the less needy would automatically win.

30.   Cf. T. D. Weldon, *The Vocabulary of Politics.* Baltimore, MD: Penguin Books, 1953, p. 76 for his distinction between "Puzzles, Problems, and Difficulties." As he argues, problems have solutions. But "we do not solve [difficulties], we surmount them, reduce them, avoid them, or ignore them."

31.   The Trade Act of 2002 (P.L. 107-210) provided for tax credits for health insurance and support services for workers displaced by foreign trade. In 2003, Sen. Grassley and Sen. Baucus, the Finance chairman and ranking Democrat, both endorsed this approach as a way of covering the working poor. A similar proposal figured in Bush administration's health proposals for the next three years, though with increasing emphasis upon Health Savings Accounts rather than Medicaid.

32.   For additional exposition and details of such a plan, see Etheredge and Moore, "A New Medicaid Program," 432-434.

33.   Premium assistance has been slow to develop because of such factors as administrative complexity, the ERISA exemption, lack of experience or reluctance of employers or state officials, and worker preference for SCHIP. But the prospect of a strong, federally supported tax credit might change that. Cf. Shirk and J Ryan, *Premium Assistance,* 3.

34.   However attractive this option might seem, a few cautionary observations may lead toward a more realistic perspective. President Bush's tax credit proposal was, initially, for $70 billion over ten years with no mention of HSAs as a preferred option. Later, the amount for Medicaid tax credits was reduced by two-thirds

while allocations for HSAs were increased four-fold. Also significant was the qualified support given by the National Governors' Association, which endorsed the tax credit proposal, but took the opportunity to say that such options "should not come at the expense of Medicaid funding." Whether either side—partisans of Medicaid or of HSAs—can collaborate in seeking common ground and resist the temptation to hijack this issue remains to be seen. Cf. *Medicaid Reform—A Preliminary Report from the National Governors' Association.* Washington, D.C.: National Governors' Association, June 2005, 9.

35.   Especially with the linking of SSI with Medicaid and the expansion of dual eligibility with the MCCA. Cf. Vladeck, "Where the Action Really Is, 91.

36.   NGA, *Medicaid Reform—A Preliminary Report,* 2, 3.

37.   Those already mentioned but also managed care, managed behavioral health care, and comprehensive disease management.

38.   Medicaid Community Attendant Services and Support Act.

39.   Frank S. Thompson and Courtney Burke, "The Promise and Peril of Executive Federalism: The Case of Medicaid Demonstration Waivers," paper prepared for APSA annual meeting in Washington, DC, 2006.

40.   The ICF/MR was an add-on to the ICF that grew beyond expectations and proved to be quite expensive. Use of RUGs for the SNF prospective payment system had the untoward result of diverting patients from nursing homes but also promoting another expensive alternative, the assisted living facility. Cf. David Barton Smith, *Reinventing Care: Assisted Living in New York City* (Nashville, Tenn.: Vanderbilt University Press, 2003), esp. ch. 3.

41.   Individual members or state delegations within Congress often intervene on behalf of their individual states, though mostly to advocate for their state or some interest within it. Committee chairmen have also requested GAO investigations which take years and tend to produced narrow, specific results: for instance, a multi-year series of investigations led, ultimately to a prohibition in the DRA against using unspent SCHIP funds to insure childless adults. This limited result took years and, of course, dealt with the abuses long after their onset.

42.   How to proceed in this matter is far from obvious. "Separation of powers" cuts both ways: the administration ought not to legislate; but neither should Congress execute or administer. In other words, legal complexities are involved, and various types of intervention, such as a "legislative veto" or "come into agreement" provisions might be unconstitutional. Nevertheless, assigning a specific oversight responsibility to the congressional oversight committees or a commission similar to ProPAC, PPRC, or MedPAC with reporting requirements by "the Secretary" would send a strong message to the administration.

43.   Another model would be the Advisory Commission on Intergovernmental Relations (ACIR) which included representation of the governors. Our view is that such a model would lead to politicizing and eventual schism. Also, the governors are already represented, perhaps too well, by the National Governors' Association.

44.   A step strongly advocated by Bruce Vladeck, to whom we are indebted.

45.   Cf. Marion Ein Lewin and Stewart Altman (eds.) *America's Health Care Safety Net.* Washington, D.C.: National Academy Press, 2000; Michael Perry and Neal Robertson, *Individual with Disabilities and their Experience with Managed Care: Results from Focus Group Research.* Washington, D.C.: Kaiser Commission on Medicaid and the Uninsured, 1999.

46.   A term employed by James Tallon among others. There is an element of perversity in the way the current FMAP is calculated. Use of the (inverse of) per capita income does help to reduce the fiscal disparity among the states. But the FMAP

formula tends to lag behind the current economic situation in a particular state. A state in recession in 2006 may have a low current FMAP because it is based on data three or more years before a time that state was more prosperous and when it might have expanded its Medicaid program. Today, it may cut back, have a relatively generous FMAP several years later and then expand once again to make up for lost ground. Smith *et. al, Making Medicaid Work,* 42-43.

47. Currently, only 17 states are above the FPL. Moreover, the SSI standard is only 74% of the FPL.

48. Smith, *et al., Making Medicaid Work,* 12-13.

49. Cf. *Crossing the Quality Chasm: A New Health System for the 21st Century.* Washington, D.C.: National Academy Press, 2001. This work deals with quality improvement generally, and not with Medicaid, but many of the approaches discussed, such as disease management, could be adapted for Medicaid.

50. Nicole Lurie, Minna Jung, and Risa Lavizzo-Mourey, "Disparities and Quality Improvement: Federal Policy Levers," *Health Affairs* Vol. 24(2)2005, 354-364.

51. Initial grants could be competitive, though federal interest in such demonstrations and the potential usefulness of technical assistance and dissemination of information would seem to call for some federal-state collaboration thereafter.

52. Cynthia Smith, Cathy Cowan, Stephen Heffler, Aaron Calin, and the National Health Accounts Team, "National Health Spending in 2004: Recent Slowdown Led by Prescription Drug Spending," *Health Affairs,* Vol. 25(1)2006, 186-196 at p. 191.

53. The point being that nursing home admissions and censuses might be tilted toward the sicker or more disabled Medicaid beneficiaries. Nursing homes would need to upgrade their medical and caring capabilities, but in turn would be entitled to a case-mix adjuster that took account of the increased severity of cases.

54. Problems such as the "woodwork" effect and loss of economies associated with institutional placement might be partly offset by the higher intensity of the nursing home census, which would increase the relative advantage of community-based placement.

55. States could tighten the income and asset tests for nursing homes. Another measure would be to screen nursing home applicants or residents to assure the appropriateness of placement in a nursing home. States impose limits on new beds—a variant of which is to allow nursing homes to "layaway" beds: shut down beds but "bank" the credit for future use. States could also set different income and eligibility standards for nursing homes and HCB services or programs which would allow them greater freedom to vary services for the HCB services. Steps already taken by the DRA of 2005 with respect to HCBS was to eliminate the requirement of a waiver (making them subject only to a plan amendment) and allow states more freedom to target special groups or limit enrollments. Cf. Smith, *et al., Making Medicaid Work,* 28-30; and Joshua M. Wiener and Jane Tilly, "Long-Term Care—Can the States Be the Engine of Reform," in John Holahan, Alan Weil, and Joshua M. Wiener, *Federalism and Health Policy.* Washington, D.C.: Urban Institute Press, 2003, 249-292 at 272-277.

56. Wiener makes the point that there is great variation in the coverage and quality of HCB services in different states and that an important reason for heavy utilization of nursing homes is the lack of an attractive alternative. *Ibid.,* 277-278.

57. Robert Master gives an example. He notes that 70% of hospital admissions for individuals with spinal cord injury, cerebral palsy, muscular dystrophy, multiple sclerosis, and spina bifida are for urinary tract infections, respiratory infections, or skin ulcers that could be prevented with simple prevention or early interven-

tion. A person living at home with spinal cord injury who sensed the recurrence of urinary tract infection could notify his plan that could, with rapid response, avoid the need for an expensive and unnecessary hospitalization. His example illustrates the need for patient education, effective communication, accurate assessment, rapid response, and system organization. "Medicaid Managed Care and Disabled Populations," in Stephen M. Davidson and Stephen A. Somers, (eds.), *Remaking Medicaid: Managed Care for the Public Good.* San Francisco: Jossey-Bass Publishers, 1998, pp. 100-117 at p. 102.

58.   *Ibid.,* p. 102.

59.   Cf. James Robinson, "Medical Management After Managed Care," *Health Affairs—Web Exclusives*, January-June 2004, pp. W4-269-280. In a study of several MCOs that purported to be merging managed care with medical management Robinson found that relatively little was invested in "medical management," and that, practically, nothing was done about physician behavior. Among the reasons were little expectation that greater effort would produce much and a desire not to irritate either physicians or patients. As for the patients, most of the management came down to urging them to adhere to their drug regimes and the doctors' orders. Widely known, though, is Robert Master's outstanding success with merging managed care and disease management in the Community Medical Alliance that provides primary and low-intensity inpatient care for HIV/AIDS patients.

60.   Victor A. Villagra, "Integrating Disease Management Into the Outpatient Delivery System During and After Managed Care, *Health Affairs—Web Exclusives*, January-June 2004, pp. W4-281-283 at p. 282. One danger with disease management is over-reliance on expensive and sophisticated programs or methodologies rather than commonsense organization, preventive care, and systematic and thoughtful use of existing personnel and protocols.

61.   Richard J. Baron, "Commentary—A Provider's View," in Davidson and Somers, *Remaking Medicaid,* 118-123, at 120-121.

10

Postscript

The months following the election of 2006 would seem an opportune time for some bipartisan efforts to reform Medicaid and to find ways of covering more of the uninsured. Democrats had retaken the Congress and gained six governorships and control of a number of state legislative assemblies. According to the National Governors' Association, 25 to 30 states were proceeding with or contemplating Medicaid/SCHIP expansions to cover the uninsured, some of them pointing toward universal coverage. And both parties needed accomplishments: Republicans to show a concern over domestic issues other than tax reduction and Democrats to demonstrate a capacity to govern.

Despite favorable auspices, significant Medicaid initiatives seemed likely to be shoved aside or stalled out—quite possibly until after 2008—because of supervening priorities or behavior of a familiar and perennial sort: larger objectives such as tax legislation or campaigning for NHI, mobilizing for the next election, partisanship and ideological differences.

The national election of 2006 was largely about the war in Iraq,[1] producing no special mandate for any domestic policy. Even though Democrats won control of both houses, their majorities were small: 51-49 in the Senate,[2] and 233 to 202 in the House—not large enough to pass any big, controversial legislation, especially with a Republican president in power—and their majorities could be easily lost with a few blunders. Several leading Democrats were already running for president, distracting attention and resources from the domestic policy agenda. Republicans needed to find a way out of the Iraq morass. But with respect to domestic policy they might do best to let the Democrats flounder with a difficult situation and, for their part, pick and choose message and policy options that played to Republican advantage.

Like the Republicans in 1994, Democrats in January of 2007 "hit the ground running," though with a "100-hour" flurry rather than a 100-day campaign. Bills were introduced that dealt with implementation of the September 11th commission recommendations; increasing the minimum wage from $5.15 per hour to $7.25; lifting the ban on funding of stem-cell research; allowing the federal government to negotiate lower prices on prescription drugs for Medicare beneficiaries; reducing interest rates on student loans; and using some of the royalties from offshore oil and gas leases to encourage alternate energy sources.[3]

The items on the 100-hour list had all been part of the campaign preceding the election. The most controversial were federal negotiation over drug prices and funding for stem-cell research. Whether enactable or not, both were good campaign issues then and for the future. Notable for their absence were any proposals related to Medicaid or expanded health coverage. For that matter, neither Medicaid nor health care were issues in the campaign.

Two measures adopted early in January by the House are important for fiscal discipline and could affect Medicaid along with other entitlement programs. One is the revival of PAYGO ("pay-as-you go") rules by the House that require expenditures or tax reductions that would increase the deficit to be offset by expenditure reductions or tax increases—a restraint that exerted a downward pressure on Medicare and Medicaid expenditures when it was in force from 1990 to 2002. Another provision—also a campaign item—requires earmarks to be identified as such, their sponsors named, and certifications made that neither the sponsors nor their spouses benefit from them. The Senate version added that sponsors must be disclosed at least 48 hours before Senate consideration. These provisions, which apply to spending, authorizing, or tax legislation, could curb expenditures and increase the transparency of procedures that have been notoriously opaque.

Several changes in committee leadership are likely to be important for Medicaid. Sen. Edward Kennedy takes over as chairman of the Health, Education, Labor and Pensions Committee, which gives him greater visibility and more power in his role as the leading Democratic champion of national health insurance, a cause that will detract some attention from Medicaid. Also important is Rep. Henry Waxman's move to the chairmanship of the House Committee on Government Reform. Known as a skillful and tenacious investigator, he is expected to direct much of his attention to contracting in Iraq, the implementation of the Deficit Reduction Act of 2005 and the Medicare pharmaceutical benefit, and Medicaid fraud and abuse, including use and misuse of waivers. He will have a large staff, with some Medicaid veterans. This shift can bring needed oversight and even exposure to some administrative activities, though it, too, could divert attention and legislative energy from Medicaid.[4]

The new Congress began with no major Medicaid issues on its agenda, but developments elsewhere soon moved Medicaid policy toward a critical juncture, with state waiver initiatives, the reauthorization of SCHIP, and the president's budget proposals for FY 2008—all three high stakes, emotionally charged issues—converging and potentially in conflict.

Distressed by budget pressures and the numbers of uninsured, a growing number of states by 2007 were responding to liberal federal waiver policies and CMS promptings by modifying their Medicaid and/or SCHIP programs, some by reducing benefits and imposing cost-sharing requirements, others by covering children above 200% of the FPL up to 300% or more and seeking ways to include parents and single adults. Some of the more venturesome states adopted goals of covering all the uninsured in poverty and a few developed schemes that would combine Medicaid and SCHIP with tax credits, premium subsidies, and mandates to achieve universal coverage. Late in 2006, the number of states considering "fundamental restructuring" of Medicaid along such lines had grown—according to report—to 25 or 30.[5]

Whether these various tendencies become a broad movement with a consensus that Medicaid in its present form is "unsustainable" and needs fundamental "restructuring" remains to be seen.[6] Also, "restructuring" is a catch-all term; and there is an important difference between making Medicaid part of a larger scheme to insure the poor and dismantling the program to cover more of the uninsured.

A major issue in covering the uninsured is money: whether it should come from diverted DSH funds, the SCHIP enhanced match, Medicare and/or Medicaid cost savings, or additional federal funds. From this perspective, the president's budget proposals were vitally important for those seeking to use Medicaid or SCHIP expansion as a way to include more of the uninsured. Governors especially hoped for a generous SCHIP reauthorization that would allow for growth beyond a bare maintenance of the program. There was also speculation among Democrats and Medicaid and SCHIP advocates that President Bush might seek some bipartisan "legacy" accomplishments in health policy. On both accounts, he disappointed them.

One proposal in the State of the Union Address in January was to make income applied to health insurance taxable, with a deduction of $7500 for an individual and $15,000 for families. According to the administration, this measure would give the self-employed and workers in small industries the same benefit available to those in large firms and would tax rich, "gold-plated" plans that increased aggregate costs by insulating individuals from the consequences of their health care decisions. Another purpose, according to Secretary Leavitt, was to help states interested in expanding coverage for the uninsured—though Sen. Debbie Stabenow (D., Mich.), a member of the Senate Finance Committee, observed that a tax credit would be much more helpful.[7] Others expressed a fear that the scheme would undermine employer-supported insurance; and Pete Stark, chairman of the Ways and Means health subcommittee, said that he "did not intend to consider the proposal," though he would be happy to meet with the president "to consider alternative ideas."[8]

The president's budget, delivered to Congress early in February, further aggrieved supporters of Medicaid and SCHIP because of the amounts allotted, the implicit shifting of burdens from the federal government to the states, and the low priority given to the states' concerns. None of these should have been surprising, since they were staples of administration policy, but this budget seemed to health care liberals like hunkering down for a protracted struggle, not seeking to "work together."

The Medicaid provisions sought $27.4 billion in savings over the next five years ($60.9 billion in ten years)--a large sum, 86% of which would come from the states. Not only was this burdensome, but some of the provisions seemed mean-spirited or counterproductive.[9] One in particular, "the Affordable Choices Initiative," has major long-term policy significance. A companion piece to the administration's capped individual tax deduction, it would encourage states to use their DSH money and other funds to pay for "basic private health insurance" for the uninsured and give legislative sanction to a CMS strategy of diverting DSH money from the safety-net providers to the purchase of *private* insurance. This would favor private insurance, such as HSAs, over state Medicaid programs and raise squarely an issue of safety-net providers and how they were to be financed.

The president's budget included a five-year reauthorization of SCHIP, but with amounts recommended and provisions that were intended to return the focus of the program to children in families with incomes below 200% of the FPL. In essence, the budget proposal would continue funding at its current baseline figure of $5 billion a year and use unexpended SCHIP funds and a global fund of $4.8 billion to compensate shortfalls in states that spent beyond their allocations. The second element was a selective reduction of the SCHIP enhanced federal match from approximately 70% back to the Medicaid matching rate for children in families above 200% of poverty or for coverage of adults or parents.

One argument for these measures is that they would move SCHIP back toward its original statutory intent.[10] They might also remove some of the incentives to choose SCHIP-related ventures over traditional Medicaid. And with 17 states over 200% of poverty and 11 states above 300% all getting an enhanced match, it seems legitimate to question how much of this burden the federal government should carry.

Nevertheless, the administration's proposal dashed expectations, could inflict much pain, and seemed procrustean. As pointed out by the Center on Budget and Policy Priorities, funding at current levels made no allowance for enrollment campaigns aimed at the nine million uninsured U.S. children already eligible for Medicaid or SCHIP. With current program levels the administration's baseline funding plus shortfall allocations would leave a $7 billion deficit over the five-year period presenting states with the unpleasant alternatives of cutting back on enrollments, taking money from other programs, or raising taxes.

Among casualties of this budget, if enacted, may be some of the innovative attempts at the state level to combine Medicaid, SCHIP funds, and tax credits to reach all the poverty level uninsured or move beyond that toward universal coverage. Most of these schemes have relied—in addition to one-time DSH conversions—upon SCHIP coverage above 200% of the FPL. The Bush budget would undermine such efforts by pegging SCHIP to its current baseline as well as eliminating the enhanced match for adults, parents, and children in families over 200% of the FPL. More venturesome states, such as Massachusetts and California, that seek to use tax credits as well as DSH and SCHIP funds to create model programs of national significance would be further discouraged by the striking omission of federal health insurance tax credits from this budget, a step backward from previous years that seems oddly at variance with the president's own offer of tax credits for insurance purchased from HSAs.[11]

Robert Pear of the *New York Times*, in describing these developments, stated that the Bush administration and the states "appear to be on a collision course."[12] Yet the states and the federal government have often appeared to be on collision courses that have been averted or reduced in momentum. And this could be similar to earlier shoving and shouting matches over Medicaid financing, with gains and losses, and a resolution of sorts.

An indication that the Bush administration might be flexible on some of these issues came shortly after the NGA's winter meeting during which great distress was expressed over the budget proposals, and especially the SCHIP budget, the numbers of uninsured, and the inadequacy of federal aid.[13] Shortly thereafter, Secretary Leavitt asked the governors to indicate more specifically what they might have in mind and indicated that a number of waivers employing tax credits to expand health insurance might be open to consideration. This outcome may indicate that the tax credit is still an option, though probably on a back burner.

A larger and more controversial issue is the reauthorization of SCHIP, which expires on September 30, 2007. It is controversial because of the stakes involved, the complexity of the issues, and the intensity of partisan sentiment. Many Democrats would like to cover all children to 300% of the FPL and all parents and single adults in poverty. They see SCHIP expansion as a way of achieving this goal and as a step toward national health insurance. Republicans object to the growing cost of the program, its creep toward a new entitlement, and its enlistment in the NHI campaign. Less visible but controversial are such issues as allocation and reallocation formulas, limits on family coverage, prevention of "crowd-out," changes in benchmark requirements, and mandates or other protections for the beneficiaries. Another complicating factor is the renewal of PAYGO, which will require offsets for increases in the SCHIP authorization. Finally, the presidential campaign has already begun and child health is a hot issue.[14]

How hot this issue could become is illustrated by the introduction of a bill, jointly sponsored by John Dingell, chairman of the House Energy and Commerce Committee, and Sen. Hillary Rodham Clinton (D., NY), a presidential aspirant. This bill, which would triple spending on SCHIP over the next five years and increase health spending by $50 billion or more, would cover children up to four times the FPL and allow parents, employers, and small businesses to buy into the program. Sen. Clinton described the bill as a step toward universal coverage.[15]

As House and Senate Democrats began drafting their budget resolutions, they said they would not accept President Bush's cuts in health care and education, adding that they would keep taxes low and eliminate the deficit by 2012. On the revenue side, they proposed to freeze the alternate minimum tax for two years—an estimated cost of $200 billion. To pay for these items they would add "tax reforms" such as rolling back some of President Bush's tax cuts, reducing tax shelters and collecting on unreported income, and eliminating tax breaks for oil companies and other corporations.[16]

These early moves were the preliminaries to actual budgeting, though they raised a serious question of how such indulgence could be paid for—especially with the renewal of PAYGO—short of laying on a full-scale budget reconciliation. With its action-forcing and coordinating procedures and immunity from a Senate filibuster, a reconciliation can deal with big and politically charged issues as well as minute and intricate ones. It would be a good vehicle for aligning expenditures and revenues as well as for incremental changes in Medicare and Medicaid and aligning subsidies and tax benefits with Medicaid and SCHIP policies.

The other side of a major reconciliation, though, is that it takes enormous collective effort, puts many eggs in one basket, stresses majority unity, and can be delayed, stall out, or face a presidential veto. There is reason enough for Democratic reluctance to go this way at present, even though a major reconciliation may be necessary in the future. Past experience indicates that a reconciliation can force agreement on some tax and spending numbers, but seldom resolves underlying differences.

Much of the action in the immediate future is likely to center on SCHIP renewal and positioning with respect to NHI, both of which are important for the future of Medicaid but divert attention from it now. That may not be bad: a lull in the political warfare over the Medicaid entitlement could be a time for taking stock, making small repairs, planning for the future, and bipartisan collaboration on peaceful steps to reform the program.

Notes

1. Other domestic issues that figured to a lesser extent were immigration reform and the federal government's response to the Katrina hurricane disaster. Some of the "values" issues such as gay marriage and abortion had less effect than in the previous elections.
2. Even before the new Congress assembled, Sen. Tim Johnson's possible death or long-term disability because of a brain hemorrhage underscored the tenuous nature of the Democrat's hold on power.
3. *Congressional Quarterly Weekly,* January 8, 2007, 122.
4. At the same time, Henry Waxman is still a member of the health subcommittee and has a large and strong staff to deploy in his new position. Also, John Dingell, chairman of the parent Energy and Commerce Committee, has often taken a strong lead on Medicaid, is a fearsome investigator, and works well with Waxman. Rep.

Pete Stark, a strong champion of Medicaid, remains as chairman of the health subcommittee of Ways and Means. In the Senate, Max Baucus, who succeeds Charles Grassley as the new chairman of Senate Finance, is not known as a strong leader or especially interested in Medicaid. At the same time, both Grassley and Gordon Smith are generally favorable to Medicaid. Also Sen. Debbie Stabenow (D., Mich.), who has joined the Finance Committee, has a strong interest in health issues including Medicare and Medicaid. In a word, people are in different chairs and Medicaid legislative leadership may suffer, but Medicaid will have some effective defenders and may get positive action on some reform items.

5.   The number of 25 was attributed to Raymond Sheppach, executive director of the NGA. By 2007, the estimate had grown to 30. Matthew Salo, telephone interview by Smith, February 15, 2007.

6.   The "unsustainable" characterization appears in the report of the Medicaid Commission and in an article by John K. Iglehart, "Medicaid Revisited—Skirmishes over a Vast Public Enterprise," *New England Journal of Medicine,* Vol. 356(7), Feb. 15, 2007, 734-740. Late in February, *Health Affairs* published a "Web Exclusive" citing statistics that Medicaid was not only sustainable but that its share of health expenditures would stay at about the same percentage (16.5%) through 2025 and then increase slowly to 19% by 2045. Whether the program is "sustainable" or not would seem to depend in large measure upon where one sits. Cf. Richard Kronick and David Rousseau, "Is Medicaid Sustainable? Spending Projections For The Program's Second Forty Years," *Health Affairs Web Exclusive*, 23 February 2007, w271-w287.

7.   President Bush did not renew his earlier inclusion of tax credits in his budget proposal for FY 2008.

8.   *Congressional Quarterly Weekly,* Jan. 29, 2007, 325.

9.   For instance, eliminating Medicaid funds for IDEA children; or reducing the match on MMIS, nursing home inspections, and independent review organizations.

10.   A number of states were already above 200% of poverty at the time SCHIP was enacted and were "grandfathered" in with rates up to 250% of poverty, so this characterization is not strictly accurate.

11.   At the time, a dozen states were strongly considering this option and Gov. Mitt Romney of Massachusetts stated his intention to run for president touting the Massachusetts health care reform as a model for the nation. According to a government source, President Bush had originally favored inclusion of tax credits in the amount of $4800 for individuals and $9600 for families. He reportedly changed his mind and backed the much less expensive tax deductions because persuaded by advisers that this level of support for tax credits would be too redistributive and too expensive. Another indication of the administration's ambivalence about this matter may be the fact that the White House description of the president's health policy still includes a tax credit proposal with $3000 as the basic level of support.

12.   "States and U.S. at Odds on Aid for Uninsured," *New York Times*, Feb. 13, 2007, A1, 18.

13.   *New York Times,* Feb. 27, 2007, Al, 14.

14.   Cf. "The Next Big Health Care Battle," *New York Times,* Mar. 12, 2007, A-23.

15.   *New York Times,* Mar. 14, 2007, A-16.

16.   *Ibid.*

Glossary

Actuarily Sound. A requirement that capitation payments made by the state to an at-risk managed care plan be financially sound in relation to the insurance risk.

Adverse Selection. When an insurer or health plan is selected by a disproportionate number of high-risk enrollees.

Amount, Duration, and Scope. States are required to specify the amount, duration, and scope of benefits required. The benefits so specified must be adequate to accomplish the purposes of the Medicaid Act; and states cannot discriminate arbitrarily between categories of recipients.

Assignment. Agreement by a physician or provider to "assign" his fee or charge and accept Medicaid (or Medicare) payment and not seek the balance from the beneficiary.

Authorization. An act of Congress, required by Article I of the U.S. Constitution, that provides the legal authority for appropriations. Important especially in relation to entitlements, such as Medicare or Medicaid, that are permanent rather than periodic authorizations.

Baseline. Projection of future spending and revenues under assumed economic conditions and participation rates, with no change in current policy; usually projected annually and for five years by the CBO, with amendments during the year.

Block Grant. A grant typically awarded to a state or local government, distributed according to formulas established by law, to support broadly categorical activities or programs and usually with a minimum of restrictions, set-asides, or mandates; often contrasted with more narrowly defined or targeted "categorical" or "project" grants.

Boren Amendment. Named after Sen. David Boren (D., Okla.). Enacted in 1980 to allow states more flexibility in developing their own payment methods for nursing homes, but requiring that rates be "reasonable and adequate" to meet the costs of "effective and efficient operation." This legislation was extended in 1981 to include hospitals and require that payments for them take into account a "disproportionate share of low income patients with special needs." The term "Boren Amendment" is often used to refer to both the 1980 and the 1981 legislation and gave rise to a large number of lawsuits. It was resented by many governors and was repealed by BBA 1997.

Budget Resolution. Annual resolution by Congress setting forth spending, revenue, and deficit targets for the next five fiscal years; the first year is binding and guides, in principle, the activities of all other congressional committees. Also, in principle, this resolution outlines the tasks and major priorities that guide the reconciliation process.

Capitation. Payment of a fixed amount per person for a period of time rather than compensating by salary or fees for specific services or procedures.

Capped Entitlement. A benefit available to all who are eligible, but for which the government limits the amount it will contribute. Capped entitlement were proposed by the Reagan administration and again in 1995.

Categorical Eligibility. Eligible for Medicaid because meeting the qualifications for a specific category, such as aged, disabled, or a pregnant woman meeting prescribed income and asset tests.

Civil Monetary Penalty (CMP). An intermediate penalty established as an alternative to exclusion from participation in the program or criminal sanctions—penalties that were not used.

Comparability. A requirement that services provided to any category of needy beneficiary must be generally equal or "comparable" in amount, duration, and scope to those provided to any other categorically needy beneficiary. Some obvious exceptions are made for age and sex.

Cost Reimbursement. Payment on the basis of audited costs rather than "charges" or a rate set or negotiated in advance.

Disproportionate Share Hospital (DSH) Payments. Payments to hospitals that states designate as serving a disproportionate share of low-income or uninsured patients.

Dual Eligible. A person eligible both for Medicare coverage (because of age or disability) and for full Medicaid coverage.

Early and Periodic Screening, Diagnostic, and Treatment (EPSDT) Services. A Medicaid benefit established in 1967, EPSDT mandates certain services for "categorically needy" persons under 21 years of age, and includes screening for physical or mental conditions or illnesses and treatment for those conditions or illnesses discovered; a federal mandate that provides preventive and comprehensive services for children but was (and still is) considered onerous by some states and has proven difficult to enforce.

Encounter Data. Description of the diagnoses or services provided under a health plan to a member. Such information is vital for monitoring the activity of MCOs and for risk adjustment.

Entitlement Program. A program that requires the payment of benefits to all who meet the eligibility requirements, such as Medicare, Medicaid, Social Security, and veterans' pensions. These particular entitlements are not subject to periodic reauthorization and carry with them the presumption that the numbers entitled determine the expenditures rather than the budget process determining who can receive the benefits.

Employee Retirement Income Security Act (ERISA). Enacted in 1974, primarily to protect pension benefits, ERISA was extended to health plans. Under the so-called ERISA pre-emption, jurisdiction is divided between the state and federal governments so that some managed care plans and activities are exempted, a factor that adds both complexity and uncertainty to attempts to legislate or seek judicial redress and limits state oversight and regulation of employer-based health insurance.

Federal Financial Participation. (FFP) Federal matching support for state Medicaid expenditures.

Federal Medical Assistance Percentage (FMAP). Federal share (percentage) of a state's expenses that will be paid by the federal government. In the original Medicaid statute, the payment limits for covered services were to vary according to per capita income within the state and be not less than 50% nor more than 83%. For administrative costs the payments were 50% and 75% depending upon the activity.

Federal Poverty Level. Initially, devised as a statistical construct, the FPL was gradually associated with the setting of income standards for eligibility. Often referred to as "Federal Poverty Line."

Federally Qualified Health Center (FHQC). Health center in a medically underserved underserved area that is eligible for Medicare and Medicaid cost reimbursement. Rural Health Centers are similar versions for rural areas.

Freedom of Choice. Usually refers to the beneficiary's right to choose any participating provider. In addition, both the beneficiary and the provider have the right to participate or not. Also refers to the Sec. 1915(b) "Freedom of Choice" Waiver., which permits a waiver of this requirement in order to participate in an MCO.

Gramm-Rudman-Hollings. Popular title for the Balanced Budget and Emergency Deficit Control Act of 1985, important for providing mandatory procedures for budget deficit reduction, targeting Medicare and Medicaid among other programs.

Health Insurance Flexibility and Accountability (HIFA) Waivers. A waiver program, announced by the Bush administration in August 2001, intended to encourage states to initiate comprehensive efforts by the states to increase Medicaid or SCHIP coverage within current expenditure limits.

Home and Community-Based Waivers. Sec. 1915(c) waivers enacted as part of OBRA 1981.

Hyde Amendment. Named after Henry Hyde (R., IL). Passed in 1976 as an amendment to the Labor and HEW appropriations bill, it prohibits use of federal matching funds for abortions, except where the pregnancy results from rape or incest or would endanger the woman's life. This ban has been renewed each year since then.

Institution for Mental Diseases (IMD). A facility that is "primarily engaged" in providing "diagnosis, treatment, or care" for persons with mental diseases. The original legislation made IMDs, along with tuberculosis hospitals, ineligible for federal Medicaid matching payments. Eventually, the term was legislatively restricted to facilities with more than 16 beds.

Intergovernmental Transfers (IGTs). One of several "Medicaid maximization schemes" employed by states to augment their Medicaid matching funds. States would make inflated payments for categories of Medicaid expenses and, in turn, receive back transferred funds that they could use for a variety of purposes, including other health programs or additional matching funds. Other similar measures were provider donations or taxes and increased Medicaid DSH payments.

Intermediate Care Facility (ICF). First established as an alternative to the nursing home, the ICF benefit was soon modified to included the mentally retarded (ICF/MR) and others with disabilities. It provides a level of care intermediate between a nursing home and the hospital or a skilled nursing facility.

Katie Beckett Waiver. A waiver that allows a child with disabilities severe enough to require a level of treatment provided by a hospital, nursing home, or ICF/MR to be treated at home, even though that child only qualified for Medicaid because of institutionalization. Named after the child that first benefited from this waiver.

Mandate (federal). Enforceable federal requirement imposed upon a state, local government, or private party.

Mandatory Categories, Services. States that participate in the Medicaid program are required to cover specified categories and provide, at a minimum, certain services to all members within those categories—as distinguished from optional categories and optional services. Markup (Mark). Legislative state at which the text of a bill is discussed and amended. The committee or subcommittee chair normally decides which bill to consider, which then becomes the "chairman's mark."

Means Tests. Income and asset limits originally linked to state cash assistance welfare programs. They have been gradually liberalized, but still apply to both Medicaid and SCHIP.

Medicaid Fraud Control Unit (MCFU). States are required by federal law to establish MCFUs or similar units organized independently from their Medicaid agencies.

Medicaid Management Information System (MMIS). State computerized systems that track claims, help detect fraud and abuse, and aid management and program planning.

Medically Needy. Persons whose incomes would be too high to qualify for Medicaid but whose medical expenses reduce the income left to them to a level low enough to qualify.

Notice and Comment. A state in the rulemaking process that follows the Notice of Proposed Rulemaking (NPRM) during which parties may comment on the proposed rule. Especially important in law are the quality and responsiveness of the explanations and justifications the agency gives in response to comments received.

Peer Review Organization. Organizations that contract with HCFA/CMS and with the states to review Medicare and Medicaid service quality or utilization. They have been renamed "Quality Improvement Organizations" by CMS.

Per Capita Cap (PCC). A proposed cap on expenditures per Medicaid beneficiary, as opposed to an aggregate cap for a whole area. Proposed in the Reagan administration and later in 1995 and 1997, it would have limited the Medicaid rate of increase using beneficiary categories such as age, sex, disability, and poverty level.

Pre-admission Screening and Annual Resident Review (PASARR).
A requirement that states must provide a pre-admission screening and annual review for those with a mental illness or mentally retarded to be admitted to a Medicaid long-term care nursing facility.

Program of All-Inclusive Care for the Elderly (PACE). A program that provides comprehensive care for elderly Medicare and Medicaid beneficiaries.

Qualified Medicare Beneficiary (QMB). A Medicare beneficiary whose income is too high to qualify as a dual eligible, but whose income is below the federal poverty level with assets that do not exceed $4000. Medicaid pays a part of the Medicare premium and copays, depending on income.

Quality Assurance Reform Initiative (QARI). A project initiated in 1993 that helped develop quality measures for the Medicaid program. The QARI project also contributed to the subsequent development of the Quality Improvement System for Managed Care (QISMC) that provided the conceptual foundations for the Medicare managed care quality improvement provisions of BBA '97.

Quality Control. Term commonly used for Medicaid Eligibility Quality Control (MEQC), a program derived from public assistance providing penalties for error rates in eligibility determinations that exceeded a specified percentage level.

Reconciliation. Process by which Congress requires committees to make the changes in legislation and appropriations to conform with the limits, allocations, and instructions contained in the budget resolution.

Risk Adjuster. Measure or technique used to adjust payments to compensate for health care expenses expected to result from differences in the health status of enrollees in separate health plans.

Rulemaking. Process by which implementing regulations are developed within the executive branch agencies or by independent regulatory agencies.

Section 209(b). An exception to the requirement established by the Social Security Amendments of 1972 that persons qualifying for Supplemental Security Income (SSI) automatically became eligible for Medicaid. Under Sec. 209(b) states were given the option of continuing to use their already established eligibility standards (which were lower) and some eleven or twelve did so.

Skilled Nursing Facility (SNF). A facility that meets certification for skilled nursing and provides mostly inpatient nursing and rehabilitation services to patients discharged from hospitals.

Specified Low Income Medicare Beneficiary (SLMB). A Medicare beneficiary whose income is above 100% but not more than 120% of the Federal Poverty Level. They qualify for payment of their Medicare premiums but not for the cost-sharing obligations.

Spend-Down. Enables a Medicaid applicant with income above the eligibility level to qualify for medically needy coverage by deducting medical or medically related expenditures over a period of time so that the income level within the particular state is met.

State Plan Amendment. A state wishing to change eligibility, benefits, or provider reimbursement must file a state plan amendment, which is subject to approval by CMS. This approval process was historically less difficult than a waiver application and approval.

Statewideness. A requirement that states operate their Medicaid programs uniformly throughout the state and not exclude particular regions, counties, or municipalities or groups living within them.

Supplemental Security Income (SSI). This provision of the Social Security Amendments of 1972 "nationalized" the adult categories of aged, blind, and disabled with national cash-assistance payments. In most states, those receiving SSI were automatically eligible for Medicaid.

Temporary Assistance for Needy Families (TANF). Title of the program that succeeded the Aid to Families with Dependent Children (AFDC). TANF led to important changes in Medicaid categorical eligibility both for those participating in TANF and for those leaving the program.

Upper Payment Limit (UPL). A requirement that the upper limits on Medicaid payments for provider categories could not exceed those established for Medicare. A provision that figured prominently in Medicaid maximization practices.

Voucher. A fixed subsidy or grant, typically made to a n individual or family head and limited to the purchase of a specific good, such as food, education, or health care.

Waiver. Approval of the "waiving" of a specific statutory or administrative provision. Waivers were especially prominent in efforts at welfare reform and for both Medicare and Medicaid. One important distinction is that between "demonstration" and "program" waivers—the first intended to demonstrate a possibility or results and the latter to make program changes as such.

Bibliography

Abraham, Laura Kaye. *Mama Might Be Better Off Dead—The Failure of Health Care in America.* Chicago, Ill.: University of Chicago Press. 1993.

Advisory Commission on Intergovernmental Relations. *Intergovernmental Problems in Medicaid.* Washington, DC: 1968.

Altmeyer, Arthur J. *The Formative Years of Social Security.* Madison, Wisc: University of Wisconsin. 1966.

Artiga, Samantha and Cindy Mann. *New Directions for Medicaid Section 1115 Waivers: Policy Implications of Recent Waiver Activity.* Washington, DC: Kaiser Commission on Medicaid and the Uninsured, 2005.

Ball, Robert M. "Report to the SSA Staff on the Implications of the Social Security Amendments of 1965," Reprinted by the National Academy of Social Insurance in *Reflections on Implementing Medicare,* Washington, DC. 1993, 1-11.

Benda, Peter M. and Charles H. Levine. "Reagan and the Bureaucracy: The Bequest, the Promise, and the Legacy," in Charles O. Jones (ed.), *The Reagan Legacy: Promise and Performance,* 102-142. Chatham, NJ: Chatham House. 1999.

Berenson, Robert A. and Walter A. Zelman. *The Managed Care Blues and How to Cure Them.* Washington, DC: Georgetown University Press. 1998.

Berkowitz, Edward D. *Disabled Policy—America's Programs for the Handicapped.* New York: Cambridge University. 1987.

____. *Mr. Social Security—The Life of Wilbur J. Cohen.* Lawrence, Kans.: University Press of Kansas. 1995.

Blatt, Barton and Fred Kaplan. *Christmas in Purgatory: A Photographic Essay on Mental Retardation.* Boston, Mass.: Allyn and Bacon. 1966.

Brown, Lawrence D. *Politics and Health Care Organization—HMOs as Federal Policy.* Washington, DC: Brookings Institution. 1983.

Califano, Joseph A., Jr. *Governing America.* New York: Simon and Schuster. 1981.

Center for American Progress. *Medicaid: The Best Safety-Net for Katrina Survivors and States.* Washington, DC: Author. 2005.

Clinton, William J. *My Life.* New York: Vintage. 2005.

Cohen, Wilbur J. "Reflections on the Enactment of Medicare and Medicaid." *Health Care Financing Review* Annual Supplement, 1985. 3-11.

Coughlin, Teresa A, Leighton Ku, and Johnny Kim. "Reforming the Medicaid Disproportionate Share Hospital Program." *Health Care Financing Review* 22(2) 2000. 137-57.

Coughlin, Teresa A. and David Liska. "Changing State and Federal Payment Policies for Medicaid Disproportionate Share Hospitals," *Health Affairs* 17(3) 1998. 118-36.

_____. *The Medicaid Disproportionate Share Hospital Payment Program: Background and Issues.* Washington, DC: Urban Institute. 1998.

Cromwell, Jerry and Sylvia Hurdle (1987). *Impact of Demonstration Projects on Medicaid and General Health Care Policy.* Waltham, Mass.: Health Policy Research Consortium. 1987.

Cromwell, Jerry, Sylvia Hurdle, Janice Singer, and Margaret MacAdam. *Impact of Demonstration Projects on Medicaid and General Health Policy.* Waltham, Mass.: Health Policy Research Center-Cooperative Research Center. 1987.

Crowley, Jeffrey S. *An Overview of the Independence Plus Initiative to Promote Consumer Direction of Services in Medicaid.* Washington, DC: Kaiser Family Foundation. 2003.

David, Sheri. *With Dignity: The Search for Medicare and Medicaid.* Westport, Conn: Greenwood. 1985.

Davidson, Stephen M. and Stephen A. Somers, eds. *Remaking Medicaid: Managed Care for the Public Good.* San Francisco: Jossey-Bass. 1998.

deParle, Jason. *American Dream.* New York: Viking. 2005.

Department of Health, Education, and Welfare. *Report of the Task Force on Medicaid and Related Programs* (McNerney Report). Washington, DC: Author. 1970.

_____. Social Rehabilitation Service. *Handbook of Public Assistance, Supplement D, Medical Assistance Program.* Washington, DC: Author. 1966.

Department of Health and Human Services, Substance Abuse and Mental Health Services Administration. *Achieving the Promise: Transforming Mental Health Care in America.* Author. 2003.

Derthick, Martha. *Policymaking for Social Security.* Washington, DC: Brookings Institution. 1979.

Donohue, John D. *Divided States.* New York: Basic Books. 1997.

Draper, Debra A., Robert E. Hurley, and Ashley C. Short. "Medicaid Managed Care: The Last Bastion of the HMO?" *Health Affairs* 23(2)155-167. 2004.

Drew, Elizabeth. *Showdown: The Struggle between the Gingrich Congress and the Clinton White House.* New York: Simon and Schuster. 1996.

Engel, Jonathan. *Poor People's Medicine: Medicaid and American Charity Care Since 1965.* Durham, NC: Duke University. 2006.

Epstein, Steven. *Impure Science—AIDS, Activism, and the Politics of Knowledge.* Berkeley, Cal.: University of California. 1996.

Etheredge, Lynn and Judith Moore. "A New Medicaid Program." *Health Affairs—Web Exclusives,* July-Dec., W3-426-439. 2003.

Falkson, Joseph F. *HMOs and the Politics of Health Services Reform.* Chicago: American Hospital Association. 1980.

Feder, Judith M. *Medicare: The Politics of Federal Hospital Insurance.* Lexington, Mass.: D.C. Heath. 1977.

Fenno, Richard E., Jr. *Learning to Govern: An Institutional View of the 104th Congress.* Washington, D.C.: Brookings Institution. 1997.

Foltz, Anne-Marie. *An Ounce of Prevention: Child Health Politics under Medicaid.* Cambridge, Mass.: MIT. 1982.

Fox, Daniel M. *Health Policies, Health Politics—The British and America Experience, 1911-1965.* Princeton, NJ: Princeton University. 1986.

Frank, Richard G., Howard H. Goldman, and Michael. "Medicaid and Mental Health: Be Careful What You Wish For." *Health Affairs* 22(1)101-113. 2003.

Geller, Jeffrey L. "Excluding Institutions for Mental Disorders from Federal Reimbursement for Services—Strategy or Tragedy?" *Psychiatric Services* 50: 1397-1403. 2000.

Gordon, Colin. *Dead on Arrival: The Politics of Health Care in Twentieth Century America.* Princeton, NJ: Princeton University. 2003.

Gordon, Linda (1994). *Pitied but Not Entitled—Single Mothers and the History of Welfare.* New York: Free Press. 1994.

Gostin, Lawrence O. *The AIDS Pandemic: Complacency, Injustice, and Unfulfilled Expectations.* Chapel Hill, NC: University of North Carolina. 2004.

Greenberg, Jay, Walter Leutz, Bruce Spitz, and Stanley Wallack. *A Historical Note on Medicare and Medicaid Waivers.* Waltham Mass.: Health Policy Consortium. 1983.

Grob, Gerald N. *The Mad among Us.* New York: Free Press. 1994.

Harris, Richard. *A Sacred Trust.* Baltimore, MD: Penguin. 1969.

Health Care Financing Administration. *Health Care Financing Administration—Strategic Plan.* Washington, DC: GPO. 1994.

_____. *Supporting Families in Transition: A Guide to Expanding Health Coverage in the Post-Welfare Reform World.* Author. ND.

Heclo, Hugh (1978) "Issue Networks and the Executive Establishment," in Anthony King. ed. *The New American Political System.* 87-124. Washington, DC: American Enterprise Institute. 1978.

Hegner, Richard E. *Dual Eligibility for Medicaid and Medicare: Options for Creating a Continuum of Care.* Washington, DC, National Health Policy Forum. 1997.

Holahan, John and Joel W. Cohen. *Medicaid: The Trade-Off between Cost Containment and Access to Care.* Washington, DC: Urban Institute. 1986.

_____, James Bell, and Gerald A. Adler. eds. *Medicaid Program Evaluation.* 1987. *Final Report.* Baltimore, MD: Health Care Financing Administration.

_____, Teresa Coughlin, Leighton Ku, David Heslam, and Colin Winterbottom (1993). "Understanding the Recent Growth in Medicaid Spending," in Rowland, Feder, and Salganicoff, eds. *Medicaid Financing Crisis: Balancing Responsibilities Priorities, and Dollars.* 23-42. Washington, DC: AAAS Press. 1993.

_____, Teresa Coughlin, Leighton Ku, Debra J. Lipson and Shruti Rajan. "Insuring the Poor through Medicaid 1115 Waivers." *Health Affairs* 14(1)155-161. 1995.

_____, Stephen Zuckerman, Alison Evans, and Suresh Rangarajan. "Medicaid Management in 13 States." *Health Affairs* 17(3): 43-63. 1998.

_____, *Restructuring Medicaid Financing: Implications of the NGA Proposal.* Washington, DC: Kaiser Family Foundation. 2001.

_____, "Variation in Health Insurance Coverage and Medical Expenditures: How Much is Too Much?" in John Holahan, Alan Weil, and Joshua M. Wiener, *Federalism and Health Policy.* 111-143. Washington, DC: Urban Institute. 2003.

Hurley, Robert E. "Medicaid Confronts a Changed Managed Care Marketplace," *Health Affairs* 14(1)11-25. 1992.

_____ and Michael McCue. *Medicaid and Commercial HMOs: An At Risk Relationship.* Princeton, NJ: Center for Health Strategies. 1998.

Institute of Medicine. *Improving the Quality of Care in Nursing Homes.* Washington, DC: Author. 1968.

_____, *Crossing the Quality Chasm—A New Health System for the 21st Century.* Washington, D.C.: Author. 2001.

Joe, Thomas C.W., Judith Meltzer, and Peter Yu. "Arbitrary Access to Care: The Case for Reforming Medicaid." *Health Affairs* 4(1): 59-74. 1985.

Jost, Timothy Stolzfus. *Disentitlement? The Threat Facing Our Public Health Care Programs and a Rights-Based Response.* New York: Oxford University. 2003.

Kaiser Commission on Medicaid and the Uninsured. *Deficit Reduction Act of 2005: Implications for Medicaid.* Washington, DC: Author. 2006.

Kent, Christine. "Cover Story—Cash and Counseling, The Way of the Future." *State Health Notes.* 26(#450) August 8. 2005.

Kerwin, C.M. *Rulemaking: How Government Agencies Write Laws and Make Policy* (2nd ed.). Washington, DC: CQ. 1999.

Koyanagi, Chris and Harold H. Goldman. "The Quiet Success of the National Plan for the Chronically Mentally Ill," *Hospital and Community Psychiatry* 42(9): 899-905.

Ku, Leighton. *The Medicare/Medicaid Link: State Medicaid Programs are Shouldering a Greater Share of the Costs of Care for the Dual Eligibles.* Washington, DC: Center on Budget and Policy Priorities. 2003.

_____. *The Slowdown in Medicaid Expenditure Growth.* Washington, DC: Center on Budget and Policy Priorities. 2006.

_____ and Vikki Wachino. *The Potential Impact of Eliminating TennCare and Reverting to Medicaid: A Preliminary Analysis.* Washington, DC: Center on Budget and Policy Priorities. 2004.

Lambrew, Jeanne. *Section 1115 Waivers in Medicaid and the State Children's Health Insurance Program: An Overview.* Washington, DC: Kaiser Commission on Medicaid and the Uninsured. 2001.

_____. *The State Children's Health Insurance Program: Past, Present, and Future.* Washington, DC: National Health Policy Forum. 2006.

Leblanc, Allen J. and M. Christine Tonner. "Medicaid 1915(c) Home and Community-Based Services Waivers Across the States," *Health Care Financing Review* 22(1)159-174. 2000.

Lewin, Marion Ein and Stuart Altman. *America's Health Care Safety Net.* Washington, DC: National Academy. 2000.

Lindblom, Charles E. "The Science of Muddling Through," *Public Administration Review* 19:79-99. 1950.

Ling, Sharon K., Teresa A. Coughlin, and Stephanie Kendall. "Access to Care Among Disabled Adults on Medicaid," *Health Care Financing Review* 23(4)157-173. 2002.

Lurie, Nicole, Minna Jung, and Risa Lavizzo-Mourey. "Disparities and Quality Improvement: Federal Policy Levers." *Health Affairs* 24(2)354-364. 2005.

Mann, Cindy and Elizabeth Kenny. *Differences That Make a Difference: Comparing Medicaid and the State Children's Health Program: An Overview.* Washington, DC: Kaiser Commission on Medicaid and the Uninsured. 2005.

Marmor, Theodore R. *The Politics of Medicare,* 2d ed. Hawthorne, NY: Aldine deGruyter. 2000.

Master, Robert J. "Medicaid Managed Care and Disabled Populations," in Davidson and Somers, *Remaking Medicaid,* 100-17. 1998.

Matherlee, Karen. *The Federal-State Medicaid Match: An Ongoing Tug-of-War Over Practice and Policy.* Washington, DC: National Health Policy Forum. 2000.

McCormack, Thomas P. *The AIDS Benefits Handbook.* New Haven, Conn.: Yale University. 1990.

Mechanic, Robert E. *Medicaid's Disproportionate Share Hospital Program: Complex Structure, Critical Payments.* Washington, DC: National Health Policy Forum. 2004.

Moore, Judith D. *SCHIP in the Formative Years, an Update.* Washington, D.C.: National Health Policy Forum. 2000.

_____ and David G. Smith (2006). "Legislating Medicaid: Considering Medicaid and Its Origins," *Health Care Financing Review* 27(2)45-52. 2006.

Myers, Robert J. *Medicare.* Homewood, IL: Irwin. 1970.

Nathan, Richard P. *The Administrative Presidency.* New York: Wiley. 1983.

_____ and Fred C. Doolittle and Associates. *Reagan and the States.* Princeton, NJ: Princeton University. 1987.

_____. "Federalism and Health Policy." *Health Affairs* 24(6)1459-66. 2005.

National Governors' Association. *Health Care Reform Policy.* NGA Policy Position HR-32. Washington, DC: Author. 2001.

_____. *Short-Run Medicaid Reform from the National Governors' Association.* Washington, DC: Author. 2005.

Neustadt, Richard E. and Harvey Fineberg. *The Epidemic that Never Was—Policy Making and the "Swine Flu" Scare.* New York: Random House. 1982.

Newland, Chester A. "Executive Policy Apparatus: Enforcing the Reagan Agenda," in Lester A. Salamon and Michael S. Lund, eds. *The Reagan Presidency and the Governing of America.* 135-168. Washington, DC: Urban Institute. 1985.

Oberg, Charles N. and Cynthia Polich. "Medicaid: Entering the Third Decade." *Health Affairs* 9(3): 83-96. 1998.

Offner, Paul. *Medicaid and the States.* New York: Century Foundation. 1999.

O'Shaughnessy, Carol and Richard Price. *Medicaid "176" Waivers for Home and Community-Based Care.* Congressional Research Service (mimeo). 1985.

Panem, Sandra. *The AIDS Bureaucracy.* Cambridge, Mass.: Harvard University.1988.

Park, Edwin. *Failing to Deliver: Administration's Waiver Policy Excludes Many Katrina Survivors and Provides No Guarantee of Full Federal Financing.* Washington, DC: Center on Budget and Policy Priorities. 2005.

Pear, Robert. *New York Times.* February 24, 2003. A1.

_____. "Governors Seek Aid from Congress and Decline to Back Medicaid Plan." *New York Times*, February 26, 2003. A-14.

Pelrine, Alice (1992). "The Art of the Deal: Health Policy Making on the Fly." *Journal of American Health Policy*, May/June. 23-28. 1992.

Perry, Michael and Neal Robertson. *Individuals with Disabilities and Their Experience with Managed Care.* Washington, DC: Kaiser Commission on Medicaid and the Uninsured. 1999.

Peters, Christie Provost. *EPSDT: Medicaid's Critical but Controversial Benefits Program for Children.* Washington, DC: National Health Policy Forum, November, 2006.

Peterson, Mark A. ed. *Health Markets? The New Competition in Medical Care.* NC: Duke University. 1998.

Reichley, A. James (1981). *Conservatives in an Age of Change.* (Washington, DC: Brookings Institution. 1981.

Robinson, James C. (2001). "The End of Managed Care." *Journal of the American Medical Association* 285(20):222-28. 2001.

_____. "Management after Managed Care." *Health Affairs—Web Exclusives,* Jan.-June W4-269-280. 2004.

Rockman, Bert A. (1988). "The Style and Organization of the Reagan Presidency," in Charles O. Jones. ed. *The Reagan Legacy: Promise and Performance.* 3-29. Chatham, NJ: Chatham House.

Rodwin, Marc A. "Consumer Protection and Managed Care: the Need for Organized Consumers." *Health Affairs* 15(3):110-23. 1996.

Rosenbaum, Sara. "Negotiating the New Health System—A Nationwide Analysis of Medicaid Managed Care Contracts," in Davidson and Somers, *Remaking Medicaid* 1998. 197-218.

_____ and Julie Darnall. *Medicaid Managed Care: An Analysis of the HCFA's Notice of Proposed Rule Making.* Washington, DC: Center for Health Policy Research. 1998. Also, reports under same title issued since 1997 by the Center for Health Policy Research.

_____. *The Olmstead Decision: Implications for Medicaid.* Washington, DC: Kaiser Commission on Medicaid and the Uninsured. 2000.

_____. *Medical Necessity under the EPSDT Program: When Is Coverage Required.* Washington, DC: George Washington University, School of Public Health and Health Services. 2002.

_____. *Defined-Contribution Plans and Limited-Benefit Arrangements: Implications for Medicaid Beneficiaries*. Washington, DC: George Washington School of Public Health and Health Services, September, 2006.

Ross, Donna Cohen and Laura Cox. *In a Time of Growing Need: State Choices Influence Health Coverage Access for Children and Families*. Washington, DC: Kaiser Family Foundation. 2003, Rowland, Diane, Judith Feder, and Alina *Salgonicoff*. eds. *Medicaid Financing Crisis: Balancing Responsibilities, Priorities, and Dollars*. Washington, DC: AAAS Press. 1993.

_____ and Rachel Garfield. "Health Care for the Poor: Medicaid at 35," in *Health Care Financing Review* 18(1): 1-8. 2000.

Ryan, Jennifer and Nora Super (2003). *Dually Eligible for Medicare and Medicaid: Two for One or Double Jeopardy?* Washington, DC: National Health Policy Forum.

Ryan, Jennifer. *Medicaid in 2006: A Trip down the Yellow Brick Road?* Washington, DC: National Health Policy Forum. 2006.

Rymer, Marilyn and Gerald Adler. *Short-Term Evaluation of Medicaid: Selected Issues*. Health Care Financing Administration, Office of Research and Demonstrations. 1982.

Schick, Allen. *The Federal Budget: Politics, Policy, and Process*. Washington, DC: Brookings Institution. 1995.

Schneider, Andy, Victoria Strohmeyer, and Risa Ellberger (2000). *Medicaid Eligibility for Individuals with Disabilities*. Washington, DC: Kaiser Commission on Medicaid and the Uninsured. 2000.

_____ with Risa Elias, Rachel Garfield, David Rousseau, and Victoria Wachina. *The Medicaid Resource Book*. Washington, DC: Kaiser Commission on Medicaid and the Uninsured. 2002.

_____ Leighton Ku, and Judith Solomon. *The Administration's Medicaid Proposals Would Shift Federal Costs to the States*. Washington, DC: Center on Budget and Policy Priorities. 2006.

Shirk, Cynthia. *Rebalancing Long-Term Care: The Role of the Medicaid HCBS Waiver Program*. Washington, DC: National Health Policy Forum. 2006.

_____ and Jennifer Ryan. *Premium Assistance in Medicaid and SCHIP: Ace in the Hole or House of Cards?* Washington, DC: National Health Policy Forum. 2006.

Smith, David Barton. *Health Care Divided: Race and Healing a Nation*. Ann Arbor, Mich.: University of Michigan. 1999.

_____. *Reinventing Care: Assisted Living in New York City*. Nashville, Tenn.: Vanderbilt University. 2002.

Smith, David G. *Paying for Medicare: The Politics of Reform*. Hawthorne, NY: Aldine deGruyter. 1992.

_____. *Entitlement Politics: Medicare and Medicaid, 1995-2001*. Hawthorne, NY: Aldine deGruyter. 2002.

Smith, Vernon K., Neva Kaye, Debbie Chang, Jeanne Bonney, Charles Milligan, Dann Milne, Robert Mollica, and Cynthia Chang. *Making Medicaid Work for the 21st Century*. Washington, DC: National Academy for State Health Policy. 2004.

_____ and Gregg Moody, *Medicaid in 2005: Principles and Proposals for Reform.* Chicago, Ill.: Health Management Associates. 2005.

Sorian, Richard. *The Bitter Pill—Tough Choices in America's Health Policy.* New York: McGraw-Hill. 1998.

Sparer, Michael S. "Devolution of Power: An Interim Report Card." *Health Affairs* 17(3):7-16. 1998.

Stevens, Robert and Rosemary Stevens. *Welfare Medicine in America—A Case Study of Medicaid.* New York: Free Press. 1974.

Stockman, David A. *Triumph of Politics: How the Reagan Revolution Failed.* New York: Harper & Row. 1986.

Thompson, Frank and John DiIulio, Jr. eds. *Medicaid and Devolution: A View from the States.* Washington, DC: Brookings Institution. 1998.

Thompson, Penny. *Medicaid's Federal-State Partnership: Alternatives for Improving Fiscal Integrity.* Washington, DC: Kaiser Family Foundation. 2004.

Tilly, Jane. "Long-Term Care—Can the States Be the Engine of Reform?" in John Holahan, Alan Weil, and Joshua M. Wiener, *Federalism and Health Policy.* Washington, DC: Urban Institute. 2003.

Trent, James W. Jr. *Inventing the Feeble Mind—A History of Mental Retardation in the United States.* Berkeley, Cal.: University of California. 1994.

U.S. Congress. *Performance of the States—Eighteen Months of Experience with the Medical Assistance for the Aged (Kerr-Mills) Program.* Senate Special Committee on the Aging, Committee Print, June 15, 1962.

_____. *Limitations on Federal Participation under Title XIX of the Social Security Act.* House of Representatives, 89th Congress, 2d Session, Rpt. No. 2224. 1966.

_____. *Social Security Amendments of 1967.* 90th Congress, 1st Session, Senate Rpt. No. 744. 1967.

_____. *Medical Assistance for the Aging—The Kerr-Mills Program, 1960-1963.* Senate Special Committee on the Aging, Committee Print, October 1968.

_____. *Medicare and Medicaid—Problems, Issues, and Alternatives.* Report of the Staff to the Senate Committee on Finance, Committee Print, 91st Congress, 1st Session. February 9, 1970.

_____. *Social Security Amendments of 1972.* 92nd Congress, 2nd Session, Senate Report 1230. 1972.

_____. *Prepaid Health Plans.* Hearings, Permanent Subcommittee on Investigations of the Committee on Governmental Affairs, Senate, 94th Congress, 1st Session. 1975.

_____. *Medicaid Management Information Systems (MMIS).* Hearings before the Permanent Subcommittee on Investigations of the Committee on Government Operations, House of Representatives, 94th Congress, 1st Session. 1976.

_____. *Child Health Assessment Act.* Hearings before the Subcommittee on Health and Environment of the Committee on Commerce, House of Representatives, 95th Congress, 1st Session. 1977.

_____. *Medicare Community Care Act of 1980*. Hearing before the Subcommittee on Health and the Environment of the Committee on Interstate and Foreign Commerce, House of Representatives, 96th Congress, 2nd Session. 1980.

_____. *Current Conditions of American Federalism*. Hearings before the Committee on Government Operations, House of Representatives, 97th Congress, 1st Session. 1981.

_____. *Omnibus Budget Reconciliation Act of 1981*. Report of the Committee on the Budget to Accompany H.R. 3981, House of Representatives, 97th Congress, 1st Session, Rpt. 158. 1981.

_____. *Infant Mortality,* Report prepared by the Congressional Research Service for the Subcommittee on Health and the Environment of the Committee on Energy and Commerce. House of Representatives, Committee Print 98-J, 98th Congress, 1st Session. 1983.

_____. *Omnibus Budget Reconciliation Act of 1987*. House of Representatives, Rpt. 495, 100th Congress, 2nd Session. 1987.

_____. *Medicaid Source Book: Background Data and Analysis*. "The Yellow Book." Report prepared by the Congressional Research Service for the Subcommittee on Health and the Environment of the Committee on Energy and Commerce Cmte Print 103-A, 103rd Congress, 1st Session. 1993

_____. *Transformation of the Medicaid Program*, Hearings before the Subcommittee on Health and Environment of the Committee on Commerce, 104th Congress, 1st Session, 3 parts, June 8, 15, 21, 22, July 26, and August 1, 1995.

_____. *Special Supplement—Conference Managers Explanation of Medicaid Child Health Agreements.* 105th Congress, 1st Session, Sen. Rpt. 211. 1997.

_____. *Living without Health Insurance*. Hearings, Committee on Finance. Senate. 107th Congress, 1st Session. 2001.

U.S. General Accounting Office. *Medicaid and SCHIP—Recent HHS Approvals of Demonstration Waiver Projects Raise Concerns*. Report to the Committee on Finance, U.S. Senate. GAO-02-817. 2002.

_____. *Major Management Challenges and Program Risks: Department of Health and Human Services*. GAO-03-01. 2003.

U.S. Government Accountability Office. *Medicaid—Improved Federal Oversight of State Financing Schemes Is Needed*. GAO-04-228. 2004. (The title, "General Accounting Office" was changed to "Government Accountability Office" in July 2004).

Villagra, Victor A. "Integrating Disease Management into the Outpatient Delivery System during and after Managed Care." *Health Affairs—Web Exclusives*, Jan-June W4-281-283. 2004.

Vladeck, Bruce C. *Unloving Care: The Nursing Home Tragedy*. New York: Basic Books. 1980.

_____. "Where the Action Really Is: Medicaid and the Disabled." *Health Affairs* 22(1): 90-100. 2003.

Wachino, Victoria, Leighton Ku, Edwin Park, and Judith Solomon. *Medicaid Provisions of the House Reconciliation Bill Both Harmful and Unnecessary.* Washington, DC: Center on Budget and Policy Priorities. 2005.

Waller, Douglas. "How VA Hospitals Became the Best." *Time*, September 4, 2006, 36-37.

Weil, Alan. "There's Something about Medicaid," *Health Affairs* 22(1)13-30. 2003.

Weissert, Carol S. and William G. Weissert *Governing Health: The Politics of Health Policy.* Baltimore, Md.: Johns Hopkins. 1996.

Weldon, T.D. (1953). *The Vocabulary of Politics.* Baltimore, Md.: Penguin. 1953.

Wiener, Joshua M. and David G. Stevenson . "State Policy on Long-Term Care for the Elderly," *Health Affairs.* 17(3) 81-100. 1998.

Witte, Edwin E. *The Development of the Social Security Act.* Madison, Wisc.: University of Wisconsin. 1962.

Zubkoff, Michael (ed.) *Health: A Victim or Cause of Inflation.* New York: Milbank Memorial Fund. 1976.

Index

Access to care, 13, 35, 37, 49-50, 77, 79, 119-121, 132-133, 165-166, 192, 259, 357, 374-375, 377
Adler, Gerald, 361n31
Adult categories (Aged, Blind, Disabled)
    expenses for, 172
    "federalizing" of, 104
    SSI and, 104
"Affordable Choices" initiative, 408
Aggregation (as legislative strategy), 369, 409
    see also, "incrementalism"
Aging and Disability Resource Centers, 290-291
Aging, Subcommittee on (Senate), 36
Agricultural workers, 32
Aid to Families with Dependent Children (AFDC), 46
    Aid to Dependent Children, 11, 12, 32
AIDS, see HIV/AIDS
Alcohol and drug abuse, 193
    Medicaid support for, 194
Alcohol, Drug Abuse and Mental Health Administration (ADAMHA), 190
Alternative delivery systems (ADS), 99, 10, 165 ff, 386 ff
Altmeyer, Arthur, 23, 24, 26, 34, 42
American Medical Association
    political activities of, 23, 36, 42, 113
    vendor payments and, 13
American Public Welfare Association, 68
Americans With Disabilities Act (1990), 188, 190, 191, 285-286
    and HIV/AIDS, 199-200
Armey, Dick, 229

AZT (zidovudine), 200-201

Balanced Budget Act of 1995, 228, 230
    American Hospital Association and, 235-236
    budget Resolution and, 231
    Chafee, John and, 240
    Chafee-Rockefeller bill and, 241
    Clinton veto and government shutdown, 243
    Democrats and defensive tactics, 233
        informal task force, 233
        effectiveness of, 234-235
    formula fight, 237-239
    Medicaid program, 243
        latent political strengths, 232, 243
    Medicaid Transformation Act, 232
    National Governors' Association, 231, 281
    percentage caps, 231
    safety-net institutions and, 235
    Senate Finance Committee, 239-240
    Senate version (S1357), 240-242
    "Snow birds," 240
    veto and government shutdown, 232, 242
Balanced Budget Act of 1997, 248 ff
    additional funds and, 250
    budget "summit," 250
    CBO "scoring," 257
    Chafee-Rockefeller bill, 262
    Child Health Assistance Program (CHAP), 263
    contrasted with BBA '95, 250-251
    DSH cuts and, 257
    fraud and abuse provisions, 259-260

HMOs and managed care reforms,
254-256, 258-259
implementation, regulative, 265 ff
managed care regulation, 267-269
withdrawn, 268
SCHIP steering committee, 266
Q&As, 267
pre-shopping of provisions, 249
SCHIP legislation, 261-265
Ball, Robert, 27, 34, 85
Barbour, Haley, 355
Beckett, Julie, 191
Bed capacity and "cold bed" tests,
340-341
Bellmon, Henry, 104, 129
Benchmarks
SCHIP and, 264-265
Benefits, optional, 48, 110
Bennett, Wallace, 329
Bentsen, Lloyd, 175, 294
Beveridge Plan, 24
Bipartisan Commission on Medicaid,
303-304, 313
Block grants
OBRA '81 and, 160 ff.
Waxman, Henry and 159, 163-164
"Boll Weevil" (Democrats), 147, 159,
172
"Boom and bust" cycles, 390
Boren Amendment, 129-130
expansion of, 130
legislative text, 130
Lloyd Rader and, 129
Origins, 129
"reasonably cost related" require-
ment, 128-129
repeal of, 252, 257
Waxman amendments, 130-131
Bowen, Otis and MCCA, 202-203
Bredeson, Phil, 355
Budget and Impoundment Act of 1974,
115
major provisions, 116
significance, 116
Budget Enforcement Act (1990), 183
PAYGO and, 183
Budget neutrality (see "Neutrality,
budget")
Budget, president's
1995, 233
1997, 249-250

2007, Affordable Choices Initiative
and SCHIP reauthorization, 208-
209
Budget reconciliation, as a political
process, 212
Budget resolution of 1996
Medicaid-welfare link, 245-246
three-part strategy, 244 ff.
Budget working group, 158
Bureau of Family Services, 63, 65, 82
Burke, Sheila, 103
Bush, George H. W., 185
Bush, George W., 286
Bush v. Gore, 279
Byrd, Harry, 10, 84
Byrne, John, 45

Caps, Medicaid, 76-77, 107
5% cap, 146, 157, 231, 236-237
capped entitlement, 15, 159-160,
231
Carnegie, Andrew
on philanthropy, 18n7
Carter, Jimmy,
administration, 117 ff
Categorical eligibility, 1, 3, 14, 30,
47-48
elderly and disabled, 179
liberalizing, 173-74
pregnant women and children,
170-183
"Cash and Counseling," 289
Center for Medicare and Medicaid
Services (CMS), 284
administrative activities, 357 ff
GAO reports, 285, 353
"terms and conditions," 368n142
Chang, Deborah, 266
Charities, private, 3
philanthropy and, 17n7
public assistance and, 3-4
Child Health Assurance Program, 119-
120, 173
de-linking provision, 120
Medicaid expansion and, 119
NHI and, 119-147
origins, Child Health Assessment
Program and, 119
relation to EPSDT, 148
Childrens' Bureau, 5
Childrens' Defense Fund, 120, 121,
147, 173

Chronic and severe illnesses, conditions
   expenses for, 172
   treatment strategies, 167-168, 337-343, 375-376
Civil monetary penalties
   fraud and abuse and, 169, 259
Civil Rights Act of 1964, 83
   Title VI and, 83-84
"Clawback"and Medicare Modernization Act of 2003, 295, 386
Clinton, William, 233, 243, 249, 264
Cohen, Howard, 232
Cohen, Wilbur, 21, 27, 31, 36, 38, 42, 50
   incrementalism and, 33, 34
   Kerr-Mills and, 34-35
Committee on Economic Security, 7-12
12
Committee on the Costs of Medical Care, 27
Community health centers, 28, 202
Comparability, 47, 414
"Compassionate Conservatism," 286
Comprehensive care
   Medicaid requirement, sec. 1903(e), 50, 66, 100
   Repealed, 119-110
Congress
   Congressional Budget Office, 116
   freshmen members, 229-230
   leadership, 229
   reorganization, 116, 229
Consolidated Omnibus Budget Reconciliation Act of 1995 (COBRA), 172, 176
Constantine, Jay, 103
Consumer Bill of Rights and Responsibilities, 268
Contract with America, 229 ff.
   evaluation, 230
Coordinating committee, see "Interdepartmental Committee to Coordinate Health and Welfare"
Costs, Medicaid, 75, 96, 150, 375-376
   early assumptions and, 68
Coverage, Medicaid
   expansion, 22, 97, 150, 370, 381
   gaps and inequities, 372
   poor, 149
   unemployed, 10, 147, 171
   uninsured, 119, 385, 407-408

Crippled childrens' services, 77
Crowd-out, 390, 395

Davis, Carolyne, 142
Dean, Howard, 281
"Deeming," 218n10
Deficit Reduction Act of 2005 (DRA), 300-304, 307-313
   "benchmark" provisions, 309
   EPSDT, vulnerable groups, 309-310
   House bill, 308
   managed care stabilization fund, 385n100
   NGA and, 301
   Senate amendments, 308-30
   Gordon Smith and, 301-303
   significance, 310-312, 384-385
Deinstitutionalization, 132, 188, 190
Denton, Jeremiah and "family planning," 164
Derzon, Robert, 123
Desegregation, hospitals, 84
   efforts to achieve, 84 ff
   Medicaid and, 86 ff
   nursing homes and, 87
   physicians and, 86
   Title VI, 83 ff
Devolution, 254, 323
   antecedents, 324-330
   appraisal, 344-345, 358-359
   aspects of, 323-324
   Bush administration and, 284-285, 356-358
   Clinton administration and, 349, 352-352
   managed care and HCBS waivers, 331-345
   "marginal centralization" and, 316-331
   SCHIP and, 345-347
   Sec. 1115 waivers 349-359
Dingell, John, 159, 234
Disability
   Insurance, 32
   definition of, 191, 200
   "permanent and total," 33
   persons with, x, 95
Discrimination, racial, 83 ff
   see "desegregation," also "disparities"
Disease management, 395-397

Disparities, 373, 374
Disproportionate Share Hospital Allowance (DSH), 151, 168, 207ff
    Boren amendment(s), 130-131
    remedial legislation, 209-210
    see also "Medicaid Maximizing"
Divided government, 30, 95
Division of Medicaid Services, 61, 82
Dole, Robert, 158, 181, 245
Domenici, Pete, 156, 250
Domestic workers, 32
Drugs (pharmaceutical)
    coverage for, 150, 295
    Medicaid rebate program, 297
Dual eligibles, 207, 415
    QMBs, 205
    SLMBs, 206, 374-375

Early and Periodic Screening, Diagnostic, and Treatment Services (EPSDT), 77
    amendments, 181-182
    penalty, 110, 120
    repeal, 169
    regulatory implications, 78, 110
Earned Income Tax Credit (EITC), 261, 385
Economy, state of
    1971-74, 113
    1981-83, 171-173
    1996-97, 248
    2001-2002, 280, 293
Eisenhower, Dwight D.
    opposition to NHI, 27, 29
"Eldercare," 45
Elections(s)—results, significance
    1948, 31
    1964, 44
    1968, 96
    1976, 117-118
    1982, 172-173
    1994, 227, 229
    1996, 248
    2000, 279
    2002, 292-293
    2004, 299-300
    2006, 312-313, 405
Eligibility, 3
    categorical, 1, 3, 14, 16, 30, 47-48, 391
    citizenship, residency requirements, 32, 308

gaps and inequities, 372-373
    non-categorical, income based, 391
Employer sponsored insurance (ESI), 73, 74, 125-128
Enforcement, 73, 74, 125-128
    fraud and abuse sanctions, 126-128, 259-260
    alternatives to, 81, 107-108, 124, 133, 259-260
    penalties
        EPSDT, 110, 120
        error rates, 330-331
Entitlement(s)
    capped, 156, 157
    Medicaid as,
        arguments for, against, 378-382
        aspects of, 378-379
        threats to, 157-158, 227, 230, 299
        "weak entitlement," Medicaid as, viii, 370, 379-380, 390
    Roosevelt, Franklin on, 7
    temporary, 171
    "welfare" entitlements, 145, 157
Ewing, Oscar (plan), 26, 36
"Exceptionalism" (American), 1-3, 18-19
Executive Orders
    12291 (1983), regulatory review, 154
    12498 (1985), regulatory planning process, 154
    13217 (2001) community-based alternatives, 286-287

Factoring, 108
Falk, Isadore, 27
Family Assistance Plan (FAP), 95, 100-102, 114
    description, 101
Family Health Insurance Plan, 114
Family Opportunity Act, 309
Family planning
    Denton, Jeremiah, 178
    Hyde, Henry, 255, 275n90
Family Support Act of 1988 (partial de-linking of Medicaid and welfare), 181
Federal Security Agency, 26
"Federalizing," 95, 98, 104
Federally Qualified Health Centers, 257
Federal-state relations
    "antagonistic cooperation," 377

cycles, 377
Finance Committee, Senate, 118, 239
    bipartisan traditions and, 177
    health policy and, 177, 239-240
    HMOs and, 106
    Subcommittee on Medicaid, 290
Fiscal crises, Medicaid and
    1981-82, 172-173
    1990-92, 227
    2002-03, 293, 303
        Bush administration and, 293-294
        state responses, 293
Fishbein, Morris, 8
Flexibility proposals, 46, 165
Forand, Aime, 36, 38
Ford, Gerald, 119
"Formula fights," 237-39
Fraud and abuse, remedial measures
    development
        Social Security Amendments of
            1972, 102, 106, 108
        Medicare/Medicaid Anti-Fraud
            and Abuse Amendments of
            1977, 124-129
        BBA '97 and, 259-260
        Medicaid management and in-
            formation systems, 70, 107,
            125 ff
        program integrity, assuring, 124,
            133
        state Medicaid fraud and control
            units, 128
        technical assistance, 128
"Freedom of choice" waivers, 165, 167
Fullerton, William, 103

Gage, Larry, 298
Government Accountability Office
    (GAO)—formerly "General Ac-
    counting Office"
        Medicaid "at risk" 296
        Report on HIFA waivers, 285, 353
Graham, Bob, 259, 276n103
Gramm, Phil, 160, 261
Gramm-Latta budget proposals, 156,
    160
Gramm-Rudman-Hollings amendment
    (1985), 176
        sequester, 176
Granny's lawyer, 260
Great Society programs, 96, 119
Gregg, Judd, 303

"Gypsy moth" (Republicans), 160

Hatch, Orrin, 162, 261
Health Care Financing Administration
    (HCFA), 121
        Califano, Joseph and, 123-124
        NHI and, 124
        origins, 121 ff
            Talmadge subcommittee and,
                121-122
        title, 124
Health care reform
    Clinton administration and, 228
Health Insurance and Accountability
    Demonstration Waiver (HIFA), 281
        GAO adverse report on, 285
        NGA proposal and, 282-284
        response to, 284-285
Health Insurance Association of
    America, 114
Health Insurance Benefits Advisory
    Council (HIBAC), 244
Health Insurance Portability and Ac
    countability Act (HIPAA), 244
        three-part reconciliation and, 244-
            245
Health Maintenance Organizations
    (HMOs)
        amendments of 1976, 115, 131
        HMO Act of 1973, 114
        interest in, for Medicaid, 99, 106,
            165-167, 333-335
        see also, "managed care"
Health Security Act, 228
Heckler, Margaret, 196-197, 203
Helms, Jesse, 201
Hess, Arthur, 97
Hill-Burton (Hospital and Construction
    Act), 28, 184
HIV/AIDS, 195 ff
    Americans with Disabilities Act
        and, 199
    appraisal of efforts, 196-197
    background, 195-196
    Brandt, Edward, 196-197
    disability, issue of, 200
    Gallo, Robert, 196
    Heckler, Margaret, 197, 203
    legislation, 198-202
    Medicaid coverage and, 200, 202
    Reagan, Ronald and, 298, 223n207
    Ryan White CARE Act, 201, 202

Waxman, Henry and, 197
Hospital Cost Containment Act, 120
Holahan, John, 284
Hurricane, Katrina, see "Katrina"
Hyde, Henry (amendment), 255,
    275n90

Immigrant benefits, 260
Incrementalism
    Categorical, 3, 5
    as political strategy, 26, 42, 148-
        149, 151, 177
Indigent, medically, see "medically
    indigent, "needy"
Individuals with Disabilities Education
    Act, 1990 (IDEA), 311-312
Information technology (IT), 396
Infrastructure (for Medicaid)
    developing, 292, 398
    support for, 290-292, 381
    see also, "safety net"
Inspector general
    for health, 110
    for HEW, 114, 126
Institute of Medicine, nursing home
    study, 185
Institutional care
    institutional bias, of Medicaid,
        134, 146, 172, 184, 260, 374
    see also, "deinstitutionalization"
Institutions for Mental Diseases
    (IMDs), 49, 260
    exclusion, 104, 188-190, 345
    modifications of concept, 110
Integrated Hospital Plan, 27-28
Interdepartmental Committee to Coor-
    dinate Health and Welfare ("Coordi-
    nating Committee") 23
Intergovernmental Transfers (IGTs),
    209, 298
Intermediate Care Facility (ICF), 78-79
Intermediate Care Facility for the Men-
    tally Retarded (ICF/MR), 103-104,
    187-188
        HCBS waivers, 188

Jeffords, James, 279
Jennings, Christopher, 233
Johnson, Lyndon, 23

Kasich, John, 231-232, 249, 250
Katie Beckett Waiver, 191 ff

TEFRA and, 192, 193
Katrina (hurricane), 305-307
    Bush administration position, 305-
        306
    Disaster Relief Medicaid (Enzi-
        Kennedy), 306-307
    Emergency Health Care Relief Act
        of 2005 (Grassley-Baucus), 305-
        306
Kennedy, Edward (Ted), 118, 164, 192,
    204, 261, 406
Kennedy, John, 56, 79
Kennedy-Anderson bill, 42
Kennedy-Griffiths Health Security Act,
    113
Kerr, Robert, 37, 38, 39
Kerr-Mills (Medical Assistance for the
    Aged) 30-40
    abuses, 41
    benefit limitations, 40-41
    coverage, 41
    poorer states and, 40
    state participation, 61
    undesirable features, 39-40, 42

Land, Francis, 101, 112
"Layered complexity," viii, 6, 47, 398
Leadership, congressional
    changes in 1995, 229
Leadership states, 71
Leavitt, Michael, 210, 300-301, 354
LIFE Accounts Program, 291-292
Long, Russell, 100, 118
    Long amendment, 38, 48
Long-term care insurance, 395

Madison, James,
    "compound Republick," 1
Maintenance of effort, 109
Managed care, managed care organiza-
    tions, see also "HMOs"
    behavioral health managed care, 345
    case management, 166, 334
    cost containment, 167
    disease management, 395-397
    early attitudes toward, 106
    managed care reform, 254-256,
        258-259
    managed care regulation, 267, 269
    marketing standards, 256
    primary care case management
        (PCCM), 166, 334

Mandates, 150
    dual eligibles, 205-207
    EPSDT, 77
    nursing home standards, 80 185-
        187
    pregnant women and children, 148 ff
    revolt against, 162, 237
    services, 48
    SSI and, 104
    transition from welfare, 246
"Marginal centralization," 82, 135,
    326-327
Matching (federal), 33, 35, 39, 125,
    170 ff, 186, 247 ff, 231 ff, 386, 390
    ADC and, 12
    Counter-cyclical, 172, 390
    Federal Medical Assistance
        Percentage (FMAP), 416
Maternal and Child Health Program, 5,
    11-12, 77
McNerney taskforce, see "Taskforce
    on Medicaid and Related Programs,"
    97ff
Means, assets tests, 12, 13, 178-179,
    218n109, 246, 420
Medicaid (see also entries under topical
    headings)
    background and original legisla-
        tion, 21 ff
        afterthought?, 22
        as a "firewall," 42-43
        "comprehensive care" Sec.
            1903(e), 50
        beneficiary protections, 46-
            47, 49
        major provisions, 46
        mandated services, 49
        mental illness, 49
        "sleeping giant," 45
        "three-layer cake," 22
    early implementation, 59 ff
        data as problem, 70, 72
        enforcement, lack of, 73-74
        lack of time, 59, 61-62, 70-71
        miscalculations, 68, 69
        omissions, 63
        outreach and technical assistance,
            63, 69
        oversight, 72 ff.
        PREP, 72
        Quarterly Reviews, 70
        staffing, inadequate, 61, 69
    Supplement D, 64 ff
    major issues
        administrative structure, 69,
            112, 121-124, 183, 398
        categorical eligibility, 1, 3,
            13, 30, 47-48
        dual eligibles, 205-207, 374-375
        entitlement status, viii, 150 ff,
            378-382
        expansion, growth, and cost, 22,
            75, 97, 105-106, 150, 370, 381
        fiscal instability, 172-173, 227,
            293-294
        flexibility vs. protectiveness,
            180, 251-252, 383-384
        fraud and abuse, 112, 124-128,
            259-260
        gaps and inequities, 372 ff
        "institutional bias," 134, 136
        Medicaid "maximizing"
            schemes, 207-210
        National health insurance and,
            ix-x, 76, 113, 170, 228-229,
            369-370
        proposals to restructure, see
            separate heading, "Medicaid
            restructuring" unemployed, 10,
            147, 171,
        uninsured, 119, 385, 407-408
        welfare link, 16, 178, 181, 228,
            245-247
    specific topics
        comprehensive care, 50, 66, 100
        drug rebate, 297
        Medicaid advisory commis-
            sion (proposal for), 390-391
        Medicaid Bureau, 183, 335
        Medicaid Eligibility Quality
            Control ("Quality Control),"
            330-331
        Medicaid Management
            Information Systems, 70,
            107, 125ff
        sec. 209(b) (exemption from
            SSI eligibility criteria), 104
        sec. 1902(r)(2) (use of "less
            restrictive" methodologies,
            207
        sec. 1932, 246-247
        Special Needs Plans (SNPs),
            296
    Technical Advisory Groups

(TAGs), 330-331
Medicaid Community and Attendant
Services Act (MiCASSA), 289
  as template for service delivery,
  387-388
Medicaid Community Care Act,
  216n80
Medicaid directors, 101, 112, 268
Medicaid infrastructure grants, 290-
292m 381
"Medicaidization," 381, 386
Medicaid maximizing
  disproportionate share hospital
    payments (DSH), 207 ff
  hospital taxes and donations, 208
  Voluntary Contributions and Pro-
    vider-Specific Tax Amendments
    of 1991, 209
  intergovernmental transfers (IGTs),
    209, 298
  recycling, 210, 298
  remedial measures, 209
  upper payment limits (UPLs), 210-
    297
Medicaid "restructuring,"
  administrative actions, 180,270
  CMS and, 357-358
  Bush administration proposal of
    2003, 293
  responses to, 293-294
  legislative proposals, 158-164,
    230-232, 307-311
  National Governors' Association
    and, 231, 262, 281, 294-295
  the authors' "Modest List of
    Proposals," 382-398
Medical Assistance Advisory Council
  (MAAC), 80, 110
Medical Assistance for the Aging (see
  "Kerr-Mills"), 30
Medical Services Administration, 61
Medically indigent, "needy," 39, 47
  buy-in for, 82
  1967 limits, 76-77
Medicare
  buy-in, 49, 205-206
  and deficit reduction, 176
  initial legislation, 42 ff
Medicare Advantage Act, see "Medi
  care Prescription Drug, Improve-
  ment, and Modernization
  Act of 2003"

Medicare Catastrophic Coverage Act of
  1988, 150, 180, 190, 202, 205-206
  dual eligibility and (QMBs,
    SLMBs), 205-206
  income related premium, 205
  origins, 202-203
  repeal, significance of for Medic-
    aid, 206
Medicare Prescription Drug, Improve-
  ment, and Modernization Act of 2003
  ("Medicare Modernization Act"), 295
  Prescription drug and "clawback"
    feature, 295-296
Mental health, illness, 132-133, 188-
291
  IMDs, 199-190, 260
  Mental Health Systems Act of
    1980, 132, 190
  Repeal, 169-170
  State Comprehensive Mental
    Health Services Act (1986), 191
  New Freedom Commission on
    Mental Health, 287
  recovery, as treatment goal, 288
Mills, Wilbur, 37, 74
  influence, 44-45
  Medicaid and, 21, 42-44, 76
  resignation, 117
"Modernization" (of Medicaid), 280,
  293, 377, 382
"Money-follows-the-patient" initiative,
  289, 291
Mongan, James, 103
Mortality, infant, 179
Moss, Frank 79, 184
Moss Amendments, 79-80
Mothers' pensions, 12, 14, 15
Moynihan, Daniel, 194
Myers, Robert, 34, 76

National Academy of State Health
  Policy, 391
National Association of State Medicaid
  Directors
    Origins, 330-331
National Citizens' Coalition for Nurs-
  ing Home Reform, 129, 18-186,
  281-282, 298, 410
National Governors' Association
  role in BBA '95, 231
  HIFA waiver and, 281-284
  task force, 2003, 294

National Health Conference, 23
National health insurance, ix, 8-9, 25,
    38, 111-112, 117, 120, 131, 170, 369
National Health Insurance Partnership
    Act, 113, 114
National Institutes of Health, 28
    Heart-Cancer-Stroke proposal, 29
    Lasker Foundation and, 29
National Long-term Care Channeling
    Demonstration, 363n63
Nelson, Karen, 103, 232
Neutrality
    allotment, 352
    budget, 284, 357
    cost, 39, 396n64
New Federalism, 119, 170
New Freedom Commission on Mental
    Health, 287-288
    Campaign for Mental Health, 288
    "recovery" as central concept, 288
New Freedom Initiative, 285-292, 387
    appraisal, 291
    Olmstead v. L.E. ex rel Zimring
        (1999), 285
    origins, 285-288
Newman, Howard, 112
Nixon, Richard, 96
    domestic policy and, 96, 101
    election of 1968, 96
    Family Assistance Plan (FAP),
        101-102
    National Health Insurance Partner-
        ship, 113-114
    "Watergate" and impeachment
        crisis, 115
Norwood, Charles, 255
Nursing homes,
    alternatives to, 78-80,167-168,343,
        395
    development, 78-78
    reform, regulation of, 78-80, 184 ff
    reimbursement, 129
Nye, Christine, 335

Office of Management and Budget
    (OMB), 154,341-343
Olmstead v. L.E. ex rel Zimring (1999),
    285
    implementation, 290
Omnibus Budget Reconciliation Act of
    1981, 145, 155
    entitlements and, 159 ff

    importance and consequences, 145
    innovative nature, 155-156
    Senate and, 162,167
    strategy, 155-156
    successes and failures, 146, 147,
        171-172
    waivers and, 165 ff
OBRA '86 (SOBRA), 176-177, 178
OBRA '87
    EPSDT amendments, 181-182
    nursing home reforms, 184 ff
OBRA '89, 150
    repeal of MCCA, 150
OBRA '90, 194
Outreach, 63, 69
Oversight (of administration), 72-73

Panetta, Leon, 75
Parran, Thomas, 24
Partisanship, partisan politics
    "gridlock" and, 398
    partisan mobilization, 227-228
    politicizing of Medicaid, 377-378
Patients' rights (bills of rights), 254
    managed care reform, 254-256
Pay-as-you-go (PAYGO), 183
    Budget Enforcement Act of 1990,
        183
    revival of PAYGO, 406
Pear, Robert, 409
Pepper, Claude, 167, 204, 205
Personal Responsibility and Work Op-
    portunity Reconciliation Act of 1996
    (PRWORA), 244-245
    Temporary Assistance to Needy
        Families (TANF), 246
    de-linking Medicaid and welfare,
        246
    sec. 1931 and Medicaid eligibility,
        246-247
    and SCHIP, 247
Polycentrism, 145, 369
Preambles, 366
Pregnant women and children, x
    eligibility expansions, 147, 170 ff
Premium assistance, 372
Prepaid health plans (California), 131,
    142n117, 333
    Prepaid Health Research, Evalu-
        ation, and Demonstration Project
        (PHRED) 334, 362n38
Primary care case management, 166, 334

Professional Standards Review Organizations (PSROs), 107-108, 111
Professionalism
    quality improvement and, 254
Program for All-Inclusive Care of the Elderly (PACE), 294
Program integrity (see also, Fraud and Abuse)
    assuring, strengthening, 124, 133
Program Review and Evaluation Project (PREP), 72
Prudent layperson, 255
Prudent purchaser, 372
Public Assistance (welfare)
    de-linking from Medicaid, 147, 246-247
    disparities in eligibility, benefits, 13
    Kerr-Mills and, 39
    Social Security Act and 32, 35, 79
Public Health, 5
    categorical grants and, 7, 161-164
    post-war plan of PHS, 28
Public Welfare and Social Security Amendments of 1949, 31, 35

Qualified Medicare Beneficiary (QMB), 205
Quality Reform Initiative (QARI), 253

Rader, Lloyd, 38,104, 105, 122, 187
Reagan administration. 151
    administrative style, 152-153
    domestic programs and strategy, 153
    executive orders l2291, 12498, 154
    fiscal policy, 155
    Office of Management and Budget, key role, 154
    purging disability rolls, 190
    Reagan "revolution," 145
    Stockman, David, 154, 156
    Transition, 153-154
Recession(s), fiscal distress
    1981-83, impact of, 165, 170-173
    1991-93, 227
    2002-03, 292-293
    state and federal responses, 293-294
Regulatory "relief," 184
    Bush task force, 186
    Carter task force, 186

executive orders 12291 & 12498, 154
Richardson, Sally, 335

Riley, Richard, 178
Rockefeller, Nelson, 35, 75
Roe v. Wade, (1973), 172
Roosevelt, Franklin, 6-10, 12, 23-36, 161
Roper, William, 204
Rulemaking
    Medicaid managed care, 267-269
    SCHIP, 266-267
    See also, "regulatory relief"
Ryan White Comprehensive AIDS Resource Act of 1990 (CARE) Act, 201-202
    Provisions, 202

Safety-net, 235 381
    support for, 129-130, 149, 381
Scale, bringing to, 376-377
Schneider, Andy, xiv, 274n59,
Schweiker, Richard, 158
SCHIP (see "State Childrens' Health Insurance Program")
Sec. 209(b), 104
Sec. 222 (R&D authority), 105
Sec. 1122 (limits), 106
Sec. 1902(r)(2), 207
Sec. 1903(e) (comprehensive care), 50, 66, 100, 109-110
Sec. 1931, 246-247
September 11, 2001 (terrorist attack), 280
Sheppach, Raymond, 232, 237
Sheppard-Towner Act, 5
Shuptrine, Sarah, 178
Simkin v. Moses Cone Memorial Hospital (1963), 84
Skilled nursing facility (SNF), 108-109
Smith, Gordon, 302-304
Social Security Act of 1935
    categorical eligibility and, 9
    Committee on Economic Security, 6
    entitlement aspect, 7
    health insurance and, 7-8
    historic significance of, 6
    incrementalism and, 30
    maternal and child health, 6
    Medical Advisory Committee, 8
    poor and uninsured, 7, 8

political opposition to, 6
public health titles, 6
Roosevelt, Franklin and, 6, 8, 25
South and southern states, 10
titles in original act, 7
Social Security Amendments
 politics of, 30-31
  "legislative train," 32
 1950, 13, 188
 1960 (Kerr-Mills), 30
 1965 (Medicare; Medicaid), 21
 1967 74, 95
  EPSDT, 77-78
  ICFs, 78-79
  limits on Medicaid matching,
   76-77
  Work Incentive Program, 74
 1970, 103
 1972, 101 ff
  background, 101-103
  congressional staff and, 102, 103
   staff report of 1970, 103
  cost-saving provisions, 106-107
  Family Assistance Plan, 100
  Family Health Insurance Plan,
   114
  fraud and abuse, 102, 108
  infrastructure support for Medicaid, 111
  PSROs and, 107
  SNFs and, 108-109
  Supplemental Security Income,
   104
Social Security Disability Insurance,
 32, 190, 199
Social Security Disability Benefits
 Reform Act (1984), 365n99
Southern governors' initiative, 179
Special Committee on Aging (Senate),
 79, 125
Special Needs Plans (SNPs), 296
Specified Low-income Medicare Ben-
 eficiary (SLMB), 260
Spend down, 206
Spousal impoverishment, 206
State Children's Health Insurance
 Program (SCHIP), 228, 261
  as model for Medicaid restructur-
   ing, 282, 293, 354
  benchmark plans and actuarial
   equivalence, 264-265, 309
  Chafee-Rockefeller bill, 262

Child Health Assistance Program,
 263 ff
Child Health Assurance Program
 (CHAP), 119, 173
childless adults, unemployed and,
 346, 407
devolution and, 346
direct purchase issue, 265
funds for, 407-409
growth, 347
HIFA waiver and, 283
initial legislative passage, 264
reauthorization, 409
regulatory implementation, 265 ff.
Stark, Fortney (Pete), 204
State plans, 10, 65 ff.
Statewideness, 10, 420
Stevens, Robert and Rosemary, xin1,
 102
Stockman, David, 154, 156, 159-160,
 204
"Suitable home," 11, 13
Sundquist, Donald, 281
Supplement D, 64 ff
 description, 65
 application 66 ff
 comprehensive care and, 66-67

Taft, Robert
 Medicaid precursor, 13, 42
TAGs (see Technical Advisory Groups)
Talmadge, Herman, 118
TANF, see Temporary Assistance for
 Needy Families
Task Force on Medicaid and Related
 Programs (McNerney Task Force), 97 ff
  de-linking welfare proposed, 98
  federal leadership role, 98-99
  managed care and, 99
  origins and overview, 97-98
  "realigning incentives," 98
Tauke, Tom, 192
Tax credits
 Medicaid and, 398
Technical Advisory Groups (TAGs),
 330-331
  categories, 331
  origins, 330
  uses, 331
Technical assistance, 69, 128,
Temporary Assistance to Needy Fami-
 lies, 248

Tenncare, 355
Thompson, Tommy, 284, 294
Ticket to Work and Work Incentives
  Improvement Act (1999), 290
    infrastructure grants, 209
Tocqueville, Alexis de, 1-3, 15-16
"Triangulation," 250
Truman, Harry, 25, 26, 31

Unemployed, coverage for 10, 147, 171
Uninsured
  Medicaid coverage for, 119, 261,
    385, 407-408
  numbers of, ix

Voucher payments (for medical services), 42, 356

Wagner, Robert, 23-25
Wagner-Murray-Dingell bill(s), 23-25
Waivers
  Sec. 1915(b); 2175 managed care
    delayed growth, effects of, 334
    CMS and, 357 ff.
    OMB and, 341-342
  Sec. 1915(c); 2176 home and
    community-based
    bed capacity" and "cold bed"
      tests, 340-341
    cost neutrality and, 339
    HCFA and, 337 ff
    IMD exclusion and, 344
    MR/DD and, 344
    OMB and, 341-343
    nursing homes and, 343
  Sec. 1915(d), 353
  Katie Becket "model" waiver,
    191-193
  Sec. 1115 ("comprehensive")
    origins, 332
    scope of discretion conferred,
      349
    Clinton administration and,
      351

Bush administration and 352-
  354
  HIFA waiver and, 281-284;
  GAO report and, 353
  budget proposal of 2003, 354
  CMS administrative actions,
    357-358
  "special terms and condi-
    tions," 368n142
Specific examples:
  Florida, "Medicaid Reform
    Plan," 356; Healthier
  Mississippi, 355-356;
  Tenncare, 355; Utah, Primary
    Care Network," 354-355
Wartime Health and Education
  hearings) 26
Waxman, Henry, 26, 115, 158-159,162,
  171, 173, 206, 234, 406
  "two-step," 177-178
  effectiveness, 158, 174-175
Ways and Means Committee
  jurisdiction reduced, 116
  Social Security Act and 32
Welfare (see also public assistance and
  TANF)
  categorical eligibility, 1, 3, 16
  de-linking, 178, 181, 228, 245
  medical benefits and, 35
  TANF, 246
Welfare Administration, 66
  Bureau of Family Services, 63, 65
"Welfare medicine," 1, 3, 16
Wilensky, Gail, 183, 194, 335
Wilson Heather, 303
Winston, Ellen, 61-62, 68-69, 329
Witte, Edwin, 31
Womens' Bureau, 5
"Woodwork effect," 221n151, 343,
  403n
Wyatt v. Stickney; Partlow v. Stickney,
  (1970-2003), 112

"Y2K" problem, 266